Low Back Pain: Evidence-Based Prevention and Treatment

Low Back Pain: Evidence-Based Prevention and Treatment

Editor: Benjamin West

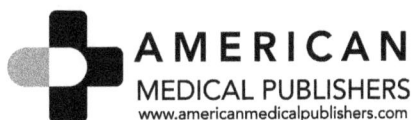

AMERICAN
MEDICAL PUBLISHERS
www.americanmedicalpublishers.com

AMERICAN
MEDICAL PUBLISHERS
www.americanmedicalpublishers.com

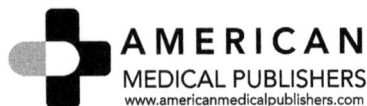

Cataloging-in-Publication Data

Low back pain : evidence-based prevention and treatment / edited by Benjamin West.
        p. cm.
Includes bibliographical references and index.
ISBN 978-1-63927-399-7
1. Backache. 2. Backache--Diagnosis. 3. Backache--Treatment. 4. Back--Diseases. 5. Pain. I. West, Benjamin.
RD771.B217 L69 2022
617.564--dc23

American Medical Publishers,
41 Flatbush Avenue,
1st Floor, New York,
NY 11217, USA

ISBN 978-1-63927-399-7 (Hardback)

Contents

Preface

Low back pain is a common condition affecting the muscles, bones and nerves of the back. It is not a specific disease but is rather a symptom of an underlying problem. It can be classified into four chief categories - musculoskeletal, infectious, inflammatory and malignant. Musculoskeletal or mechanical problems are responsible for 90% of low back pain cases. The management and prognosis of low back pain is subject to the duration of symptoms. Imaging techniques such as CT or MRI are used for the diagnosis of low back pain. Techniques such as straight leg raise test and lumbar provocative discography are used for diagnosing disc herniation and identifying the disc that is causing pain. Evidence supports the role of exercise in preventing low back pain. While acute low back pain resolves by itself, sub-chronic or chronic low back pain management requires diverse treatments comprising of NSAIDs, exercise therapy, peripheral nerve stimulation, Alexander technique and yoga, besides others. This book is a compilation of chapters that discuss the most vital concepts and emerging trends in the diagnosis and management of low back pain. Different approaches, evaluations, methodologies and advanced studies on low back pain have been included in this book. The readers would gain knowledge that would broaden their perspective about this condition.

The information contained in this book is the result of intensive hard work done by researchers in this field. All due efforts have been made to make this book serve as a complete guiding source for students and researchers. The topics in this book have been comprehensively explained to help readers understand the growing trends in the field.

I would like to thank the entire group of writers who made sincere efforts in this book and my family who supported me in my efforts of working on this book. I take this opportunity to thank all those who have been a guiding force throughout my life.

Editor

Prognostic factors of a favorable outcome following a supervised exercise program for soldiers with sub-acute and chronic low back pain

Marc Perron[1]* ⓘ, Chantal Gendron[1,2], Pierre Langevin[1,3], Jean Leblond[4], Marianne Roos[1] and Jean-Sébastien Roy[1,4]

Abstract

Background: Low back pain (LBP) encompasses heterogeneous patients unlikely to respond to a unique treatment. Identifying sub-groups of LBP may help to improve treatment outcomes. This is a hypothesis-setting study designed to create a clinical prediction rule (CPR) that will predict favorable outcomes in soldiers with sub-acute and chronic LBP participating in a multi-station exercise program.

Methods: Military members with LBP participated in a supervised program comprising 7 stations each consisting of exercises of increasing difficulty. Demographic, impairment and disability data were collected at baseline. The modified Oswestry Disability Index (ODI) was administered at baseline and following the 6-week program. An improvement of 50% in the initial ODI score was considered the reference standard to determine a favorable outcome. Univariate associations with favorable outcome were tested using chi-square or paired t-tests. Variables that showed between-group (favorable/unfavorable) differences were entered into a logistic regression after determining the sampling adequacy. Finally, continuous variables were dichotomized and the sensitivity, specificity and positive and negative likelihood ratios were determined for the model and for each variable.

Results: A sample of 85 participants was included in analyses. Five variables contributed to prediction of a favorable outcome: no pain in lying down ($p = 0.017$), no use of antidepressants ($p = 0.061$), FABQ work score < 22.5 ($p = 0.061$), fewer than 5 physiotherapy sessions before entering the program ($p = 0.144$) and less than 6 months' work restriction ($p = 0.161$). This model yielded a sensitivity of 0.78, specificity of 0.80, LR+ of 3.88, and LR- of 0.28. A 77.5% probability of favorable outcome can be predicted by the presence of more than three of the five variables, while an 80% probability of unfavorable outcome can be expected if only three or fewer variables are present.

Conclusion: The use of prognostic factors may guide clinicians in identifying soldiers with LBP most likely to have a favorable outcome. Further validation studies are needed to determine if the variables identified in our study are treatment effect modifiers that can predict success following participation in the multi-station exercise program.

Keywords: Low back pain, Clinical prediction rule, Exercises

* Correspondence: marc.perron@fmed.ulaval.ca
[1]Department of Rehabilitation, Faculty of Medicine, Université Laval, Pavillon Ferdinand-Vandry, Local 4445, 1050, avenue de la Médecine, Québec, QC G1V 0A6, Canada
Full list of author information is available at the end of the article

Background

Attempts to treat low back pain (LBP) have typically had limited success [1–4]. These difficulties are believed to be due, in part, to the fact that the cause of the pain is rarely known, leaving approximately 85% of individuals with LBP to be included in a "non-specific LBP" group [4, 5]. However, LBP is a complex condition influenced by a range of psychosocial, physical and activity-related factors that differ from person to person [6–9], rendering the non-specific LBP group heterogeneous, and unlikely to respond to the same treatment approach. It has thus been suggested that classification of LBP subjects into subgroups, followed by specific treatment of each subgroup according to their needs, is necessary in order to efficiently treat this condition [9]. Different classification systems, in which LBP subjects are assigned according to personal and clinical characteristics, have therefore been created and modified over the past 20 years [10, 11]. However, more conclusions on how to classify LBP sufferers and how to treat each subgroup are needed [12, 13]. Recent literature reviews still examine studies implementing interventions in non-specific, unclassified LBP populations. The most recent reviews evaluating the efficiency of exercise programs in the treatment of chronic LBP, for example, did not discuss LBP subgroups but treated the subjects as a homogenous population [4, 14]. Searle et al.'s review [4] confirmed the previously-held belief that stabilization and strengthening exercise programs decrease chronic LBP, but with only small effects. It remains to be examined whether division of the LBP population into subgroups will allow researchers and clinicians to obtain larger treatment effects when using exercise program interventions [2, 4, 15].

In order to accurately classify LBP patients into subgroups to which a specific intervention is assigned, valid clinical prediction rules (CPR) need to be developed [16, 17]. These rules are sets of data obtained from the history and physical evaluation of each patient, as well as from auto-administered questionnaires, that indicate which subgroup of patients will likely respond to a specific intervention. In 2011, a multi-station full-body supervised exercise program was created for soldiers with LBP and implemented at a military base of the Canadian Armed Forces. Although the program has enjoyed some clinical success, as subjectively reported by a number of soldiers, it is of great importance to maximize the efficacy of the program by determining the LBP subgroup most susceptible to benefit from it.

The development of CPR typically follows a three-step process: derivation, validation and impact analysis [16, 18, 19]. Derivation is the early hypothesis generation step in which prognostic factors are identified from a set of clinical variables that are believed to have predictive value, based on clinical experience or previous research. Kent et al. [20] recommended subdividing the derivation step into two sub-steps: hypothesis-setting, which represents the exploratory phase in which data from cohort studies may generate hypotheses about potential treatment effect modifiers, and hypothesis-testing, which is the confirmation sub-step in which pre-specified (a priori) hypotheses are tested more rigorously on subgrouping effects in samples of people similar to those who participated in the hypothesis-setting study. Subsequently, a validation step is required to identify treatment effect modifiers by testing subgroups/treatment interaction effects in randomized controlled trials involving samples of people with characteristics that are similar to (narrow validation) or different from (broad validation) those in the hypothesis-testing study. Lastly, the impact analysis aims to verify the usefulness of the CPR in improving outcomes and patient satisfaction and in decreasing costs once it is implemented in clinical practice.

According to this development framework, the present study is at the early hypothesis-setting step. Our objective was therefore to identify variables associated with a favorable outcome in soldiers with sub-acute and chronic LBP participating in a multi-station full-body supervised exercise program. The results obtained may permit generation of potential treatment effect modifiers that will eventually have to be validated before being recommended for clinical practice.

Methods

Participants

Military members consulting at Valcartier Health Centre for LBP were consecutively recruited. To be included, potential participants had to be aged 18 and older and present with an episode of subacute or chronic LBP with or without radiation to the lower limbs. Potential participants were also required to have a minimal score of 17% on the Modified Oswestry Disability Index (ODI) at the initial evaluation (based on the clinically important difference of this test [21]). Patients were excluded in the following circumstances: previous surgery to the spinal column, lumber spine injection in the past two weeks, signs of upper motor neuron lesions (bilateral paresthesia, hyperreflexia or spasticity), serious medical conditions (e.g. tumor, fracture, rheumatoid arthritis, osteoporosis) and unavailability to participate in the 6-week exercise program. Patients admitted to the clinic with acute LBP (e.g. onset of constant and intense pain [> 5/10] < 7 days, severely limited lumbar range of motion [more than 50% in at least 2 directions], obvious lateral shift) were first treated by their physiotherapist and then referred to the project coordinator, once the risk of harm associated with participation in the program was deemed low (e.g. when the indicators of acute LBP were no longer present). Participation in the study was voluntary, and informed consent forms were signed by all subjects. This study was approved by the ethics committee of the CIUSSS de la Capitale-Nationale (Quebec Rehabilitation Institute).

Previous CPR developed for rehabilitation programs in LBP populations [15, 22, 23] included 5 predictors or fewer in their final model. According to the formula suggested by Green [24] for regression analysis (50 + [8 x number of prognostic factors]), and considering the expected 5 variables in the final model, as well as an estimated 20% dropout rate, the ideal sample size was 108.

Study design

All participants took part in the 6-week exercise program, as well as in the two evaluation sessions (pre- and post- exercise program). At the initial evaluation, subjects completed forms and questionnaires on sociodemographics, symptomatology, comorbidities, work restrictions, pain and functional limitations and fear-avoidance beliefs. A physiotherapist measured their lumbar and hip mobility, conducted diagnostic and pain provocation tests and assessed endurance of the trunk muscles. Following the initial evaluation, subjects took part in the 6-week multi-station full-body supervised exercise program (2 to 3 sessions per week). The ODI was completed at the initial and at the final evaluations. The change in ODI score following the program was considered the principal measure reflecting favorable or unfavorable outcome.

Evaluations and variables

The initial evaluation was carried out by four experienced physiotherapists who completed a three-hour training session in order to standardize the evaluation protocol. Selection of the variables included in the clinical examination was based on the results of previous studies that aimed to develop preliminary CPR in patients with LBP [15, 22, 23]. The following clinical variables were collected.

Standardized subjective clinical questionnaire

This questionnaire documented participants' personal and occupational characteristics, personal medical history, current and past episodes of LBP, a detailed description of their symptoms (low back and lower limb pain mapping), pain behaviour (aggravating or relieving factors such as sitting, bending, standing, supine, walking, lifting) [25] and other characteristics such as work restrictions and number of treatments received before the initial evaluation.

Modified Oswestry disability index

The ODI is a self-administered questionnaire whose purpose is to evaluate the severity of the limitations and restrictions suffered by patients with LBP. It consists of 10 items that assess the interference of LBP with activities of daily living. Each item is scored on a categorical scale

from 0 to 5, with higher values representing greater disability. The score out of 50 is multiplied by two and expressed as a percentage. The reliability (ICC = 0.86), construct validity and sensitivity to change of this questionnaire have previously been demonstrated [26]. The minimal detectable change in persons with non-specific LBP is 10 points [21, 27, 28], while the minimal clinically important difference ranges from 10 to 19 [21, 26, 29]. Patients who experienced an improvement of at least 50% on the ODI were categorized as having a favorable outcome [15, 22, 23].

Fear-avoidance beliefs questionnaire (FABQ)

The FABQ is a self-administered questionnaire that consists of 16 questions pertaining to patients' beliefs regarding the effect of their physical activities and work on their LBP [30]. It comprises a physical activity subscale (5 questions) and a work subscale (11 questions). Each item is scored from 0 to 6, with higher scores indicating higher levels of fear-avoidance behavior. Moderate to high test-retest reliability was found respectively for the Physical Activity subscale (ICC = 0.72 to 0.90) and the Work subscale (ICC = 0.8 to 0.91) [31].

Numeric pain rating scale (NPRS)

This tool was used to document the worst and average LBP experienced by participants in the 48 h preceding the initial evaluation. Pain intensity was rated on a scale from 0 to 10, where 10 is the worst pain imaginable. Its reliability is moderate (ICC = 0.76) [32].

Lumbar and hip mobility

Lumbar range of motion (ROM) was evaluated by measuring the distance between the third fingertip and the floor in trunk forward and lateral flexions (ICC = 0.91–0.99) [33]. The single inclinometer method was used to measure trunk extension (ICC = 0.61–0.95) [34]. Passive hip ROM was measured bilaterally using a goniometer or an inclinometer (ICC = 0.56–0.99) [35] and included internal rotation, external rotation, flexion and extension.

Signs of instability

Aberrant lumbar movement patterns during forward flexion that are believed to be associated with instability were documented. These patterns include a painful arc, Gower's sign (thigh climbing), brisk movement (instability catch) or an inverted lumbar pelvic rhythm [36].

The response to the following clinical screening, diagnostic or performance tests was also documented: 1) The Straight Leg Raise, used to screen for herniated discs and to verify neural sensitivity (ICC = 0.93–0.97) [37]. The amplitude of the leg raise was measured with an inclinometer placed on the subject's tibia. 2) The Biering-Sorensen, McGill and lateral plank tests, designed to measure muscle endurance in trunk extension, flexion and lateral flexion (ICC = 0,89–0.98) [33], respectively. 3) The Prone Instability Test, used to identify patients with lumbar instability, and which has been shown to have predictive value for the stabilization group of the Treatment-Based Classification (TBC) [11] (ICC = 0.74–1.00) [36]. 4) Central posterior to anterior pressure techniques were executed to evaluate pain provocation and segmental mobility of the lumbar spine in prone position. Segment mobility was classified as hypomobile, normal or hypermobile by applying a posterior to anterior force on the spinous process of each lumbar vertebra with the hypothenar eminence. Pain was rated as present or absent. The interrater reliability of this technique is good for the identification of the least mobile segment (agreement = 82.8%, kappa = 0.71, 95% CI = 0.48 to 0.94), but poor for determining the most mobile segment (kappa = 0.29, 95% CI = – 0.13 to 0.71) [33]. The reliability of this procedure seems higher to assess pain provocation than segmental mobility [38].

Intervention

Each participant took part in the 6-week multi-station full-body supervised exercise program, which consisted of two to three sessions per week (45 to 60 min each) and was supervised by a physiotherapist. The exercise program is composed of 7 stations, each consisting of numerous exercises of increasing difficulty. The exercises were grouped together as follows: Hip strengthening and control (Station 1); The squat and its variants (Station 2); Elastic bands and the Bodyblade (Station 3); Abdominal planks and their variants (Station 4); Abdominal strengthening (Station 5); Back extensor strengthening (Station 6); and Lifting techniques (Station 7). Each of the exercises in the program is shown in an Additional file 1. The basic principal applied for all exercises was the maintenance of natural lordosis, regardless of the weight or external forces imposed on the body. Exercise parameters were chosen to increase strength, endurance and neuromuscular control. In accordance with recognized motor learning principles [39], participants were encouraged to complete a large variety of exercises and to focus on the quality, rather than the quantity, of their movements. Progression in the program led to the execution of exercises that simulated functional and occupational tasks (task-oriented approach). The initial difficulty level and choice of exercises were determined by the supervising physiotherapist according to 3 principal criteria: severity of the condition (constant or non-constant pain, disturbed sleep, limitation and restriction level according to the ODI results), the most limited plane of motion (as the prescribed exercises were primarily carried out in the planes of motion that showed limited mobility or aberrant movements) and the quality of exercise execution. The physiotherapist adjusted the difficulty level of the exercises in order to prompt maximal effort without jeopardizing the quality of the movements. Exercises were paused or stopped when fatigue led to the deterioration of the quality of movements. See the summary table of principles on exercise selection and progression in the Additional file 1. Individual interventions such as manual therapy and other physiotherapy treatment modalities were not performed during the course of the study.

Data analysis

Based on their favorable (50% improvement in the ODI score) or unfavorable outcome following participation in the program, subjects were classified into two subgroups. A first screening of the potential prognostic factors of outcome was done using univariate analyses by looking at statistical differences between groups on characteristics, questionnaires and physical examination data at baseline (Tables 1, 2 and 3). Independent t-tests (continuous variables) and chi-square tests (categorical variables) were used. A potential prognostic factor was retained when the p-value was lower or equal to 0.1.

Before entering the potential prognostic factors into a multiple logistic regression, the Kaiser-Meyer-Olkin (KMO) index was calculated on the set of variables that included all the potential prognostic factors and the group variable. The KMO index and measures of sampling adequacy (MSA) were used to determine collinearity. When the KMO index is greater or equal to 0.6, the logistic regression may be performed with all the potential prognostic factors. When the MSA are below 0.6, the associated potential prognostic factor must be removed.

The first multiple logistic regression included all valid prognostic factors. Considering that the useful information brought by one prognostic factor may be entirely offered by another, prognostic factors with very high p-values (p > .50) were removed from the model even though they had significant p-values with the univariate tests. The aim was to obtain the most efficient prognostic factors. A second multiple logistic regression was then calculated on a model that included only prognostic factors that had p-values below 0.50. From a clinical perspective, continuous factors are often impractical. Discrete criteria are better suited to clinical use. For this reason, the continuous variables retained by the second model were dichotomized based on thresholds determined by recursive partitioning analysis (SPSS, proc. TREE). Then, a third and final multiple logistic regression was calculated with the dichotomized version of the set of prognostic factors from the second model. The anti-image and inverse of the correlation matrix, drawn from factor analyses with and without the dependent variable, were used to test for collinearity

Table 1 Baseline participants' characteristics

Variables	All Subjects (N = 85)	Favorable outcome (N = 40)	Unfavorable outcome (N = 45)
Age (years)	37.22 ± 9.35	36.51 ± 10.40	37.83 ± 8.38
Gender (% men)	88.2	85.0	91.1
Weight (kg)	86.27 ± 18.57	83.82 ± 16.78	88.46 ± 19.96
Height (m)	1.74 ± 0.08	1.74 ± 0.08	1.74 ± 0.07
Body mass index (kg/m^2)	27.93 ± 5.93	27.51 ± 4.65	28.29 ± 6.90
Number of months in the army	158.30 ± 111.58	147.25 ± 112.34	168.34 ± 111.21
History of LBP (%)	74.1	70.0	77.8
Number of months since last onset of LBP	16.28 ± 32.19	12.12 ± 20.34	19.69 ± 39.38
Number of treatments received before first evaluation*	4.94 ± 5.81	3.14 ± 3.81	6.85 ± 6.92
Referred pain in lower limb (%)	31.8	22.5	40.0
Work restriction (%)*	51.8	40.0	62.2
Work restriction of 6 months or more (%)*	30.6	15.0	44.4
Numbness and tingling sensation (%)	23.5	22.2	26.7
Prone instability test (%)	66.2	71.4	61.1
Use of antidepressants (%)*	15.3	5.0	24.4
Use of nonsteroidal anti-inflammatories (%)	29.4	32.5	26.7
Pain in sitting position (VAS 0–100)	77.6	77.5	77.8
Pain in lying position* (VAS 0–100)	37.5	25.0	48.9
Pain in standing position (VAS 0–100)	84.7	75.0	93.3
Pain during walking (VAS 0–100)	40.0	32.5	46.7
Pain when coughing or sneezing (VAS 0–100)	28.2	25.0	31.1
Tingling or numbness in the lower limbs (VAS 0–100)	24.7	20.0	26.7

*Significant difference between the favorable outcome group and unfavorable outcome group ($p < 0.10$; univariate analyses). Continuous variables are shown as Mean ± 1 Standard Deviation, while categorical variables are shown as %

between variables included in the model. Finally, the sensitivity, specificity and the positive and negative likelihood ratios (LR+ and LR-, respectively) were determined for each variable and for the overall regression model. All analyses were conducted with SPSS software (Version 23; IBM SPSS Statistics for Mac. Armonk, NY: IBM Corp) except for the sensitivity, specificity and likelihood ratios (with 95% confidence intervals) which were estimated with the package epiR (Tools for the Analysis of Epidemiological Data, a package available for the 3.3.1 version of the R statistical software).

Results

Of the 104 individuals that were recruited, nineteen (18.3%) did not complete the 6-week program or did not take part in the final evaluation. Therefore, a constant sample of 85 participants (81.7%) was included in all analyses. The reasons given by the individuals for dropping out of the study were: difficulties in coming to the Valcartier Health Centre due to military duties ($n = 2$), medical reasons ($n = 1$), new employment outside of the military (n = 2), prolonged absence for a military exercise or mission ($n = 3$) and personal or unknown reasons

Table 2 Baseline participants' questionnaire scores

Questionnaires	All Subjects (N = 85)	Favorable outcome (N = 40)	Unfavorable outcome (N = 45)
FABQ Work subscale (0–42)*	21.04 ± 10.75	16.63 ± 9.43	25.05 ± 10.38
FABQ Physical Activity subscale (0–24)	13.23 ± 5.03	12.57 ± 5.08	13.8 ± 5.0
Worst LBP perceived in the last 48* hours (1 to 10 scale)	4.65 ± 1.94	4.28 ± 1.94	4.98 ± 1.90
Mean LBP perceived in the last 48 h (1 to 10 scale)	2.96 ± 1.30	2.73 ± 1.26	3.18 ± 1.31
Modified Oswestry Disability Index (0–100)	32.1 ± 12.1	32.1 ± 12.7	32.2 ± 11.8

*Significant difference between the favorable outcome group and unfavorable outcome group ($p < 0.10$; univariate analyses). Continuous variables are shown as Mean ± 1 Standard Deviation, while categorical variables are shown as %

Table 3 Performance in the clinical tests at baseline

Variables	All Subjects (N = 85)	Favorable outcome (N = 40)	Unfavorable outcome (N = 45)
Mean distance fingertip to ground in trunk flexion (cm)	10.67 ± 10.87	10.96 ± 10.51	10.41 ± 11.29
Mean distance fingertip to ground in trunk lateral flexion (cm)	48.18 ± 4.52	48.28 ± 4.22	48.08 ± 4.81
Trunk lateral flexion discrepancy (R-L, cm)	2.37 ± 2.27	2.21 ± 1.87	2.51 ± 2.59
Worst trunk lateral flexion (cm)	46.99 ± 4.60	47.17 ± 4.38	46.83 ± 4.84
Mean trunk extension (deg)	24.23 ± 9.91	24.82 ± 9.79	23.71 ± 10.10
Mean hip internal rotation (deg)	30.84 ± 9.54	5.97 ± 7.25	5.97 ± 4.68
Hip internal rotation discrepancy (R-L, deg)	7.54 ± 6.33	28.32 ± 9.23	27.42 ± 10.17
Worst hip internal rotation (deg)	27.84 ± 9.69	31.31 ± 9.02	30.41 ± 10.06
Mean hip external rotation (deg)	45.12 ± 10.87	45.76 ± 11.26	44.55 ± 10.59
Hip external rotation discrepancy (R-L, deg)	5.97 ± 5.99	7.22 ± 6.65	7.82 ± 6.09
Worst hip external rotation (deg)	41.35 ± 11.81	42.15 ± 12.53	40.64 ± 11.23
Mean hip flexion (deg)	111.08 ± 8.87	111.33 ± 10.38	110.84 ± 7.64
Hip flexion discrepancy (R-L, deg)	4.36 ± 3.24	4.55 ± 3.13	4.20 ± 3.36
Worst hip flexion (deg)	106.45 ± 11.04	108.47 ± 11.32	104.66 ± 10.58
Mean hip extension (deg)	11.15 ± 11.05	11.07 ± 11.95	11.22 ± 10.31
Hip extension discrepancy (R-L, deg)	3.08 ± 2.76	2.90 ± 2.53	3.24 ± 2.97
Worst hip extension (deg)	9.61 ± 10.99	9.62 ± 12.04	9.60 ± 10.10
Mean lateral plank (sec)	65.72 ± 35.46	66.79 ± 30.58	64.76 ± 39.61
Lateral plank discrepancy (R-L, sec)	14.00 ± 12.74	14.62 ± 14.07	13.45 ± 11.56
Worst lateral plank (sec)	58.57 ± 33.75	57.86 ± 26.26	59.14 ± 39.11
Mean score on Biering-Sorensen test (sec)	84.19 ± 44.12	95.10 ± 47.09	74.48 ± 39.33
Mean score on McGill abdominal test (sec)	101.96 ± 56.29	112.07 ± 58.65	92.97 ± 53.15
Mean Straight Leg Raise (deg)	72.85 ± 10.95	72.55 ± 10.59	73.12 ± 11.36
Straight Leg Raise discrepancy (R-L, deg)	4.76 ± 4.78	4.40 ± 4.04	5.08 ± 5.38
Worst Straight Leg Raise (deg)	70.47 ± 11.46	70.35 ± 10.77	70.57 ± 12.16

sec: second, deg.: degree, cm: centimeter. All measurements are shown as Mean ± 1 Standard Deviation. None of the clinical variables showed a significant difference (univariate analyses)

($n = 11$). The individuals who dropped out had higher scores on the numerical pain rating scale evaluating worst and mean LBP perceived in the last 48 h when compared to the participants included in the final analyses ($p < 0.05$). No other differences were found. Subjects retained for analyses participated in 14.4 ± 2.6 sessions on average during the 6-week program (a mean of 2.34 sessions/week).

The mean baseline ODI score for the whole sample was 32.1 ± 12.1, considered as a moderate disability level [26]. Forty participants (47%) were categorized as having favorable outcome based on the ODI criterion, and 45 participants (53%) as unfavorable. The mean ODI change was 23.9 ± 11.0 for the group with favorable outcome and 3.4 ± 10.3 for the group with unfavorable outcome.

Tables 1, 2 and 3 present the clinical variables at baseline for the whole sample, as well as for both groups with favorable/unfavorable outcome. Notably, 74 % of the participants had previous episodes of LBP, and the time elapsed since the last episode varied from 1 to 200 months (mean 16.3 ± 32.2 months). Thirty-two percent ($n = 27$) had referred pain to the lower limbs. Finally, 51.8% of the participants ($n = 44$) had work restrictions.

The univariate tests identified seven potential prognostic factors with a KMO index of .692. As all MSA were above .600, no potential prognostic factors needed to be removed. The first multiple logistic regression indicated that two prognostic factors (work restrictions because of LBP and worst LBP perceived in the last 48 h) brought no unique information, with p-values respectively of .843 and .813, and were thus removed from the model. The second set of five factors with the group variable had a KMO index of .635. Although two prognostic factors had a MSA value very slightly below .6, all were kept in the model as these MSA were above .6 when the seven prognostic factors were used. [40] Furthermore, when the prognostic factors were dichotomized (see below), these MSA rose respectively to .60 and .62, and all five MSA were above or equal to .6. The model of the second multiple logistic regression had a highly significant (p = .00011) moderate capacity (Nagelkerke R^2 = .412) to predict the program outcome (favorable outcome: 86% correct; unfavorable outcome: 70% correct; global: 78% correct). This set of five variables included: (1) "no pain in lying down" [dichotomous], (2) "no use of antidepressants" [dichotomous], (3) "FABQ Work subscale" [continuous], (4) "number of treatments received before the first evaluation" [continuous], and (5) "no work restriction of 6 months or more" [dichotomous]. Individually, only variables 1 and 4 had p-values below .05 (respectively of .017 and .030). Since we were at the hypothesis-setting step of CPR development and since it is possible that beyond our sample these variables contain unique information that can predict the favorable or unfavorable outcomes, we decided to continue with the full set of five variables.

The FABQ Work subscale was dichotomized with the help of a recursive partitioning technique that indicated an optimal cutoff point of 22.5. Then, the potential dichotomized prognostic factor of a favorable outcome was set at a score below 22.5 on the FABQ Work subscale. The recursive partitioning technique did not successfully dichotomize the number of previous treatments. Therefore, this variable was dichotomized based on the threshold that led to the model yielding the best accuracy in predicting outcome. A criterion of 4 previous treatments or fewer was set as a potential dichotomized prognostic factor of favorable outcome.

The results of the third and final multiple logistic regression are shown in Tables 4 and 5. The model has a significant (p = .00004) moderate capacity (Nagelkerke R^2 = .370) to predict the program outcome (favorable outcome: 78% correct; unfavorable outcome: 80% correct; global: 79% correct). Furthermore, as the five variables had an odds ratio above 2.0 in this final regression, we decided to retain all variables in the final model. Even though the Nagelkerke R^2 may be lower, the outcome classification appears almost identical if not very slightly better. There was no sign of multicollinearity between variables included in the model. As seen in Table 4, only the first variable has a p-value below .05 (p = .017; Odds ratio = 3.7 [1.3–10.6]). It is also noteworthy that two variables have p-values of .061: (a) "no use of anti-depressants" (Odds ratio: 5.2 [0.9–29.4]), and (b) "FABQ Work below 22.5" (Odds ratio: 2.9 [0.9–8.6]).

In sum, for a patient or client presenting with all five criteria, the prognostic factors have low sensitivity and high specificity. The sensitivity improves to 0.78 for individuals presenting at least four of the five criteria. However, this increase in sensitivity comes at the expense of a decrease in specificity. Table 6 reports the prediction rate of a favorable outcome according to the number of criteria fulfilled. The satisfaction of four out of five criteria appears to be the best compromise between sensitivity and specificity.

Discussion

This study identified five variables of a favorable outcome in patients with LBP who participated in a multi-station full-body supervised exercise program. Clinicians may anticipate a favorable outcome when their initial assessment identifies 4 or 5 variables included in our model. On the other hand, a less favorable outcome is expected if 3 or fewer variables are present, since the expected failure rate would be 80%. It is to be noted that these findings were established for a 50% improvement on the ODI and different variables would likely have been obtained had a different ODI threshold or other outcomes been used. Furthermore, the LR+ (3.9) and LR- (0.28) were relatively low [35], suggesting that the predictive capability of the model is limited. In comparison, Hicks et al. [15] found similar LR+ (LR+ 4.0), but higher LR- (LR- 0.18), with their preliminary CPR. Rabin et al. could not, however, validate this preliminary CPR in a subsequent study [13]. In contrast, Stolze et al. [23] reported a LR+ of 10.6 (95% confidence interval [CI]: 3. 52, 32.14) in a CPR deviation study created to generate potential treatment effect modifiers of pilates exercises.

Three of the five variables included in our model had already been identified as prognostic factors of favorable outcomes for individuals with LBP in previous studies. We found that a score below 22.5 on the FABQ work subscale predicted a favorable outcome, which is in agreement with previous studies in which fears and beliefs about work were associated with poor recovery in patients with work-related LBP [41]. The FABQ work score was

Table 4 Predictive capacity of individual variables obtained in the multiple logistic regression

Variables	Sig.	Sensitivity	Specificity	LR+	LR-	Odd Ratio
No pain in lying down	0.017	0.75 [0.58–0.87]	0.49 [0.34–0.64]	1.47 [1.05–2.06]	0.51 [0.29–0.92]	3.65 [1.3–10.6]
No use of antidepressants	0.061	0.95 [0.82–0.99]	0.24 [0.13–0.40]	1.26 [1.05–1.51]	0.20 [0.05–0.90]	5.2 [0.9–29.4]
FABQ Work < 22.5	0.061	0.73 [0.56–0.85]	0.67 [0.51–0.80]	2.18 [1.38–3.43]	0.41 [0.24–0.70]	2.9 [0.9–8.6]
Number of previous treatments < 5	0.144	0.68 [0.51–0.81]	0.58 [0.42–0.72]	1.60 [1.07–2.39]	0.56 [0.35–0.91]	2.2 [0.8–6.3]
Work restriction < 6 months	0.161	0.85 [0.69–0.94]	0.44 [0.30–0.60]	1.53 [1.14–2.05]	0.34 [0.15–0.75]	2.48 [0.7–8.8]

Numbers in square brackets represent the 95% confidence interval

Table 5 Predictive capacity according to the number of criteria present

Number of Prognostic factors	Sensitivity	Specificity	LR+	LR-
One or more	1.00 [0.89–1.00]	0.02 [0.001–0.13]	1.02 [0.98–1.07]	N/A
Two or more	0.95 [0.82–0.99]	0.18 [0.09–0.33]	1.16 [0.99–1.35]	0.28 [0.06–1.33]
Three or more	0.90 [0.75–0.96]	0.49 [0.34–0.64]	1.76 [1.30–2.39]	0.20 [0.07–0.54]
Four or more	0.78 [0.61–0.89]	0.80 [0.65–0.90]	3.88 [2.11–7.12]	0.28 [0.16–0.50]
Five	0.33 [0.19–0.49]	0.93 [0.81–0.98]	4.88 [1.50–15.88]	0.72 [0.58–0.90]

Numbers in square brackets represent the 95% confidence interval

not identified as a predictor in CPRs developed by Hicks et al. [15] and Stolze et al.[23]. However, a score of less than 19 on the FABQ work subscale was considered a treatment effect modifier in the CPR developed by Flynn et al. [22], later validated by Childs et al., [42] whose aim was to identify patients likely to benefit from lumbar manipulation. As in the current study, participants in Flynn and Child's studies were recruited from care facilities within the military, suggesting that fear-avoidance beliefs about military tasks may be of particular concern in soldiers with LBP. We also found that patients who do not use antidepressant medication were more likely to have a better outcome. This finding suggests that patients requiring antidepressants had less favorable outcomes, an observation which concords with the literature showing that patients with LBP in a depressive state are predisposed to longer recovery time and to the development of chronicity [43, 44]. A third prognostic factor of outcome in our model was "no work restriction of six months or more". In the military context, a work restriction of fewer than six months should be interpreted as a temporary modification of regular duties for a non-chronic health condition, in contrast to a six-month medical category which is attributed to people for whom slow recovery or permanent health problems are anticipated. This finding is in agreement with previous studies that identified prolonged absence from work and the number of days of reduced activity as predictors of slower recovery in patients with LBP [41, 43]. "No pain when lying down" and "having had fewer than five physiotherapy treatments before the baseline evaluation", that were both identified as prognostic factors in our model, have, to our knowledge, never been associated with the outcome of LBP. It is to be noted that the cutoff criteria for two of the prognostic factors (FABQ Work subscale and number of previous treatments) are actually tied to our sample and must be confirmed by future studies.

This single-arm study was the preliminary step of a process aiming to develop a CPR that can be used to identify patients most likely to benefit from the proposed exercise program. Three of the five variables identified in our final model are generally recognized as prognostic factors in people with LBP and only one of these has been validated as a treatment effect modifier within a CPR aiming to predict patients likely to benefit from lumbar manipulation. The methodological approach used in our study was deliberately liberal. To minimize the possibility of missing potential prognostic factors, we set the p value for retaining variables at 0.1 and, as suggested in hypothesis-setting studies, [20] we did not perform corrections for multiple comparisons. Investigating a high number of variables (more than 50) in a relatively small sample, as we did in the present study, increases the likelihood of finding significant associations by chance (type 1 error), which can be considered a limitation. However, only one prognostic factor was below the generally accepted level of significance of 0.05 and our final model has only a limited predictive capability. Thus, before continuing to the validation step, our results need to be confirmed in a hypothesis-testing study in which a limited number of a priori hypotheses will be tested and appropriate adjustments for multiple comparisons will be made. Any subsequent validation study should also be conducted with non-military groups (broad validation), as the present results may not be generalizable to the greater population. On the other hand, the well-standardized multivariate protocol and the acceptable dropout rate represent strengths of this study. Finally, the targeted sample size of 90 participants to be included in the statistical analyses was not met, as only 85 of the 104 participants took part in both evaluation sessions.

Conclusion

The present study established five variables to identify patients most likely to have a favorable outcome, regardless of their participation in the exercise program. Careful use of these variables is mandatory for clinical

Table 6 Prediction rate of a favorable outcome according to the number of criteria fulfilled

Number of variables	0	1	2	3	4	5	0 to 3	4 or 5
Favorable outcome	0.0%	22.2%	12.5%	26.3%	75.0%	81.3%	20.0%	77.5%
Unfavorable outcome	100%	77.8%	87.5%	73.7%	25.0%	18.7%	80.0%	22.5%

purposes as this study is at the early stage of CPR development. Future validation studies should be carried out with other populations to confirm this CPR and subsequently, to verify whether some of these factors may be considered treatment effect modifiers.

Abbreviations

CI: Confidence interval; CPR: Clinical prediction rule; FABQ: Fear-avoidance beliefs questionnaire; ICC: Intraclass correlation coefficient; KMO: Kaiser-Meyer-Olkin; LBP: Low back pain; LR: Likelihood ratio; MSA: Measure of sampling adequacy; NPRS: Numeric pain rating scale; ODI: Modified Oswestry disability index; ROM: Lumbar range of motion; TBC: Treatment-based classification

Acknowledgments

The authors wish to thank Sophie Bernard, Nathalie Fortier, Pierre-Marc Vézina and Alex Volant, physiotherapists, and Hélène Simard, physiotherapist-assistant, for their contribution to the data collection, as well as Samuel Camiré-Bernier for his technical assistance. We also thank Dany Ducharme for having consented to the publication of photos illustrating the exercises included in our program.

Funding

This study was supported by a grant from the *Ordre professionnel de la physiothérapie du Québec* and the Quebec Rehabilitation Research Network partnership program.

Authors' contributions

MP - Coordination of the study, study design and writing of the protocol, training of research assistants, data analysis and interpretation, writing of the article, final approval of the version to be published; CG - Study design and writing of the protocol, training of research assistants, data collection and interpretation, critical revision of the article, final approval of the version to be published; PL- Study design and writing of the protocol, training of research assistants, data interpretation, critical revision of the article, final approval of the version to be published; JL - Data analysis and interpretation, writing of the article, final approval of the version to be published; MR - Data collection and interpretation, writing and critical revision of the article, final approval of the version to be published; JSR - Design and writing of the protocol, training of research assistants, data analysis and interpretation, writing of the article, final approval of the version to be published.

Consent for publication

Consent for publication was obtained from the person appearing in images included in the additional file.

Competing interests

The authors declare that they have no competing interests.

Author details

[1]Department of Rehabilitation, Faculty of Medicine, Université Laval, Pavillon Ferdinand-Vandry, Local 4445, 1050, avenue de la Médecine, Québec, QC G1V 0A6, Canada. [2]Canadian Forces Health Services Group, Valcartier Garison, Quebec City, Canada. [3]Physio Interactive, Quebec City, Canada. [4]Centre for Interdisciplinary Research in Rehabilitation and Social Integration (CIRRIS), Quebec City, Canada.

References

1. Bogduk N. Management of chronic low back pain. Med J Aust. 2004;180(2):79–83.
2. Geneen LJ, Moore RA, Clarke C, Martin D, Colvin LA, Smith BH. Physical activity and exercise for chronic pain in adults: an overview of Cochrane reviews. Cochrane Database Syst Rev. 2017;4:CD011279.
3. Rubinstein SM, van Middelkoop M, Assendelft WJ, de Boer MR, van Tulder MW. Spinal manipulative therapy for chronic low-back pain: an update of a Cochrane review. Spine (Phila Pa 1976). 2011;36(13):E825–46.
4. Searle A, Spink M, Ho A, Chuter V. Exercise interventions for the treatment of chronic low back pain: a systematic review and meta-analysis of randomised controlled trials. Clin Rehabil. 2015;29(12):1155–67.
5. Deyo RA, Phillips WR. Low back pain. A primary care challenge. Spine (Phila Pa 1976). 1996;21(24):2826–32.
6. Huijnen IP, Rusu AC, Scholich S, Meloto CB, Diatchenko L. Subgrouping of low back pain patients for targeting treatments: evidence from genetic, psychological, and activity-related behavioral approaches. Clin J Pain. 2015;31(2):123–32.
7. Pincus T, Burton AK, Vogel S, Field APA. Systematic review of psychological factors as predictors of chronicity/disability in prospective cohorts of low back pain. Spine (Phila Pa 1976). 2002;27(5):E109–20.
8. Ramond A, Bouton C, Richard I, Roquelaure Y, Baufreton C, Legrand E, Huez JF. Psychosocial risk factors for chronic low back pain in primary care–a systematic review. Fam Pract. 2011;28(1):12–21.
9. Vassilaki M, Hurwitz EL. Insights in public health: perspectives on pain in the low back and neck: global burden, epidemiology, and management. Hawaii J Med Public Health. 2014;73(4):122–6.
10. Delitto A, Erhard RE, Bowling RW. A treatment-based classification approach to low back syndrome: identifying and staging patients for conservative treatment. Phys Ther. 1995;75(6):470–85. discussion 485-479
11. Fritz JM, Cleland JA, Childs JD. Subgrouping patients with low back pain: evolution of a classification approach to physical therapy. J Orthop Sports Phys Ther. 2007a;37(6):290–302.
12. Fritz JM, Lindsay W, Matheson JW, Brennan GP, Hunter SJ, Moffit SD, Swalberg A, Rodriquez B. Is There a subgroup of patients with low back pain likely to benefit from mechanical traction? Results of a randomized clinical trial and subgrouping analysis. Spine (Phila Pa 1976). 2007b;32(26):E793–800.
13. Rabin A, Shashua A, Pizem K, Dickstein R, Dar G. A clinical prediction rule to identify patients with low back pain who are likely to experience short-term success following lumbar stabilization exercises: a randomized controlled validation study. J Orthop Sports Phys Ther. 2014;44(1):6–B13.
14. Wang XQ, Zheng JJ, Yu ZW, Bi X, Lou SJ, Liu J, Cai B, Hua YH, Wu M, Wei ML, et al. A meta-analysis of core stability exercise versus general exercise for chronic low back pain. PLoS One. 2012;7(12):e52082.
15. Hicks GE, Fritz JM, Delitto A, McGill SM. Preliminary development of a clinical prediction rule for determining which patients with low back pain will respond to a stabilization exercise program. Arch Phys Med Rehabil. 2005;86(9):1753–62.
16. Childs JD, Cleland JA. Development and application of clinical prediction rules to improve decision making in physical therapist practice. Phys Ther. 2006;86(1):122–31.
17. Laupacis A, Sekar N, Stiell IG. Clinical prediction rules. A review and suggested modifications of methodological standards. JAMA. 1997;277(6):488–94.
18. Haskins R, Osmotherly PG, Rivett DA. Validation and impact analysis of prognostic clinical prediction rules for low back pain is needed: a systematic review. J Clin Epidemiol. 2015;68(7):821–32.
19. McGinn TG, Guyatt GH, Wyer PC, Naylor CD, Stiell IG, Users RWS. Guides to the medical literature: XXII: how to use articles about clinical decision rules. Evidence-based medicine working group. JAMA. 2000;284(1):79–84.
20. Kent P, Keating JL, Leboeuf-Yde C. Research methods for subgrouping low back pain. BMC Med Res Methodol. 2010;10:62.
21. Maughan EF, Lewis JS. Outcome measures in chronic low back pain. Eur Spine J. 2010;19(9):1484–94.
22. Flynn T, Fritz J, Whitman J, Wainner R, Magel J, Rendeiro D, Butler B, Garber M, Allison SA. Clinical prediction rule for classifying patients with low back pain who demonstrate short-term improvement with spinal manipulation. Spine (Phila Pa 1976). 2002;27(24):2835–43.
23. Stolze LR, Allison SC, Childs JD. Derivation of a preliminary clinical prediction rule for identifying a subgroup of patients with low back pain likely to benefit from Pilates-based exercise. J Orthop Sports Phys Ther. 2012;42(5):425–36.
24. Green SB. How many subjects does it take to do a regression analysis. Multivariate Behav Res. 1991;26(3):499–510.
25. Goodman Cavallaro C, Snyder Kelly TE. Differential diagnosis for physical therapists: screening for referral. 5th ed. St-Louis: Elsevier-Saunders; 2013.
26. Smeets R, Koke A, Lin CW, Ferreira M, Demoulin C. Measures of function in low back pain/disorders: low back pain rating scale (LBPRS), Oswestry disability index (ODI), progressive Isoinertial lifting evaluation (PILE), Quebec back pain disability scale (QBPDS), and Roland-Morris disability questionnaire (RDQ). Arthritis Care Res (Hoboken). 2011;63(Suppl 11):S158–73.

27. Fritz JM, Irrgang JJ. A comparison of a modified Oswestry low back pain disability questionnaire and the Quebec back pain disability scale. Phys Ther. 2001;81(2):776–88.

28. Ostelo RW, Deyo RA, Stratford P, Waddell G, Croft P, Von Korff M, Bouter LM, de Vet HC. Interpreting change scores for pain and functional status in low back pain: towards international consensus regarding minimal important change. Spine (Phila Pa 1976). 2008;33(1):90–4.

29. Davidson M, Keating JL. A comparison of five low back disability questionnaires: reliability and responsiveness. Phys Ther. 2002;82(1):8–24.

30. Waddell G, Newton M, Henderson I, Somerville D, Main CJA. Fear-avoidance beliefs questionnaire (FABQ) and the role of fear-avoidance beliefs in chronic low back pain and disability. Pain. 1993;52(2):157–68.

31. Williamson E. Fear Avoidance Beliefs Questionnaire (FABQ). Aust J Physiother. 2006;52(2):149.

32. Cleland JA, Childs JD, Whitman JM. Psychometric properties of the neck disability index and numeric pain rating scale in patients with mechanical neck pain. Arch Phys Med Rehabil. 2008;89(1):69–74.

33. Lindell O, Eriksson L, Strender LE. The reliability of a 10-test package for patients with prolonged back and neck pain: could an examiner without formal medical education be used without loss of quality? A methodological study. BMC Musculoskelet Disord. 2007;8:31.

34. Fritz JM, Brennan GP, Clifford SN, Hunter SJ, Thackeray A. An examination of the reliability of a classification algorithm for subgrouping patients with low back pain. Spine (Phila Pa 1976). 2006;31(1):77–82.

35. Cleland JA, Koppenhaver S. Netter's orthopaedic clinical examination: an evidence basec approach. 2nd ed. Philadelphia: Saunders-Elsevier; 2011.

36. Hicks GE, Fritz JM, Delitto A, Mishock J. Interrater reliability of clinical examination measures for identification of lumbar segmental instability. Arch Phys Med Rehabil. 2003;84(12):1858–64.

37. Neto T, Jacobsohn L, Carita AI, Oliveira R. Reliability of the Active-Knee-Extension and Straight-Leg-Raise Tests in Subjects With Flexibility Deficits. J Sport Rehabil. 2015;Technical Notes;17:2014–0220.

38. Stochkendahl MJ, Christensen HW, Hartvigsen J, Vach W, Haas M, Hestbaek L, Adams A, Bronfort G. Manual examination of the spine: a systematic critical literature review of reproducibility. J Manipulative Physiol Ther. 2006;29(6):475–85. 485 e471–410

39. Shumway-Cook A, Woollacott MH. Motor control: translating research into clinical practice. 4th ed. Philadelphia: Wilkins LW; 2012.

40. Dziuban CD, Shirkey EC. When is a correlation matrix appropriate for factor analysis? Some decision rules. Psychol Bull. 1974;81(6):358–61.

41. Poitras S, Rossignol M, Dionne C, Tousignant M, Truchon M, Arsenault B, Allard P, Cote M, Neveu A. An interdisciplinary clinical practice model for the management of low-back pain in primary care: the CLIP project. BMC Musculoskelet Disord. 2008;9:54.

42. Childs JD, Fritz JM, Flynn TW, Irrgang JJ, Johnson KK, Majkowski GR, Delitto A. A clinical prediction rule to identify patients with low back pain most likely to benefit from spinal manipulation: a validation study. Ann Intern Med. 2004;141(12):920–8.

43. Henschke N, Maher CG, Refshauge KM, Herbert RD, Cumming RG, Bleasel J, York J, Das A, McAuley JH. Prognosis in patients with recent onset low back pain in Australian primary care: inception cohort study. BMJ. 2008;337:a171.

44. Traeger AC, Henschke N, Hubscher M, Williams CM, Kamper SJ, Maher CG, Moseley GL, McAuley JH. Estimating the risk of chronic pain: development and validation of a prognostic model (PICKUP) for patients with acute low back pain. PLoS Med. 2016;13(5):e1002019.

2

Clinical classification in low back pain: best-evidence diagnostic rules based on systematic reviews

Tom Petersen[1]* (ID), Mark Laslett[2,3] and Carsten Juhl[4,5]

Abstract

Background: Clinical examination findings are used in primary care to give an initial diagnosis to patients with low back pain and related leg symptoms. The purpose of this study was to develop best evidence Clinical Diagnostic Rules (CDR) for the identification of the most common patho-anatomical disorders in the lumbar spine; i.e. intervertebral discs, sacroiliac joints, facet joints, bone, muscles, nerve roots, muscles, peripheral nerve tissue, and central nervous system sensitization.

Methods: A sensitive electronic search strategy using MEDLINE, EMBASE and CINAHL databases was combined with hand searching and citation tracking to identify eligible studies. Criteria for inclusion were: persons with low back pain with or without related leg symptoms, history or physical examination findings suitable for use in primary care, comparison with acceptable reference standards, and statistical reporting permitting calculation of diagnostic value. Quality assessments were made independently by two reviewers using the Quality Assessment of Diagnostic Accuracy Studies tool. Clinical examination findings that were investigated by at least two studies were included and results that met our predefined threshold of positive likelihood ratio ≥ 2 or negative likelihood ratio ≤ 0.5 were considered for the CDR.

Results: Sixty-four studies satisfied our eligible criteria. We were able to construct promising CDRs for symptomatic intervertebral disc, sacroiliac joint, spondylolisthesis, disc herniation with nerve root involvement, and spinal stenosis. Single clinical test appear not to be as useful as clusters of tests that are more closely in line with clinical decision making.

Conclusions: This is the first comprehensive systematic review of diagnostic accuracy studies that evaluate clinical examination findings for their ability to identify the most common patho-anatomical disorders in the lumbar spine. In some diagnostic categories we have sufficient evidence to recommend a CDR. In others, we have only preliminary evidence that needs testing in future studies. Most findings were tested in secondary or tertiary care. Thus, the accuracy of the findings in a primary care setting has yet to be confirmed.

Keywords: Diagnostic accuracy, Sensitivity and specificity, Clinical examination, Low back pain classification, Clinical decision making

* Correspondence: tompet@mail.tele.dk
[1]Back Center Copenhagen, Mimersgade 41, 2200 Copenhagen N, Denmark
Full list of author information is available at the end of the article

Background

Identifying diagnostic, prognostic and treatment orientated subgroups of patients with low back pain (LBP) has been on the research agenda for many years [1, 2]. Diagnostic reasoning with a structural/pathoanatomical focus is common among clinicians [3], and it is regarded as an essential component of the biopsychosocial model [4–6]. Within this model, emphasis has been on the role of psychosocial considerations and how these factors can interfere with recovery. Indeed, there is good quality evidence for the predictive value of a set of psychosocial factors for poorer outcome in patients with LBP [7, 8]. These factors are multifactorial, interrelated, and only weakly associated to the development and prognosis of LBP [9], which might be one of the explanations why effects of treatments targeting those risk factors has been reported to be small, mostly short term, and there was little evidence that psychosocial treatments were superior to other active treatments [7, 10].

Maybe it is time to swing the pendulum towards the "bio" in the biopsychosocial model. There are many examples in medicine where the pathology has been identified prior to any effective treatments being developed making it an ongoing challenge to generate new diagnostic knowledge on which to base more effective treatment strategies in the future. Alongside clinicians, many researchers within the field of LBP feel that choosing the most effective treatment for the individual patient is not possible without better understanding of the biological component of the biopsychosocial model [4].

In 2003 the present authors suggested a diagnostic LBP classification system based on a review of the literature [11, 12]. This system has been fully or partly used in prognostic and outcome studies by other research groups [13–15]. The present study is driven by the obvious need for an update based on recent evidence. The relevance of an updated diagnostic classification is as follows:

First, diagnostic patterns of signs and symptoms from history and physical examination may assist the clinician in explaining the origin of pain to the patient and in directing treatment at the painful structure. Patients with persistent LBP often have misconceptions about what is going on [16], and may have been given all sorts of speculative explanations for their symptoms resulting in anxiety and confusion. These patients often seek an explanation about what is wrong [17], and new evidence suggests that offering clear explanations and information about aetiology, prognosis and interventions may improve patient outcomes [7]. Giving an explanation based on best evidence may contribute to 1) reducing the patient's confusion and conceptual chaos, 2) reassurance that the clinician knows what is going on, 3) visualizing the potential benefit of treatment directed at the painful structure (mental imagery has been suggested to have potential in pain management [18, 19], 4) provided that the above efforts are successful, motivating the patient to open a therapeutic window.

Second, the need for studies testing the effect of treatment strategies for subgroups of patients with LBP in primary care has been emphasized in consensus-papers [1, 20] as well as current European guidelines [21]. Targeting treatment to classifications merely based on prognostic patient characteristics has not been convincingly successful in finding treatment modalities that are more beneficial than others [22]. A diagnostic classification may assist in generating hypotheses as to which treatment modalities are more likely to target the pain source for future testing in randomized trials.

Finally, an evidence-based clinical diagnosis with acceptable accuracy will reduce the need for invasive or expensive diagnostic methods (often with substantial waiting time and expense).

The focus of this review is to outline the diagnostic value of signs and symptoms for use in primary care without access to confirmatory paraclinical methods. The clinician must not mislead the patient, so it is important to distinguish between diagnostic labels that can be given to patients with reasonable confidence and those only suggesting suspected best evidence pathoanatomy. Therefore, it is of interest to identify signs and symptoms with the potential to diagnose common sources and causes of LBP i.e. intervertebral discs, sacroiliac joints, facet joints, bones, nerve roots, muscles, peripheral nerve tissue, and central nervous system sensitization.

Throughout this review, we use the term Clinical Diagnostic Rule (CDR) meaning that we have applied a clinical decision rule to the field of clinical diagnostics. A clinical decision rule "is a clinical tool that quantifies the individual contributions that various components of the history, physical examination, and basic laboratory results make toward the diagnosis, prognosis, or likely response to treatment in a patient. Clinical decision rules attempt to formally test, simplify, and increase the accuracy of clinicians' diagnostic and prognostic assessments" [23].

The aim of this paper was to develop multi-faceted Clinical Diagnostic Rules (CDRs) for the lumbar spine using individual diagnostic accuracy scores based on best evidence for use in primary care clinical practice and research. If possible, single clinical examination findings would be clustered in CDRs based on well-defined criteria.

Methods

The reporting of this review was based on the Preferred Reporting Items for Systematic reviews and Meta-analyses statement (PRISMA) [24].

Eligibility criteria and study selection

To be included studies were required to meet the following criteria:

1) Participants had LBP with or without leg pain
2) Use of an appropriate reference standard as listed in Table 1.
3) Evaluation of at least one clinical finding available to primary care clinicians.
4) Presentation of data enabling calculation of sensitivity and specificity.

For some diagnostic categories, recent systematic reviews were found covering our topic. These were included if they complied with the principles recommended by the Cochrane Collaboration [25]. In other categories, where searches in included systematic reviews were terminated before 2011, our searches were performed up to May 2015 from the date where the search of those reviews was terminated. In categories where no systematic reviews were found, we conducted systematic searches in the electronic databases PubMed, Embase, and CINAHL. Details of the search strategy are presented in Additional files 1, 2, 3 and 4. One of the authors (TP) reviewed the search results from the databases (titles and abstracts). Any titles and abstracts from studies that appeared to compare the results of clinical examination findings on patients with LBP with those of diagnostic reference standards were selected for full text review. Reference lists of selected studies were reviewed for additional studies. If necessary, authors were contacted for clarification of unclear reporting. The data extraction from the selected studies was prepared by one author (TP) and the second author (ML) reviewed the complete data extraction form for accuracy. Any disagreements were resolved by discussion. In diagnostic findings where no studies presenting sensitivity and specificity were found, studies presenting predictive values (sensitivity only) were included. We extracted values of diagnostic accuracy for clinical examination findings that were investigated by at least two studies.

Reference standards

In this review, we used the best available reference standards for diagnosis of the relevant source and cause of LBP. See Table 1. Index tests results were reported if they were investigated in at least two studies using the best available reference standard.

Quality assessment

Original studies were retrieved in full text and independently scored for quality and risk of bias using Quality Assessment of Diagnostic Accuracy Studies (QUADAS) in accordance with the recommendations of the Cochrane Handbook for Systematic Reviews of DTA [26]. Any disagreements were resolved by discussion. In a few cases, one of the present authors were co-authoring a paper or we were not able to acquire the original papers included in previous reviews. In these cases the results of QUADAS were transferred from the review in question to the present paper.

Grading of recommendations

There is currently no consensus regarding criteria to assess the quality of evidence of diagnostic tests [27]. In this study, diagnostic values that were in agreement in more than two thirds of studies were included in our final recommendations. Downgrading of recommendations from strong to weak was made in cases with serious risk of bias due to verification bias, partial verification bias, differential verification, incorporation bias, or test review bias.

Diagnostic accuracy measures

In order to be clinically useful, we considered the cut-off for a clinical finding to rule in the disorder to be a positive likelihood ratio (LR) above 2.0 [28], meaning that a

Table 1 Reference standards for painful lumbosacral spine structures

Structure	Reference standard	References
Intervertebral disc	Provocation discography with control disc verification	[171]
Facet joint	Double block procedure in joint space or at nerve supply	[148]
Sacroiliac joint	Double block procedure in joint space	[172]
Nerve root involvement	Magnetic resonance imaging, myelography, or surgical findings with or without clinical findings	[173]
Spinal stenosis	Expert opinion based on radiographs, magnetic resonance imaging or surgical findings with or without clinical findings	[75, 174]
Spondylolisthesis	Sagittal plane rotation or translation movement on functional radiograph or translation on static radiograph	[152, 155]
Fracture	Radiographs, computed tomography or magnetic resonance imaging	[155]
Myofascial structures	None available.	
Peripheral nerve	None available.	
Central sensitization	Expert consensus	

positive index test will at least double the ratio of having the disorder compared to not having the disorder. This means that if the pretest probability is 0.3, the pretest odds is 0.3/0.7 = 0.43 and if the LR is 2.0 the posttest odds is 2*0.43 = 0.86 and the posttest probability can then be estimated to 0.46. For a useful clinical finding to rule out the disorder, we considered the cut-off to be a negative LR below 0.5 [28], meaning that a negative index test will reduce the odds of having the disorder at least by half compared to not having the disorder. Overall, the change from pretest to posttest chance of having the disorder in question depends on the pretest probability.

In summary, clinical examination findings that were investigated by at least two studies were included. Diagnostic values that were in agreement in more than two thirds of studies and met our predefined threshold of positive likelihood ratio ≥ 2 or negative likelihood ratio ≤ 0.5 were considered for the CDR.

Statistics
A meta-analysis was considered if evidence of clinical homogeneity could be established. Clinical heterogeneity was assessed by comparing the similarity of patient samples, performance of tests, and reference standards. However, a qualitative synthesis of studies according to principles of best-evidence synthesis [29] was performed if studies were clinically heterogeneous.

Results
Table 2 outlines the findings in each of the diagnostic categories that are supported by more than one study. Characteristics of the included studies are presented in Additional file 5. Results of the quality assessments are presented in Additional file 6. Results of the searches of the literature are presented in Additional files 7, 8, 9, 10, 1, 2, 3 and 4.

Because of heterogeneous study populations, performance of index tests, and choice of reference standards, only descriptive statistics were used to summarize findings across studies. The diagnostic value of findings in each category is presented below.

Intervertebral disc
A previous systematic review of clinical diagnosis of lumbar intervertebral discs (ID) has terminated the literature search at February 2006 [30], Therefore, databases were searched by the present authors from that date up to May 2015. The results of the search are presented in Additional file 7. Three studies [31–33] from the Hancock review and one study [34] from our updated search were included (Table 2).

The evidence is sufficient to constitute a Clinical Diagnostic Rule (CDR). We recommend the use of centralization of symptoms during physical examination. Two studies using strict criteria for centralization (change of pain in the furthermost whole body region) reported high levels of positive LR [32, 33], meaning that a positive test is useful for ruling in the diagnosis. One study using less strict criteria for centralization (change in any furthermost extent of pain) [31], However, a positive LR of 2.1 even in this study indicates the presence of relatively few false positive tests.

Facet joint
A previous systematic review of clinical diagnosis of facet joints (FJ) terminated the literature search at February 2006 [30]. The current search started from that date up to May 2015. The results are presented in Additional file 7. Seven studies [32, 35–40] from the Hancock review and three studies [41–43] from our updated search were included in this review (Table 2).

The evidence is insufficient to constitute a CDR. No studies supporting Revel's suggested rule [35] or part thereof were identified.

The only negative findings from studies with single block reference standards that appeared potentially useful for ruling out FJ pain were centralization [32, 39] and no relief with recumbency [37, 38].

Sacroiliac joint
A previous systematic review of clinical diagnosis of sacroiliac joints (SIJ) terminated the literature search at February 2006 [30]. The current search started from that date up to May 2015. Results are presented in Additional file 7. Four studies [32, 44–46] from the Hancock review and three studies [47–49] from our updated search were included (Table 2).

The evidence is sufficient to constitute a CDR. We recommend the use of the Laslett rule [44] comprising at least 3 positive out of 5 of the following findings from physical examination: distraction, compression, thigh thrust, Gaenslen's test, or sacral thrust.

The rule was supported by two additional studies where composites of at least 3 positive out of 5 tests resulted in high levels of positive LR [45, 48]. There is only a slight difference in tests included in the composites.

We recommend the addition of no centralization from the "Laslett composite" to the CDR as it increases the positive LR without compromising the negative LR. The value of centralization for screening out SIJ pain was supported by one more study with single block reference standards reporting an acceptable negative LR [32].

Furthermore, we recommend the use of the physical examination finding dominant pain the posterior superior iliac crest (PSIS) area. This finding was only investigated in one study using the double block standard [49]. However, the usefulness is supported by the fact that all included studies comprised patients with pain location in the PSIS area and it is a logical assumption that a

Table 2 Diagnostic accuracy of clinical tests for lumbar diagnoses that are investigated by more than one study

Structure	Sensitivity (95% CI)	Specificity (95% CI)	Positive LR (95% CI)	Negative LR (95% CI)
Intervertebral disc				
Studies supporting a diagnostic rule				
Centralization (P) Donelson 1997 [31]	0.64 (0.46–0.79)	0.70 (0.50–0.86)	2.1 (1.2–3.9)	0.52 (0.32–0.86)
Centralization (P)[a] Young 2003 [32]	0.47 (0.22–0.73)	0.95 (0.62–1.0)	9.4 (0.6–146.9)	0.56 (0.35–0.91)
Centralization (P)[a] Laslett 2005 [33]	0.40 (0.28–0.54)	0.94 (0.73–0.99)	6.9 (1.0–47.3)	0.63 (0.49–0.82)
Studies not supporting a diagnostic rule				
None				
Additional findings reported by more than one study				
Pain crosses midline[a] (H) Young 2003 [32]	0.27 (0.11–0.52)	0.38 (0.14–0.69)	0.4 (0.2–1.2)	1.96 (0.76–5.03)
Midline pain only (H) Schwarzer 1995 [34]	0.03 (0.00–0.14)	—	—	—
Facet joint				
Revel's suggested rule: 5 of 7 positive findings Manchikanti 2000 [35]	0.13 (0.07–0.22)	0.84 (0.76–0.90)	0.8 (0.4–1.7)	1.03 (0.92–1.16)
Age more than 65 years (H)	0.22 (0.14–0.32)	0.85 (0.77–0.91)	1.5 (0.8–2.6)	0.92 (0.80–1.05)
Pain relieved in recumbent position (P)	0.94 (0.86–0.98)	0.17 (0.10–0.25)	1.1 (1.0–1.2)	0.39 (0.18–0.96)
Pain not increased with cough (P)	0.90 (0.82–0.95)	0.13 (0.08–0.21)	1.0 (0.9–1.1)	0.76 (0.34–1.66)
Pain not increased with forward flexion (P)	0.16 (0.09–0.25)	0.82 (0.73–0.88)	0.9 (0.5–1.6)	1.03 (0.91–1.17)
Pain not increased with rising from flexion (P)	0.55 (0.44–0.65)	0.48 (0.39–0.58)	1.1 (0.8–1.4)	0.94 (0.70–1.26)
Pain not increased with hyperextension (P)	0.10 (0.05–0.18)	0.86 (0.78–0.92)	0.7 (0.3–1.2)	1.05 (0.95–1.16)
Pain not increased with extension/rotation (P)	0.68 (0.57–0.77)	0.30 (0.22–0.40)	1.0 (0.8–1.2)	1.07 (0.71–1.61)
Studies supporting items of Revel's suggested rule				
Pain relieved in recumbent position (P) Single block Revel 1998 [38]	0.96 (0.71–1.00)	0.48 (0.30–0.67)	1.9 (1.3–2.7)	0.07 (0.01–1.15)
Pain relieved in recumbent position (P) Single block Revel 1992 [37]	0.63 (0.41–0.82)	0.76 (0.52–0.92)	2.7 (1.1–6.3)	0.48 (0.27–0.87)
Studies not supporting items of Revel's suggested rule				
Age more than 65 years (H) Manchikanti 1999 [36]	0.19 (0.10–0.32)	0.66 (0.54–0.78)	0.6 (0.3–1.1)	1.21 (0.98–1.51)
Age more than 61 years (H) Manchikanti 2008 [41]	0.19 (0.12–0.29)	0.75 (0.69–0.81)	0.8 (0.5–1.3)	1.07 (0.94–1.12)
No pain with extension/rotation (P) Schwarzer 1994 [42]	0.0 (0.0–0.13)	0.88 (0.82–0.93)	0.0 (—)	1.13 (1.07–1.20)
No pain with hyperextension (P) Fairbank 1981 [43]	0.36 (0.16–0.61)	0.36 (0.15–0.65)	0.6 (0.2–1.3)	1.77 (0.74–4.24)
Revel's suggested rule Single block[a] Laslett 2004 [40]	0.11 (0.39–2.8)	0.91 (0.83–0.95)	1.2 (0.4–4.3)	0.98 0.84–1.13
Additional findings reported by more than one study				
Traumatic onset (H) Manchikanti 2000 [35]	0.48 (0.37–0.59)	0.50 (0.41–0.59)	1.0 (0.7–1.3)	1.05 (0.80–1.37)
Traumatic onset (H) Manchikanti 1999 [36]	0.54 (0.40–0.67)	0.47 (0.35–0.60)	1.0 (0.7–1.4)	0.99 (0.67–1.44)
No centralization (P) Single block[a] Young 2003 [32]	1.00 (0.78–1.0)	0.11 (0.02–0.44)	1.3 (0.9–1.4)	NA
No centralization (P) Single block[a] Laslett 2006 [39]	1.00 (0.74–1.0)	0.17 (0.11–0.27)	1.2 (1.1–1.3)	NA
Sacroiliac joint				
Laslett composite: no centralization and 3 of 5 positive findings: distraction, compression, thigh thrust, Gaenslen's test, sacral thrust (P)[a] Laslett 2003 [44]	0.91 (0.62–0.98)	0.87 (0.68–0.95)	7.0 (2.4–20.4)	0.11 (0.02–0.68)
Laslett rule: 3 of 5 positive findings alone (P)[a] Laslett 2003 [44]	0.91 (0.62–0.98)	0.78 (0.61–0.89)	4.2 (2.1–8.2)	0.12 (0.02–0.76)
Studies supporting items of Laslett's rule				
van der Wurff composite 3 out of 5 positive findings: distraction, compression, thigh thrust, Gaenslen's test, Patrick's test (P) van der Wurff 2006 [45]	0.85 (0.72–0.99)	0.79 (0.65–0.93)	4.0 (2.0–7.9)	0.19 (0.07–0.47)

Table 2 Diagnostic accuracy of clinical tests for lumbar diagnoses that are investigated by more than one study *(Continued)*

Stanford composite 3 out of 5 positive findings: Patrick's test, thigh thrust, Gaenslen's test, compression, sacral thrust (P) Stanford 2010 [47]	0.82 (0.52–0.95)	0.57 (0.37–0.74)	1.9 (1.1–3.2)	0.32 (0.09–1.19)
Ozgocmen composite 3 out of 5 positive findings: Patrick's test, thigh thrust, Gaenslen's test, Mennell, sacral thrust (P) Ozgocmen 2008 [48]	0.45 (0.18–0.75)	0.89 (0.71–0.97)	4.4 (1.3–15.4)	0.62 (—)
No centralization (P) Single block[a] Young 2003 [32]	0.92 (0.76–0.98)	0.23 (0.12–0.41)	1.2 (1.0–1.5)	0.33 (0.08–1.45)
Studies not supporting items of Laslett's rule				
Gaenslen's test (P) Single block Dreyfuss 1996 [46]	0.67 (0.52–0.79)	0.35 (0.22–0.50)	1.0 (0.8–1.4)	0.95 (0.53–1.72)
Thigh thrust (P) Single block Dreyfuss 1996 [46]	0.42 (0.29–0.57)	0.45 (0.31–0.60)	0.8 (0.5–1.2)	1.28 (0.84–1.96)
Sacral thrust (P) Single block Dreyfuss 1996 [46]	0.51 (0.36–0.66)	0.40 (0.25–0.57)	0.9 (0.6–1.2)	1.22 (0.76–1.96)
Additional findings reported by more than one study				
Dominant pain in SIJ without tuber area (H) Van der Wurff 2006 [49]	0.89 (0.72–0.96)	0.79 (0.62–0.89)	4.2 (2.1–8.20)	0.14 (0.05–0.42)
PSIS pointing Single block Dreyfuss 1996 [46]	0.71 (0.57–0.82)	0.48 (0.33–0.63)	1.4 (1.0–1.9)	0.61 (0.35–1.07)
Disc herniation with nerve root involvement				
Hancock rule L4 nerve, 3 out of 4 positive findings: corresponding dermatomal pain location, sensory deficits, reflex and motor weakness Hancock 2011 [52]	0.50 (0.21–0.79)	0.90 (0.85–0.93)	5.0 (?)	0.01 (?)
Hancock rule L5 nerve, 3 out of 4 positive findings: Corresponding dermatomal pain location, sensory deficits, reflex and motor weakness Hancock 2011 [52]	0.37 (0.28–0.46)	0.83 (0.76–0.88)	2.2 (?)	0.76 (?)
Hancock rule S1 nerve, 3 out of 4 positive findings: corresponding dermatomal pain location, sensory deficits, reflex and motor weakness Hancock 2011 [52]	0.28 (0.21–0.35)	0.94 (0.88–0.98)	4.7 (?)	0.77 (?)
L4 dermatomal pain location only (P) L3 disc	0.39 (0.14–0.68)	0.97 (0.94–0.99)	13.0 (?)	0.63 (?)
L5 pain dermatomal location only (P) L4 disc	0.25 (0.18–0.34)	0.92 (0.86–0.96)	3.2 (?)	0.79 (?)
S1 pain dermatomal location only (P) L5 disc	0.22 (0.16–0.29)	0.98 (0.94–1.00)	11.0 (?)	0.80 (?)
L4 location sensory loss (P) L3 disc	0.42 (0.15–0.72)	0.74 (0.69–0.79)	1.6 (0.8–3.3)	0.79 (0.49–1.28)
L5 location sensory loss (P) L4 disc	0.60 (0.51–0.69)	0.54 (0.45–0.62)	1.3 (1.0–1.6)	0.75 (0.58–0.97)
S1 location sensory loss (P) L5 disc	0.59 (0.51–0.66)	0.60 (0.50–0.69)	1.5 (1.1–1.9)	0.69 (0.54–0.87)
Patellar reflex weakness (P) L3 disc	0.50 (0.21–0.79)	0. 83 (0.78–0.87)	2.9 (0.6–5.5)	0.60 (0.34–1.06)
Achilles reflex weakness (P) L5 disc	0.48 (0.40–0.56)	0.83 (0.75–0.90)	2.9 (1.8–4.5)	0.62 (0.52–0.74)
Quadriceps weakness (P) L3 disc	0.67 (0.35–0.90)	0.40 (0.34–0.46)	1.1 (0.7–1.7)	0.84 (0.37–1.89)
Tibialis anterior weakness (P) L4 disc	0.46 (0.37–0.55)	0.70 (0.63–0.77)	1.6 (1.1–2.1)	0.77 (0.63–0.93)
Peroneal weakness (P) L4 disc	0.50 (0.41–0.59)	0.68 (0.60–0.75)	1.6 (1.2–2.1)	0.73 (0.60–0.90)
Ext. hallucis longus weakness (P) L4 disc	0.54 (0.44–0.63)	0.64 (0.56–0.72)	1.5 (1.2–2.0)	0.72 (0.58–0.90)
Calf weakness (P) L5 disc	0.30 (0.23–0.38)	0.63 (0.53–0.72)	0.8 (0.6–1.1)	1.11 (0.94–1.33)
Studies supporting items of the Hancock rule				
All 3 findings positive: sensory loss, paresis, loss of reflexes (P) any nerve Vroomen 1998 [74]	0.31 (0.14–0.56)	0.93 (0.83–0.97)	4.3 (1.3–14.1)	0.74 (0.53–1.04)
Dermatomal pain location (H) any nerve Vroomen 2002 [53]	0.89 (0.84–0.93)	0.31 (0.24–0.40)	1.3 (1.1–1.5)	0.34 (0.20–0.58)
Pain location (H) corresponding S1 nerve Bertilson 2010 [54]	0.55 (0.28–0.79)	0.76 (0.63–0.86)	2.3 (1.1–4.7)	0.60 (0.31–1.16)
L5 location sensory loss (P) disc L4 Kerr 1988 [55]	0.30 (0.19–0.44)	0.86 (0.71–0.94)	2.2 (0.9–5.4)	0.81 (0.65–1.02)
S1 location sensory loss (P) disc L5 Kerr 1988 [55]	0.45 (0.31–0.59)	0.86 (0.71–0.94)	3.2 (1.3–7.7)	0.64 (0.48–0.86)
Anterior thigh sensory loss (P) L2-L4 nerves Suri 2010 [56]	0.08 (1.01–0.27)	0.96 (0.82–1.00)	2.3 (0.23–24.2)	0.95 (0.83–1.09)
Anterior thigh sensory loss (P) L2 nerve Suri 2010 [56]	0.50 (0.01–0.99)	0.96 (0.86–1.00)	12.5 (1.8–87.0)	0.52 (0.13–2.08)
Medial knee sensory loss (P) L2-L4 nerves Suri 2010 [56]	0.17 (0.05–0.37)	0.96 (0.82–1.00)	4.7 (0.6–39.00)	0.86 (0.71–1.05)

Table 2 Diagnostic accuracy of clinical tests for lumbar diagnoses that are investigated by more than one study *(Continued)*

Medial ankle sensory loss (P) L2-L4 nerves Suri 2010 [56]	0.17 (0.05–0.37)	1.00 (0.88–1.00)	NA	0.83 (0.69–1.01)
Medial ankle sensory loss (P) L4 nerve Suri 2010 [56]	0.31 (0.09–0.61)	1.00 (0.91–1.00)	NA	0.69 (0.48–0.99)
Medial foot sensory loss (P) L4 disc Gurdjian 1961 [57]	0.13 (0.11–0.16)	0.94 (0.92–0.96)	2.3 (1.5–3.3)	0.92 (0.89–0.96)
Lateral foot sensory loss (P) L5-S1 nerves Suri 2010 [56]	0.21 (0.08–0.41)	0.92 (0.73–0.99)	2.6 (0.6–11.6)	0.86 (0.68–1.08)
Lateral foot sensory loss(P) L5 disc Gurdjian 1961 [57]	0.23 (0.20–0.27)	0.90 (0.87–0.92)	2.3 (1.7–3.1)	0.85 (0.81–0.90)
S1 location sensory loss (P) L5 disc Kerr 1988 [49]	0.47 (0.33–0.61)	0.86 (0.71–0.94)	3.3 (1.4–8.0)	0.61 (0.46–0.83)
Patellar reflex weakness (P) L4 nerve Suri 2010 [56]	0.39 (0.18–0.65)	0.95 (0.84–0.99)	7.7 (1.7–35.0)	0.65 (0.42–1.00)
Patellar reflex weakness (P) L3 disc Knutsson 1961 [58]	1.00 (0.34–1.00)	0.84 (0.78–0.89)	6.4 (4.6–9.0)	NA
Achilles reflex weakness (P) L5-S1 nerves Suri 2010 [56]	0.29 (0.13–0.49)	0.96 (0.80–1.00)	7.1 (1.0–53.2)	0.74 (0.58–0.95)
Achilles reflex weakness (P) L5 nerve Suri 2010 [56]	0.33 (0.16–0.56)	0.91 (0.78–0.97)	3.9 (1.1–13.8)	0.73 (0.52–1.03)
Achilles reflex weakness (P) L5 disc Gurdjian 1961 [57]	0.56 (0.52–0.60)	0.75 (0.71–0.79)	2.3 (1.9–2.7)	0.58 (0.52–0.64)
Achilles reflex weakness (P) L5 disc Kerr 1988 [55]	0.87 (0.75–0.94)	0.89 (0.75–0.96)	7.9 (3.1–19.9)	0.14 (0.07–0.31)
Achilles reflex weakness (P) L5 disc Knutsson 1961 [58]	0.78 (0.67–0.86)	0.65 (0.55–0.73)	2.2 (1.7–2.9)	0.34 (0.22–0.54)
Reflex absence ankle/knee (P) any nerve Vroomen 2002 [53]	0.14 (0.09–0.21)	0.93 (0.88–0.97)	2.2 (1.0–4.8)	0.91 (0.84–0.99)
Sit to stand weakness (P) L3 nerve Suri 2010 [56]	0.50 (0.19–0.81)	0.77 (0.62–0.89)	2.2 (1.00–5.0)	0.65 (0.34–1.23)
Sit to stand weakness (P) L4 nerve Suri 2010 [56]	0.54 (0.25–0.81)	0.80 (0.65–0.91)	2.8 (1.2–6.1)	0.57 (0.31–1.05)
Heel raise weakness (P) L5-S1 nerves Suri 2010 [56]	0.14 (0.04–0.32)	0.96 (0.80–1.00)	3.5 (0.4–28.9)	0.90 (0.76–1.06)
Great toe ext. weakness (P) L5 nerve Suri 2010 [56]	0.61 (0.36–0.83)	0.86 (0.71–0.95)	4.4 (1.8–10.8)	0.45 (0.25–0.82)
Great toe ext. weakness (P) L4 disc Knutsson 1961 [58]	0.75 (0.65–0.83)	0.53 (0.43–0.63)	1.6 (1.3–2.1)	0.47 (0.31–0.71)
Ankle dorsiflexion weakness (P) L4 disc Kerr 1988 [55]	0.60 (0.46–0.72)	0.89 (0.75–0.96)	5.4 (2.1–13.9)	0.45 (0.31–0.64)
Ankle plantarflexion weakness (P) L5 disc Kerr 1988 [55]	0.13 (0.06–0.25)	1.00 (0.90–1.00)	NA	0.87 (0.78–0.97)
Paresis not specified (P) any nerve Vroomen 2002 [53]	0.27 (0.21–0.35)	0.93 (0.88–0.97)	4.1 (2.0–8.4)	0.78 (0.70–0.87)
Studies not supporting items of the Hancock rule				
Pain location (H) corresponding L4 nerve Bertilson 2010 [54]	0.00 (0.00–0.32)	0.85 (0.73–0.92)	0.0 (NA)	1.18 (1.05–1.32)
Pain location (H) corresponding L5 nerve Bertilson 2010 [54]	0.78 (0.55–0.91)	0.28 (0.17–0.43)	1.1 (0.79–1.47)	0.80 (0.30–2.14)
Non-specific sensory deficits (P) any disc level Stankovic 1999 [59]	0.56 (0.42–0.68)	0.40 (0.28–0.53)	0.9 (0.7–1.3)	1.12 (0.71–1.75)
Non-specific sensory deficits (P) any disc level Vucetic 1996 [60]	0.45 (0.37–0.53)	0.69 (0.39–0.91)	1.5 (0.6–3.3)	0.80 (0.54–1.18)
Sensory loss not specified (P) L3-L5 discs Kosteljanetz 1984 [63]	0.60 (0.47–0.73)	0.57 (0.41–0.72)	1.4 (0.9–2.1)	0.69 (0.46–1.05)
Sensory loss not specified (P) L3-L5 disc Knutsson 1961 [58]	0.28 (0.22–0.36)	0.65 (0.41–0.85)	0.8 (0.4–1.6)	1.10 (0.79–1.54)
Sensory loss not specified (P) L5 or S1 nerve Albeck 1996 [61]	0.67 (0.54–0.79)	0.42 (0.20–0.67)	1.2 (0.8–1.8)	0.78 (0.41–1.47)
Great toe sensory loss (P) L5-S1 nerves Suri 2010 [56]	0.18 (0.06–0.37)	0.87 (0.66–0.97)	1.4 (0.4–5.1)	0.94 (0.75–1.19)
Hypesthesia (P) any nerve Vroomen 2002 [53]	0.28 (0.21–0.36)	0.66 (0.56–0.74)	0.8 (0.6–1.2)	1.09 (0.93–1.29)
Hypalgesia (P) any nerve Vroomen 2002 [53]	0.17 (0.11–0.24)	0.84 (0.77–0.90)	1.1 (0.6–1.9)	0.98 (0.88–1.09)
Hypesthesia (P) L5 or S1 nerve (P) Albeck 1996 [61]	0.67 (0.54–0.79)	0.42 (0.20–0.67)	1.2 (0.8–1.8)	0.78 (0.41–1.47)
Disturbed touch sensibility (P) corresponding L4 nerve Bertilson 2010 [54]	0.13 (0.02–0.47)	0.75 (0.62–0.85)	0.5 (0.1–3.4)	1.16 (0.86–1.57)
Disturbed touch (P) corresponding L5 nerve Bertilson 2010 [54]	0.22 (0.09–0.45)	0.51 (0.37–0.65)	0.5 (0.2–1.1)	1.52 (1.04–2.23)
Disturbed touch sensibility (P) corresponding S1 nerve Bertilson 2010 [54]	0.36 (0.15–0.65)	0.68 (0.54–0.79)	1.1 (0.5–2.7)	0.94 (0.58–1.52)
Disturbed pain sensibility (P) corresponding L4nerve Bertilson 2010 [54]	0.00 (0.00–0.32)	0.45 (034.–0.60)	0.0 (NA)	2.1 (1.59.–2.82)
Disturbed pain sensibility (P) corresponding L5 nerve Bertilson 2010 [54]	0.44 (0.25–0.66)	0.40 (0.26–0.54)	0.7 (0.4–1.3)	1.4 (0.81.–2.45)
Disturbed pain sensibility (P) corresponding S1 nerve Bertilson 2010 [54]	0.36 (0.15–0.65)	0.58 (0.44–0.71)	0.9 (0.4–2.0)	1.10 (0.66.–1.81)
Patellar reflex weakness (P) L3 disc Gurdjian 1961 [57]	0.02 (0.00–0.12)	0.92 (0.91–0.94)	0.3 (0.0–2.2)	1.06 (1.01–1.11)
Achilles reflex weakness (P) L3-L5 disc Spangfort 1972 [62]	0.31 (0.29–0.33)	0.80 (0.76–0.84)	1.6 (1.3–2.0)	0.86 (0.81–0.91)

Table 2 Diagnostic accuracy of clinical tests for lumbar diagnoses that are investigated by more than one study *(Continued)*

Reflex weakness not specified (P) L5 or S1 nerve Albeck 1996 [61]	0.61 (0.47–0.73)	0.63 (0.38–0.84)	1.7 (0.9–3.1)	0.62 (0.39–0.99)
Disturbed reflexes not specified (P) corresponding L4 nerve Bertilson 2010 [54]	0.38 (0.14–0.69)	0.64 (0.51–0.76)	1.0 (0.4–2.7)	1.00 (0.55–1.73)
Disturbed reflexes not specified (P) corresponding L5 nerve Bertilson 2010 [54]	0.61 (0.39–0.80)	0.56 (0.41–0.70)	1.4 (0.8–2.3)	0.70 (0.37–1.32)
Disturbed reflexes not specified (P) corresponding S1 nerve Bertilson 2010 [54]	0.27 (0.10–0.57)	0.48 (0.35–0.62)	0.5 (0.2–1.4)	1.52 (0.95–2.41)
Reflex weakness not specified (P) any disc level Stankovic 1999 [59]	0.46 (0.33–0.60)	0.70 (0.56–0.80)	1.5 (0.9–2.5)	0.77 (0.57–1.05)
Reflex weakness not specified (P) any level Vucetic 1996 [60]	0.35 (0.28–0.44)	0.77 (0.46–0.95)	1.5 (0.6–4.2)	0.84 (0.61–1.16)
Heel walk weakness (P) L5-S1 nerves Suri 2010 [56]	0.14 (0.04–0.32)	0.80 (0.59–0.93)	0.7 (0.2–2.3)	1.08 (0.84–1.38)
Great toe ext. weakness (P) L5-S1 nerves Suri 2010 [56]	0.38 (0.21–0.58)	0.80 (0.59–0.93)	1.9 (0.8–4.7)	0.78 (0.55–1.10)
Ankle dorsiflexion weakness (P) any level Vucetic 1996 [60]	0.29 (0.22–0.37)	0.77 (0.46–0.95)	1.2 (0.4–3.5)	0.93 (0.68–1.27)
Foot drop (P) L4 disc Gurdjian 1961 [51]	0.01 (0.00–0.01)	0.93 (0.86–0.97)	0.1 (0.0–0.3)	1.07 (1.01–1.13)
Extensor hallucis longus weakness (P) L4 disc Gurdjian 1961 [57]	0.20 (0.17–0.23)	0.88 (0.86–0.91)	1.8 (1.3–2.3)	0.90 (0.86–0.95)
Ankle dorsiflex weakness (P) L3-L5 disc Spangfort 1972 [62]	0.30 (0.28–0.32)	0.66 (0.61–0.71)	0.9 (0.8–1.1)	1.06 (0.97–1.15)
Disturbed motor function not specified (P) corresponding L4 nerve Bertilson 2010 [54]	0.50 (0.22–0.78)	0.53 (0.40–0.66)	1.1 (0.5–2.2)	0.95 (0.45–1.98)
Disturbed motor function not specified (P) corresponding L5 nerve Bertilson 2010 [54]	0.56 (0.34–0.75)	0.42 (0.28–0.57)	1.0 (0.6–1.6)	1.06 (0.57–1.98)
Disturbed motor function not specified (P) corresponding S1nerve Bertilson 2010 [54]	0.36 (0.15–0.65)	0.62 (0.48–0.74)	1.0 (0.4–2.3)	1.03 (0.63–1.69)
Motor weakness not specified (P) L5 or S1 nerve Albeck 1996 [61]	0.34 (0.23–0.48)	0.47 (0.24–0.71)	0.7 (0.4–1.1)	1.38 (0.83–2.30)
Motor weakness not specified (P) L3-L5 disc Knutsson 1961 [58]	0.62 (0.54–0.69)	0.50 (0.27–0.73)	1.2 (0.8–2.0)	0.77 (0.70–1.49)
Motor weakness not specified (P) L3-L5 discs Kosteljanetz 1984 [63]	0.47 (0.33–0.60)	0.52 (0.36–0.68)	1.0 (0.6–1.5)	1.02 (0.46–1.05)
Motor weakness not specified (P) any disc level Stankovic 1999 [59]	0.60 (0.46–0.72)	0.38 (0.26–0.51)	1.0 (0.7–1.3)	1.07 (0.66–1.7)
Additional findings reported by more than one study				
Straight Leg Raise (P) L5 or S1 nerves Albeck 1996 [61]	0.83 (0.72–0.91)	0.21 (0.09–0.43)	1.1 (0.8–1.4)	0.78 (0.28–2.20)
Straight Leg Raise (P) L5 or S1 nerves Suri 2010 [56]	0.69 (0.51–0.83)	0.84 (0.65–0.94)	4.3 (1.7–11.0)	0.37 (0.21–0.65)
Straight Leg Raise (P) L5 nerve Suri 2010 [56]	0.67 (0.44–0.84)	0.67 (0.50–0.80)	2.0 (1.1–3.5)	0.50 (0.25–1.0)
Straight Leg Raise (P) L3-L5 discs Knutsson 1961 [58]	0.96 (0.91–0.98)	0.10 (0.03–0.30)	1.1 (0.9–1.2)	0.43 (0.10–1.94)
Straight Leg Raise (P) L3-L5 discs Spangfort 1972 [62]	0.97 (0.96–0.97)	0.11 (0.08–0.15)	1.1 (1.1–1.1)	0.29 (0.20–0.42)
Straight Leg Raise (P) L4 or L5 discs Kerr 1988 [55]	0.98 (0.93–0.99)	0.44 (0.30–0.60)	1.8 (1.3–2.4)	0.05 (0.01–0.19)
Straight Leg Raise (P) L4 or L5 discs Gurdjian 1961 [57]	0.82 (0.80–0.84)	0.45 (0.35–0.56)	1.5 (1.2–1.8)	0.40 (0.30–0.52)
Straight Leg Raise (P) L3-L5 discs Gurdjian 1961 [57]	0.81 (0.78–0.83)	0.37 (0.23–0.54)	1.2 (1.0–1.7)	0.52 (0.34–0.81)
Straight Leg Raise (P) L4-L5 discs Demircan 2002 [71]	0.97 (0.94–0.99)	0.82 (0.73–0.89)	5.4 (3.6–8.2)	0.03 (0.01–0.08)
Straight Leg Raise (P) L3-L5 discs Kosteljanetz 1984 [63]	0.79 (0.66–0.88)	0.48 (0.32–0.63)	1.5 (1.1–2.1)	0.45 (0.25–0.81)
Straight Leg Raise (P) any disc level Charnley 1951 [72]	0.78 (0.68–0.86)	0.64 (0.39–0.84)	2.2 (1.1–4.5)	0.34 (0.19–0.60)
Straight Leg Raise(P) any disc level Kosteljanetz 1988 [70]	0.89 (0.76–0.96)	0.14 (0.00–0.58)	1.0 (0.8–1.4)	0.78 (0.11–5.71)
Straight Leg Raise (P) any disc level Hakelius 1972 [64]	0.96 (0.95–0.97)	0.14 (0.11–0.18)	1.1 (1.1–1.2)	0.27 (0.19–0.38)
Straight leg raise (P) any nerve Vroomen 2002 [53]	0.64 (0.56–0.71)	0.57 (0.48–0.65)	1.5 (1.2–1.9)	0.64 (0.49–0.83)
Straight leg raise (P) any disc level Majlesi 2008 [73]	0.53 (0.37–0.67)	0.89 (0.75–0.96)	4.9 (1.8–12.9)	0.53 (0.37–0.76)
Straight leg raise (P) any disc level Haldeman 1988 [68]	0.44 (0.33–0.57)	0.78 (0.61–0.89)	2.0 (1.0–4.2)	0.71 (0.53–0.94)
Straight leg raise (P) any disc level[a] Meylemans 1988 [67]	0.35 (0.26–0.44)	1.00 (0.92–1.00)	NA	0.65 (0.57–0.75)
Crossed SLR (P) L5 or S1 nerves Suri 2010 [56]	0.07 (0.02–0.22)	0.96 (0.81–0.99)	1.7 (0.2–18.0)	0.97 (0.85–1.1)
Crossed SLR (P) L4 or L5 disc Kerr 1988 [55]	0.43 (0.34–0.53)	0.97 (0.86–0.99)	15.6 (2.2–109.1)	0.58 (0.49–0.74)

Table 2 Diagnostic accuracy of clinical tests for lumbar diagnoses that are investigated by more than one study *(Continued)*

Crossed SLR (P) L3-L5 discs Spangfort 1972 [62]	0.23 (0.21–0.25)	0.88 (0.84–0.91)	2.0 (1.5–2.6)	0.87 (0.83–0.91)
Crossed SLR (P) L3-L5 discs Knutsson 1961 [58]	0.25 (0.18–0.32)	0.95 (0.74–1.00)	4.7 (0.7–32.2)	0.80 (0.69–0.91)
Crossed SLR (P) L4-L5 discs Poiraudeau 2001 [69]	0.29 (0.16–0.45)	0.83 (0.66–0.93)	1.7 (0.7–4.0)	0.86 (0.68–1.10)
Crossed SLR (P) any disc level Kosteljanetz 1988 [70]	0.24 (0.13–0.40)	1.00 (0.59–1.00)	NA	0.76 (0.64–0.89)
Crossed SLR (P) any disc level Stankovic 1999 [59]	0.29 (0.18–0.42)	0.87 (0.75–0.93)	2.2 (1.0–4.9)	0.82 (0.67–1.00)
Slump (P) any disc level Majlesi 2008 [73]	0.84 (0.74–0.90)	0.83 (0.73–0.90)	4.9 (?)	0.19 (?)
Slump (P) any disc level Stankovic 1999 [59]	0.94 (0.84–0.98)	0.23 (0.13–0.36)	1.2 (1.0–1.4)	0. 26 (0.08–0.85)
Spinal Stenosis				
Cook rule: 3 of 5 positive findings Cook 2011 [76]	0.29 (0.27–0.31)	0.88 (0.87–0.90)	2.5 (2.0–3.1)	0.80 (0.76–0.85)
Age more than 48 years (H)	0.88 (0.85–0.89)	0.49 (0.47–0.50)	1.7 (1.6–1.8)	0.25 (0.21–0.32)
Bilateral symptoms (H)	0.03 (0.02–0.04)	0.98 (0.98–0.99)	2.3 (1.1–4.8)	0.98 (0.97–0.99)
Leg pain worse than back pain (H)	0.16 (0.14–0.18)	0.92 (0.91–0.93)	2.1 (1.5–2.8)	0.91 (0.87–0.94)
Pain with walking/standing (H)	0.67 (0.64–0.69)	0.44 (0.42–0.46)	1.2 (1.1–1.3)	0.75 (0.66–0.86)
Sitting relieves pain (H)	0.26 (0.24–0.29)	0.86 (0.84–0.88)	1.9 (1.5–2.3)	0.86 (0.82–0.91)
Studies supporting items of the Cook rule				
Age more than 50 years (H) Konno 2007 [84]	0.95 (0.90–0.98)	0.79 (0.70–0.86)	4.6 (3.10–6.81)	0.06 (0.03–0.13)
Bilateral pain (H) Ljunggren 1991 [78]	0.51 (0.40–0.62)	0.92 (0.85–0.96)	6.3 (3.15–12.74)	0.54 (0.43–0.68)
Severe leg pain (H) Katz 1995 [79]	0.65 (0.51–0.79)	0.67 (0.51–0.83)	2.0 (?)	0.52 (?)
Symptoms extending down the legs when walking (P) Jensen 1989 [80]	0.63 (0.31–0.86)	0.80 (0.55–0.93)	3.1 (0.99–9.82)	0.47 (0.19–1.19)
Leg pain or numbness (H) Konno 2007 [84]	0.94 (0.90–0.98)	0.12 (0.07–0.20)	1.1 (0.99–1.18)	0.41 (0.17–1.01)
Radiating leg pain (disc disease with spinal stenosis) (H) Roach 1997 [81]	0.94 (?)	0.21 (?)	1.2 (?)	0.29 (?)
Symptoms worse by standing (H) Konno 2007 [84]	0.85 (0.78–0.90)	0.75 (0.66–0.83)	3.4 (2.40–4.88)	0.20 (0.14–0.31)
Symptoms exacerbated when standing up (H) Sugioka 2008 [82]	0.92 (0.87–0.95)	0.21 (0.15–0.27)	1.2 (1.06–1.27)	0.39 (0.22–0.69)
Walking or standing worst posture (H) Fritz 1997 [83]	0.88 (0.71–0.96)	0.33 (0.16–0.56)	1.3 (0.93–1.89)	0.35 (0.10–1.21)
Symptoms worse walking and relieved by rest (H) Konno 2007 [84]	0.94 (0.89–0.97)	0.81 (0.73–0.88)	5.1 (3.34–7.71)	0.07 (0.04–0.14)
Pseudoclaudication (H) Roach 1997 [81]	0.63 (?)	0.71 (?)	2.2 (?)	0.52 (?)
Sitting best posture (H) Fritz 1997 [83]	0.89 (0.71–0.96)	0.39 (0.20–0.61)	1.5 (0.98–2.15)	0.29 (0.09–1.0)
Symptoms improve when seated (H) Katz 1995 [79]	0.53 (0.37–0.67)	0.83 (0.70–0.96)	3.1 (?)	0.58 (?)
Studies not supporting items of the Cook rule				
Pain below buttocks (H) Katz 1995 [79]	0.88 (0.78–0.98)	0.34 (0.18–0.50)	1.3 (?)	0.64 (?)
Leg pain with walking that is relieved by sitting (H) Fritz 1997 [83]	0.81 (0.62–0.91)	0.16 (0.55–0.38)	0.96 (0.73–1.26)	1.2 (0.33–4.49)
Pain worse when walking (H) Katz 1995 [79]	0.71 (0.57–0.85)	0.30 (0.14–0.46)	1.0 (?)	0.97 (?)
Intermittent claudication (H) Sugioka 2008 [82]	0.73 (0.66–0.79)	0.38 (0.31–0.46)	1.2 (1.02–1.38)	0.70 (0.52–0.95)
Pain occurs while walking (H) Sugioka 2008 [82]	0.83 (0.77–0.87)	0.27 (0.21–0.34)	1.1 (1.01–1.26)	0.64 (0.44–0.97)
Additional findings reported by more than one study				
Symptoms improved by bending forward (H) Konno 2007 [84]	0.72 (0.64–0.79)	0.92 (0.85–0.96)	8.8 (4.48–17.15)	0.30 (0.23–0.40)
Symptoms improved by bending forward (H) Sugioka 2008 [82]	0.43 (0.36–0.50)	0.75 (0.69–0.81)	1.7 (1.28–2.36)	0.76 (0.66–0.88)
No pain with flexion (P) Katz 1995 [79]	0.79 (0.67–0.91)	0.44 (0.27–0.61)	1.4 (?)	0.48 (?)
Walking easier bending forward (H) Sugioka 2008 [82]	0.55 (0.48–0.62)	0.61 (0.53–0.68)	1.4 (1.12–1.75)	0.74 (0.61–0.90)
Improved treadmill walking tolerance bending forward (Distinguish from PVD) (P) Dong 1989 [85]	0.58 (0.36–0.77)	0.82 (0.52–0.95)	3.2 (0.85–11.81)	0.52 (0.28–0.93)

Table 2 Diagnostic accuracy of clinical tests for lumbar diagnoses that are investigated by more than one study *(Continued)*

Earlier onset of symptoms with level treadmill walking vs inclined (P) Fritz 1997 [83]	0.65 (0.46–0.81)	0.84 (0.62–0.94)	4.1 (1.41–12.14)	0.41 (0.23–0.72)
Symptoms improved by walking uphill (Distinguish from PVD) (H) Dong 1989 [85]	0.16 (0.55–0.38)	1.0 (0.74–1.0)	NA	0.84 (0.69.–1.02)
Thigh pain with extension (P) Katz 1995 [79]	0.51 (0.36–0.66)	0.69 (0.53–0.85)	1.6 (?)	0.71 (?)
Symptoms induced by bending backward (H) Konno 2007 [84]	0.62 (0.54–0.70)	0.48 (0.39–0.58)	1.2 (0.95–1.52)	0.78 (0.58–1.05)
Gait abnormality (ataxic, wide based, poor coordination) (P) Cook 2011 [76]	0.29 (0.27–0.32)	0.81 (0.79–0.83)	1.6 (1.2–1.9)	0.87 (0.82–0.92)
Wide based gait (P) Katz 1995 [79]	0.43 (0.28–0.58)	0.97 (0.91–1.0)	14.3 (?)	0.59 (?)
Spondylolisthesis				
Studies supporting a diagnostic rule				
Manual hypermobility test positive (P) Fritz 2005 [87]	0.46 (0.30–0.64)	0.81 (0.60–0.92)	2.4 (0.9–6.4)	0.66 (0.44–0.99)
Lack of manual hypomobility test positive (P) Fritz 2005 [87]	0.43 (0.27–0.61)	0.95 (0.77–0.99)	9.0 (1.3–63.9)	0.60 (0.43–0.84)
Lack of manual hypomobility test positive and flexion ROM > 53° (P) Fritz 2005 [87]	0.29 (0.13–0.46)	0.98 (0.91–1.00)	12.8 (0.8–211.6)	0.72 (0.55–0.94)
Manual flexion hypermobility test positive (P) rotation Abbott 2005 [88]	0.05 (0.01–0.36)	0.99 (0.96–1.00)	4.1 (0.2–80.3)	0.96 (0.83–1.11)
Manual flexion hypermobility test positive (P) translation Abbott 2005 [88]	0.05 (0.01–0.22)	0.99 (0.97–1.00)	8.7 (0.6–134.7)	0.96 (0.88–1.05)
Manual extension hypermobility test positive (P) rotation Abbott 2005 [88]	0.22 (0.06–0.55)	0.97 (0.94–0.99)	8.4 (1.9–37.6)	0.80 (0.56–1.13)
Manual extension hypermobility test positive (P) translation Abbott 2005 [88]	0.16 (0.06–0.38)	0.98 (0.94–0.99)	7.1 (1.7–29.2)	0.86 (0.71–1.05)
Slipping by palpation (P) Kalpakcioglu 2009 [90]	0.88 (0.80–0.93)	1.00 (0.89–1.00)	NA	0.12 (0.07–0.20)
Slipping by palpation (P) Collaer 2006 [91]	0.60 (0.15–0.95)	0.87 (0.73–0.96)	4.7 (1.6–13.9)	0.46 (0.16–1.35)
Passive lumbar extension test (P) Kasai 2006 [89]	0.84 (0.70–0.93)	0.90 (0.82–0.95)	8.8 (4.5–17.3)	0.18 (0.08–0.37)
Passive lumbar extension test (P) Ferrari 2014 [92]	0.44 (0.29–0.59)	0.86 (0.67–0.95)	3.2 (1.1–9.7)	0.65 (0.47–0.90)
Studies not supporting a diagnostic rule				
None				
Additional findings reported by more than one study				
Slipping by inspection (P) Kalpakcioglu 2009 [90]	0.21 (0.14–0.30)	1.00 (0.89–1.00)	NA	0.79 (0.71–0.87)
Slipping and Sill sign by inspection and palpation (P) Ahn 2015 [93]	0.81 (0.65–0.91)	0.89 (0.79–0.95)	7.4 (3.6–15.2)	0.21 (0.10–0.44)
Aberrant movements (P) Fritz 2005 [87]	0.18 (0.08–0.36)	0.90 (0.71–0.97)	1.9 (0.4–8.7)	0.91 (0.73–1.13)
Aberrant movements (P) Sundell 2013 [94]	0.69 (0.42–0.87)	0.50 (0.25–0.74)	1.4 (0.7–2.7)	0.62 (0.23–1.66)
Fracture				
The Henschke rule 1 out of 3 positive findings: age >70 years, significant trauma, prolonged use of corticosteroids (H) Henschke 2009 [96]	0.88 (0.47–1.00)	0.50 (0.47–0.53)	1.8 (1.3–2.3)	0.25 (0.04–1.57)
The Henschke rule 2 out of 3 positive findings (H) Henschke 2009 [96]	0.63 (0.31–0.86)	0.96 (0.95–0.97)	15.5 (8.4–28.4)	0.39 (0.16–0.96)
Age >70 years (H)	0.50 (0.22–0.78)	0.96 (0.94–0.97)	11.2 (5.3–23.6)	0.52 (0.26–1.05)
Significant trauma (major in young, minor in elderly) (H)	0.25 (0.07–0.59)	0.98 (0.96–0.98)	10.0 (2.9–35.1)	0.77 (0.52–1.15)
Prolonged use of corticosteroids (H)	0.25 (0.07–0.29)	0.99 (0.99–1.00)	48.5 (11.5–204)	0.75 (0.51–1.13)
Studies supporting items of the Henschke rule				
Age >74 years (H) van den Bosch 2004 [97]	0.59 (0.48–0.69)	0.84 (0.82–0.86)	3.7 (3.0–4.5)	0.49 (0.38–0.63)
Trauma (H) Gibson 1992 [98]	1.00 (0.59–1.00)	0.51 (0.41–0.62)	2.1 (1.7–2.5)	0.00 (NA)
Trauma (H) Patrick 1983 [99]	0.80 (0.65–0.90)	0.55 (0.51–0.59)	1.8 (1.5–2.1)	0.36 (0.20–0.68)
Trauma (H)[a] Scavone 1981 [103]	0.65 (0.44–0.83)	0.95 (0.93–0.96)	12.8 (8.6–19.2)	0.37 (0.22–0.62)

Table 2 Diagnostic accuracy of clinical tests for lumbar diagnoses that are investigated by more than one study *(Continued)*

Studies not supporting items of the Henschke rule				
Trauma (H) Deyo 1986 [100]	0.36 (0.16–0.62)	0.90 (0.86–0.93)	3.4 (1.6–7.4)	0.71 (0.49–1.06)
Trauma (H) Reinus 1998 [101]	0.07 (0.02–0.18)	0.60 (0.56–0.65)	0.18 (0.07–0.5)	1.54 (1.38–1.71)
Using steroids (H) Deyo 1986 [100]	0.00 (0.00–0.23)	0.99 (0.98–1.00)	0.0 (NA)	1.01 (0.99–1.02)
Additional findings reported by more than one study				
The Roman rule 2 out of 5 positive findings: age >52 years, no leg pain, body mass index >22, no regular exercise, female gender (H) Roman 2010 [102]	0.95 (0.83–0.99)	0.34 (0.33–0.34)	1.4 (1.3–1.8)	0.16 (0.04–0.51)
Female gender (H) van den Bosch 2004 [97]	0.72 (0.62–0.81)	0.42 (0.41–0.45)	1.2 (1.1–1.5)	0.64 (0.46–0.92)
Female gender (H) Roman 2010 [102]	0.89 (0.75–0.97)	0.41 (0.38–0.44)	1.5 (1.3–1.7)	0.26 (0.10–0.65)
Neurological signs not specified (P) Gibson 1992 [98]	29 (0.04–0.71)	0.88 (0.80–0.94)	2.4 (0.67–8.7)	0.81 (0.51–1.30)
Neurological signs not specified (P) Reinus 1998 [101]	0.05 (0.01–0.15)	0.92 (0.89–0.94)	0.7 (0.2–2.2)	1.03 (0.96–1.10)
Sensory deficits not specified (P) Patrick 1983 [99]	0.03 (0.00–0.13)	0.98 (0.97–0.99)	1.4 (0.2–10.9)	0.99 (0.94–1.04)
Sensory deficits not specified (P)[a] Scavone 1981 [103]	0.27 (0.12–0.83)	0.88 (0.85–0.90)	2.2 (1.1–4.3)	0.83 (0.66–1.05)
Motor deficits not specified (P) Patrick 1983 [99]	0.02 (0.00–0.13)	0.99 (0.98–1.00)	3.1 (0.4–27.3)	0.98 (0.94–1.03)
Motor deficits not specified (P)[a] Scavone 1981 [103]	0.23 (0.09–0.44)	0.89 (0.87–0.91)	2.2 (1.1–4.5)	0.86 (0.70–1.06)
Deep tendon reflex abnormality not specified (P) Patrick 1983 [99]	0.08 (0.02–0.20)	0.95 (0.93–0.97)	1.5 (0.5–4.9)	0.97 (0.89–1.06)
Deep tendon reflex abnormality not specified (P)[a] Scavone 1981 [103]	0.12 (0.02–0.30)	0.89 (0.87–0.91)	1.1 (0.4–3.2)	0.99 (0.86–1.14)
Tenderness not specified (P) Patrick 1983 [99]	0.73 (0.56–0.85)	0.59 (0.54–0.63)	1.8 (1.4–2.2)	0.47 (0.28–0.78)
Tenderness not specified (P)[a] Scavone 1981 [103]	0.50 (0.32–0.68)	0.73 (0.70–0.76)	1.9 (1.3–2.8)	0.68 (0.46–1.00)
Spasm not specified (P) Patrick 1983 [99]	0.25 (0.13–0.41)	0.83 (0.79–0.86)	1.5 (0.83–2.6)	0.90 (0.75–1.09)
Spasm not specified (P)[a] Scavone 1981 [103]	0.12 (0.04–0.29)	0.91 (0.89–0.93)	1.3 (0.4–3.7)	0.98 (0.85–1.12)

(?) = No original data presented to allow for calculation of CI. (—) = Calculation not possible. Calculations are based on number of patients
H history or questionnaire finding, *P* physical examination finding, *PVD* peripheral vascular disease, *LR* likelihood ratio, *CI* confidence interval, *NA* not applicable
[a]Values transferred from previous systematic reviews

strict interpretation of pain location; i.e. dominant pain in the PSIS area opposed to any level of pain, will increase the specificity of this finding.

Disc herniation with nerve root involvement

A systematic review in the field of clinical diagnostic of disc herniation with lumbar nerve root involvement (NRI) has terminated the search of literature at October 2008 [50] and an update is in progress. [51] Therefore, no search of the literature was performed by the present authors. However, we reviewed the included studies and the reference lists of those studies for additional clinical findings. Thirteen studies [52–64] were included from the systematic review and one study was excluded due to lack of a reference standard negative population [65]. In addition, eight studies were included from the latest Cochrane review [66] and our hand search of reference lists [67–74] (Table 2). Data from original studies were reviewed and new calculations of diagnostic values were performed as appropriate.

The evidence is sufficient to constitute a CDR. We recommend initial screening by use of the straight leg raise (SLR) test in combination with the Hancock rule

[52] comprising at least 3 positive out of 4 of the following findings: dermatomal pain location in concordance with a nerve root, and corresponding sensory deficit, reflex and motor weakness.

The CDR was supported by another composite [74] who reported the diagnostic value of a combination of 3 neurological signs in patients with monoradicular pain.

The value of a negative SLR test for screening out nerve root involvement was supported by the vast majority of single studies reporting acceptable levels of negative LRs regardless of level of nerve root involvement [55–58, 62–64, 71, 72].

Furthermore, we recommend the use of crossed SLR that was supported by acceptable positive LRs in the vast majority of studies [55, 58, 59, 62, 70].

The single findings included in the Hancock rule were supported by most studies reporting diagnostic value. Findings were supported by studies reporting acceptable levels of positive LRs: dermatomal S1 pain location [54], L2-L5 sensory deficits [55–57], L4 patellar reflex weakness [56, 58], S1 Achilles reflex weakness [55–58], L4 knee extension weakness [56], L5 dorsiflexion weakness of ankle and toes [55, 56, 58], or S1 plantarflexion weakness of ankle [55, 56]. One study reported acceptable level of negative LR: any nerve dermatomal pain location [53].

The diagnostic value of dermatomal pain location in the Hancock rule was supported by only one additional study and only regarding S1 distribution [54]. However, the usefulness is supported by the fact that 11 out of 14 studies included a patient population with radicular pain location, and it is a logical assumption that a strict interpretation of radicular pain; i.e. dermatomal distribution corresponding neurological findings, will increase the specificity of this finding.

Spinal stenosis

A recently updated systematic review in the field of clinical diagnostic of lumbar spinal stenosis (SS) terminated at March 2011 [75]. Therefore, no search of the literature was performed by the present authors. Nine studies [76–84] were included from the systematic review (Table 2). Two of the nine studies included the same population [82, 84] and we chose to use values from one [82] because it reported diagnostic accuracy of questionnaire items not necessarily part of the reference standard based on physical examination and imaging. In addition, we included one study that was identified by our hand search of reference lists [85].

The evidence is sufficient to constitute a CDR. We recommend the use of the Cook rule [76] comprising at least 3 positive out of 5 of the following findings from patient history: age more than 48 years, bilateral symptoms, leg pain more than back pain, pain during walking/standing, and pain relief upon sitting (Table 2). Furthermore, we recommend the use of improved walking tolerance with the spine in flexion that was supported by two studies with acceptable levels of positive LRs [83, 85], and the patient history report of relief by forward bending that was supported by two studies with acceptable levels of positive LRs [77] or negative LRs [79].

The single findings included in the Cook rule were supported by other studies reporting diagnostic value. Some findings were supported by studies reporting high levels of positive LRs: age above 50 years [77], bilateral pain [78], severe leg pain [79], leg pain worse with walking [77, 80], pseudoclaudication [81], pain worse with standing [77], and symptoms improved when seated [79]. Other studies reported acceptable levels of negative LRs: no leg pain [77, 81], pain not worse when walking or standing [82, 83], and sitting not best posture [83].

Spondylolisthesis

A recently updated systematic review of clinical diagnosis of lumbar spondylolisthesis terminated at March 2010 [86]. Therefore, databases were searched by the present authors from that date up to May 2015. Results of the search are presented in Additional file 8. Three studies from the systematic review [87–89] and five studies from our updated search [90–94] were included (Table 2).

The evidence is sufficient to constitute a CDR. We recommend a combination of two physical examination findings positive: intervertebral slip by inspection or palpation and segmental hypermobility by use of manual passive physiological intervertebral motion test (Table 2). Furthermore, we recommend the use of the passive lumbar extension test as a supplement for the identification of degenerative spondylolisthesis in the elderly. All tests were supported by two studies with acceptable levels of positive LRs.

Fracture

An recently updated systematic review of the diagnosis of lumbar fracture terminated at March 2012 [95]. Therefore, no search of the literature was performed by the present authors. Eight studies from the systematic review [96–103] were included (Table 2).

The evidence is insufficient to constitute a CDR. Best evidence synthesis indicates the potential benefit of the Henschke rule [96] comprising at least 1 negative out of 3 of the following findings from patient history: findings: age >70 years, prolonged use of corticosteroids, and significant trauma (Table 2). This rule presented with the lowest negative LR meaning that when none of these findings are present, the clinician will be able to rule out a lumbar fracture with acceptable confidence.

Regardless of setting in which the studies were conducted, single studies provided inconsistent results, and the Henschke rule has not been validated in other studies.

Myofascial pain

There is no available evidence regarding diagnostic value. We have conducted a systematic search of the literature to May 2015 revealing that studies in the field are hampered by the lack of an adequate diagnostic reference standard. The results of the search are presented in Additional file 9. It appears that clinical criteria are in fact the reference standard. Firm manual pressure applied to the muscle and elicited feedback from the patient appears to be the only means to establish the diagnosis. However, there is considerable variability of criteria used to diagnose a Myofascial Pain Syndrome [104]. The original criteria for a myofascial trigger point (TrP) originally proposed by Travell and Simons [105], have been revised based on clinical experience and results from reliability studies, but neither have been rigorously validated [104].

We suggest a composite of four minimum criteria that support the diagnosis: 1) presence of a palpable taut band within a skeletal muscle, 2) presence of a hypersensitive spot within the taut band with or without reproduction of a distinct referred pain sensation with stimulation of the spot, 3) patient recognition of the elicited pain. These criteria are based on a strict interpretation of the nine criteria currently under debate by The International Association for the Study of Pain (IASP) [106].

We have found no accepted reference standard by which a TrP can be diagnosed. However, several methods have been suggested in order to at least demonstrate construct validity of the clinical criteria. The results of our search revealed some attempts to demonstrate construct validity when TrPs were compared to electromyography [107–111], sonoelastography [112], and quantitative sensory testing [113, 114]. Methodological quality is generally low due to lack of blinding, differences in definition of active and latent TrPs, and all studies but two [108, 113] investigated the shoulder and neck region making generalizability questionable when results are transposed to the low back.

In the absence of evidence regarding diagnostic accuracy, physical examination findings should demonstrate inter-rater reliability in order to be considered clinically meaningful. Two recent systematic reviews conclude that physical examination findings cannot identify TrPs with an acceptable degree of reliability [115, 116]. However, the authors state that if diagnostic criteria were revised to include only a palpable tender spot in the muscle that when palpated reproduces the patients' familiar pain in that spot or in a distinct pattern, then the present evidence indicates that worthwhile agreement might be achieved. This reasoning is in line with our suggestion of including three of the IASP criteria.

There are significant issues in relation to the intra- and inter-observer reliability of identifying a muscle containing a TrP, and there are no data supporting the ability of different examiners to agree on the exact location of a TrP within a specific muscle.

Taken together, no conclusions can be made based on the present evidence although our suggested criteria to be used in future diagnostic studies appear to have face validity.

Peripheral nerve

There is no available evidence regarding diagnostic value. We have conducted a systematic search of the literature up to May 2015 revealing that all studies in the field are hampered by the lack of an adequate diagnostic reference standard. The results of the search are presented in Additional file 10. It appears that clinical criteria are in fact the reference standard. We suggest the following criteria to be used in future diagnostic studies: Patient recognition of usual lumbar or leg pain with at least two stages of sensitizing maneuvers, i.e. knee extension, ankle dorsiflexion, or neck flexion during SLR or slump test.

Although it has not been possible to report rigorous diagnostic validity of our suggested criteria, they appear to have some degree of face validity across authors. However, there is considerable variability of criteria used to diagnose increased peripheral neural mechanosensitivity [117]. Most commonly used are SLR and slump, but the interpretation of a positive test response differs. Authors may put emphasis on provocation of any lumbar or leg pain, patient recognition of their usual pain, and/or restriction of movement during testing [118].

Our search identified no studies that made comparisons between peripheral nerve mechanosensitivity testing and diagnostic procedures that appear to have the potential to be considered as reference standard (i.e. nerve conduction electrodiagnostics, ultrasound imaging, or magnetic resonance neurography]. However, our literature searches identified a number of studies attempting to demonstrate construct validity of particular aspects of the clinical representation of peripheral nerve pain.

Several studies found that reduction in range of movement (ROM] during SLR or slump as criterion for increased neural mechanosensitivity had no proven value in discriminating between patients with LBP and asymptomatic persons [119–124]. Also the hypothesis, that increased muscle tension might be responsible for the changes in ROM during SLR and slump test, has been refuted by electromyographic studies [122, 125–127]. These studies found that muscle tension is an unlikely source to ROM reduction during SLR and slump, but they did not address the main concern, that is, that any fascial network in the back and legs would be a equally plausible source of pain provocation during neural sensitizing maneuvers. Taken together, the data support the view of Shacklock [118] who claimed that reproduction of the patients usual symptoms should be an integral part of the diagnostic criteria.

In the absence of an accepted reference standard, physical examination findings should demonstrate inter-rater reliability in order to be considered clinically meaningful. Our search did not identify any reviews exploring the inter-tester reliability of SLR or slump in patients with LBP. However, we found three individual studies in which the inter-tester reliability of patient recognition of lumbar or leg pain with at least two stages of sensitizing maneuvers was investigated. In all studies, Kappa values (K] indicated substantial agreement between examiners [128]. Walsh et al.[129] reported K = 0.80 (CI 0.39–0.94) for SLR and 0.71 (CI 0.33–0.71) for Slump, Philip et al. [130] reported K = 0.89 (CI 0.81–0.97) for Slump, and Petersen et al. [12] reported K = 0.59 (CI 0.39–0.79) for SLR and Slump.

To summarize, no conclusions can be made based on the present evidence although our suggested criteria to be used in future diagnostic studies appear to have face validity and acceptable level of intertester reliability.

Central sensitization

There is insufficient evidence to generate a diagnostic rule to identify patients with a condition characterized by "increased responsiveness of nociceptive neurons in the central nervous system to their normal or subthreshold afferent input" [131]. We have not conducted a systematic search of the literature inasmuch as studies in the field are hampered by the lack of an adequate diagnostic reference standard because the underlying mechanisms behind localized, regional and widespread pain are not fully understood [132, 133]. In the absence of anything better, we suggest the consensus-based Nijs rule to support the diagnosis of central sensitization (CS) [134].

The first step in the rule is to exclude a neuropathic pain source by use of the IASP criteria [135] and NeuP-SIG guidelines [136]. The next step is to make sure that the following criterion 1 is satisfied in combination with either criterion 2 or 3:

Criterion 1. Pain experience disproportionate to the nature and extent of injury or pathology, i.e. not sufficient evidence of injury, pathology, or objective dysfunctions capable of generating nociceptive input consistent with the patient's severity of pain and disability.
Criterion 2. At least one of the following patterns present:
– bilateral pain/mirror pain (i.e., symmetrical pain pattern)
– pain varying in (anatomical) location/travelling pain to anatomical locations unrelated to the presumed source of nociception e.g., hemilateral pain, large pain areas with non-segmental (i.e., neuroanatomically illogical) distribution
– widespread pain (defined as pain located axially, on the left and right side of the body and both above and below the waist)
– allodynia/hyperalgesia outside the segmental area of (presumed] nociception. These findings are based on testing of light touch by means of a swap or cold items (allodynia) as well as testing by pin prick or pressure (hyperalgesia).
Criterion 3. Hypersensitivity of senses unrelated to the muscular system. These findings are based on a score of at least 40 on the Central Sensitization Inventory [137, 138].

Our suggested criteria are based on a consensus report by researchers from different professions [134] and are in line with other experts in neurophysiology [139–141]. Thus, although it has not been possible to report diagnostic value of the criteria, and only aspects of construct validity have been reported [142], they appear to have face validity. Results of systematic reviews are not consistent with respect to prevalence of generalized or widespread sensitization after quantitative sensory testing as stand-alone tests in patients with chronic LBP [142, 143]. However, a composite of criteria fairly similar to those of the Nijs rule for separating CS from nociceptive and peripheral neuropathic pain sources have been reported to have acceptable levels of inter-tester reliability (K = 0.77, CI 0.57–0.96) [144] and discriminative validity (positive LR 40.6, CI 20.4–80.8) [145].

Taken together, no conclusions can be made based on the present evidence although our suggested criteria to be used in future diagnostic studies appear to have face validity, and promising aspects of construct validity and level of intertester reliability has been reported.

Discussion

We found no composites of clinical findings that were able to fully substitute for the respective reference standards. Thus, in cases where a patho-anatomical diagnosis is of crucial importance for the clinician or the patient, the patient must be referred for more sophisticated diagnostic procedures, which may include high tech imaging or minimally invasive, controlled and guided injection procedures.

Intervertebral disc

Our recommendation for the disc CDR is strong due to risks of partial verification bias in only one [32] of the three studies investigating the finding of centralization. In all studies, a high risk of selection bias is present, because they included patients from secondary care referred for diagnostic invasive procedures. Consequently, the studies are likely to overestimate the diagnostic gain of using the CDR in comparison to primary care settings where the prevalence is somewhat lower.

In addition to the discography studies, our search identified two studies reporting the diagnostic value of centralization for identifying patients with MRI findings of extruded or sequestrated discs [146, 147] Results of these studies were not in concordance and warrant further investigation.

Facet joint

It was not possible to constitute a CDR for the identification of painful FJ. Double block procedure in joint space or at nerve supply was judged to be acceptable as reference standard when at least one of the following criteria were satisfied: a positive controlled block, i.e. the anesthetic block definitely reduced the pain from the injected joint, where as a block in a non-painful joint had no marked effect on pain, a positive confirmatory block, the anesthetic block definitely reduced the pain from the injected joint at two separate occasions 1 to 2 weeks apart, or a positive comparative dual block, i.e. a short- followed by a long lasting anesthetic significantly reduced pain in the predicted time periods [148].

The only negative findings from studies with single block reference standards that supported single tests of the Revel rule for ruling out FJ pain was no relief with recumbency [37, 38]. However, the quality of evidence for this finding was downgraded due to serious risk of test review bias in both studies.

We found two additional single block studies investigating diagnostic value of non-centralization using a single block reference standard [32, 39]. Both studies reported acceptable levels of sensitivity (0.96 and 0.97 respectively) and negative LRs (0.22 and 0.28 respectively). However, the quality of evidence for this finding was downgraded due to risk of partial- or differential bias in the two studies. Although validated with only a single block reference standard, a finding of centralization might have preliminary merit for ruling out a symptomatic facet joint because there is no point in giving patients with a negative screening block a second block, even if the second block was positive the same conclusion is reached, non-FJ pain. The same reasoning applies to the value of no relief in recumbency.

The results regarding no relief with recumbency and non-centralization appear promising, but they need verification in future studies.

It is unclear whether the three studies by Manchikanti et al. [35, 36, 41] might include the same populations. However, this issue would have no influence on the conclusion.

Sacroiliac joint

Our recommendation for the SIJ CDR is strong. Only one out of three studies supporting the diagnostic value of the composite of tests displayed risk of differential bias [44]. In all studies, however, a high risk of selection bias is present, because they included patients from secondary or tertiary care referred for diagnostic invasive procedures. The CDR is supported by an additional two out of three studies where composites of at least 3 positive out of 5 tests resulted in high levels of positive LRs [45, 48]. Although the content of the composites are comparable there is a slight difference in the use Patrick's PABER test and Mennell's test. The fact that one study did not support the rule [47], might be explained by the fact that the double block were performed only 30 min apart, which increases the risk of false positive findings. Furthermore, the quality of this study suffered from the risk of test review bias.

The recommendation of no centralization during physical examination was weak based on two studies [32, 44]. One of those was reporting an acceptable level of negative LR for centralization using a single block reference standard, making non-centralization useful for ruling out a symptomatic SIJ [32]. However, both studies suffered from risk of partial verification bias leading to a downgrading of the quality of evidence.

We found two additional studies investigating diagnostic value of SIJ area pointing, without indication of whether or not the pain was dominant, using insufficient reference standard in terms of a single or periarticular SIJ blocks [46, 149]. The results were not in concordance and warrant further investigation.

Nerve root involvement

The strength of our recommendation for the CDR is weak based on mediocre methodological quality in most of the studies. Studies revealed serious risk of bias in relation to differential verification, incorporation, or test review.

The studies included used surgical or imaging findings as a reference standard. We found no differences in diagnostic values when results from surgical and imaging studies were compared, which indicates that the findings are similar across reference standards used. Readers, interesting in results from pooling of studies exclusively using surgery as reference standard, are referred to the most recent systematic reviews [50, 66].

The reference standards have an influence on the diagnostic value of index tests. Studies using surgery means that results were obtained in a patient population with high prevalence of severe disc herniations, and thus results cannot be generalized to primary care populations where prevalence is much lower. Studies using imaging may display prevalence more like what is found in primary care, however at the expense of more false positive findings [150]. Consequently, uncertainty remains as to the generalizability of the results in primary care settings. Only two studies [53] and [68] included patients representative of those seen in primary care.

As suggested by others [66] we have tried to increase the performance of tests in clinical practice by recommending a CDR using a combination of tests with high levels of sensitivity and specificity. Other combinations of tests have been suggested [53, 69, 72, 151], but these are not summarized in the format of CDRs and they are not supported as well by single studies as the Hancock rule.

When possible, we chose to report one level disc or nerve root as reference standard in order to reduce the number of false positives due to noise from other non-relevant levels. This choice reflects the clinical reasoning process in daily practice. The clinician needs to compare dermatomal pain distribution with corresponding motor or reflex weakness in order to make a meaningful diagnostic pattern.

Spinal stenosis

The strength of our recommendation for the CDR is weak, based on low methodological quality of studies. Many of the quality items revealed serious risks of bias. First, the index test was part of the reference standard (incorporation bias) in all studies resulting in a high risk of overestimation of the diagnostic value of findings. Most studies used expert opinion based on a combination of physical examination findings and imaging even though data suggest that imaging is probably not sufficient as a reference standard in comparison with surgical findings [150]. Only two studies used surgical verification of diagnosis as part of the reference standard [77, 78]. Second, the majority of studies had problematic reporting of blinding (test review bias) i.e. whether the reference standard result was interpreted blind to those of the index test and vice versa [76–78, 82, 83, 85]. Third, all studies included patients from secondary or tertiary settings with a high prevalence of patients with SS. Consequently, there is a high risk of selection bias that is likely to overestimate the diagnostic gain of using the CDR in comparison to primary care settings where the prevalence is dramatically lower.

Spondylolisthesis

The strength of our recommendation for the CDR is strong based on the methodological quality of studies. Although several of the studies displayed risk of disease progression bias and poor description of index tests, the quality items reveal serious risks of bias in few cases [90, 94].

In the present review, functional dynamic radiographs were accepted to identify segmental instability if index tests were pain provocation or movement tests and plain static radiographs if index tests were palpation of slip.

Flexion-extension functional radiographs are considered the "gold standard" in degenerative spondylolisthesis, and a disc angle change >10° or change in translation > 3 mm are generally used as cut-offs [152]. Plain radiographs with lateral views are useful in the initial investigation of isthmic spondylolisthesis [153]. A slip of > 3 mm has been suggested as cut-off [154], but the literature is lacking as to what degree of slip is significant [153]. Instead, the descriptive Meyerding classification [154] is often reported.

All studies used a definition of spondylolisthesis similar to the above, except Abbott et al. [88] that used a cut-off of 2 standard deviations beyond the mean of a sample of pain free individuals.

Even though the positive LRs across single studies are only of moderate levels, the magnitude of LRs will probably rise to a level sufficient to be useful in clinical practice when they are used in combination.

All studies, except one [88] were performed in tertiary settings resulting in high risk of selection bias that is likely to overestimate the diagnostic gain of using the CDR when applied to primary care.

Fracture

It was not possible to constitute a CDR for the identification of a painful fracture. Results of single studies were not in concurrence and the majority of studies had serious risks of bias with respect to differential verification, test review, and uninterpretable results/withdrawals.

A symptomatic fracture is considered a 'red flag' warranting referral to secondary care. Consequently we have emphasized findings that are able to exclude patients with this condition.

The Henschke rule [96] has the potential to be a useful screening tool in primary care. However, the results need confirmation in future studies as the results of the only other primary care study included in this review were not in concordance [100]. Overall, the results from these two studies did not differ markedly from the rest.

Trauma (major in young persons and minor in the elderly] is a highly plausible mechanism that can lead to fracture and a highly increased prevalence of osteoporotic fractures are seen in patients, mainly female, with age above 75 years [97]. Both of these features contribute to the diagnostic value of the rule although not validated as stand-alone findings.

The inconsistency of results may be influenced by the method of imaging. Radiography was used in all studies with the addition of CT-scan in only one study [102]. No study used MRI. Radiographs may be adequately sensitive, but their ability to distinguish acute from chronic fractures is poor. MRI is more specific because it identifies marrow edema or an associated hematoma, which may indicate a symptomatic fracture [155].

Myofascial pain

The suggested criteria should be regarded as the first step in defining a common set of diagnostic criteria for selection of patients to be included in future reliability and validity studies.

Our literature searches identified a number of studies attempting to demonstrate construct validity, but we did not perform a systematic search for additional studies in reference lists. Therefore, the included studies must be regarded as important examples of attempts of validation rather than a systematic review of this type of literature. The studies used TrPs found by manual palpation as the reference standard, meaning that the purpose of these studies were to identify the underlying physiological mechanisms behind the presence of TrPs rather than a diagnostic validation of palpation findings. Several hypothetical theories have been suggested in order to explain the formation and persistence of TrPs [156].

It is a matter of controversy whether TrPs should be regarded as stand-alone entities that are a primary pain source or whether they are secondary to other painful disorders [106, 157]. Consequently, a myofascial pain syndrome may coexist with several other syndromes in our proposed classification system. It is essential to exclude underlying disorders capable of causing reproduction of a referred pain sensation with stimulation of a hypersensitive spot in the muscle before a conclusion can be made as to whether the myofascial TrP is the dominant source of the patient's pain.

Peripheral nerve

While diagnostic value of the SLR and slump is demonstrated in patients with lumbar radiculopathy, the value in relation to painful peripheral nerve tissue is unknown. Our search did not identify any studies investigating the ability of these tests to discriminate patients with peripheral nerve pain from other competing disorders. The suggested criteria should be regarded as an attempt to define a common set of diagnostic criteria for selection of patients to be included in future validity studies.

The spread of sensitizing effects along the nerve is a plausible explanation for why movement of a distant body part can change sensory responses. However, it has been argued that the fascial network in the back and legs and may account for positive findings in terms of pain and limited range of movement during SLR and slump test [127, 158]. Therefore, structural differentiation between neural tissues as opposed to musculoskeletal connective tissues has been proposed. When lumbar or leg pain increase during the SLR test with dorsiflexion of the ankle or flexion of the neck, a neural pain source is alleged to be identified [118]. Likewise, regarding the slump test, with the addition that the pain decrease with the release of neck flexion [118, 159]. Our search of the literature did not identify any studies that specifically tested this hypothesis.

In line with other authors [160, 161], we suggest the term "Increased neural mechanosensitivity" to describe a condition where the patient's usual pain is reproduced by sensitizing maneuvers. Increased neural mechanosensitivity has been given several other labels, i.e. adverse neural tension, neurodynamics, and neural tension dysfunction [118, 160].

The issues discussed in the myofascial pain section above, concerning coexistence with several other syndromes in our proposed classification system, apply to peripheral nerve as a pain source as well.

Central sensitization

Although the Nijs rule is the result of a consensus process, caution is warranted because the participating experts are a selective sample within the field of neuroscience. Therefore, the suggested criteria should be regarded as an attempt to define a common set of diagnostic criteria for selection of patients to be included in future validity studies. A possible use of the Nijs rule in clinical practice has been exemplified in a recent paper [162].

CS might be explained by an amplification of neural signaling within the central nervous system that elicits pain hypersensitivity" [139] However, controversy exists as to the nature of CS and whether it is possible to identify this condition in clinical practice [140, 163].

The pathophysiological mechanisms are not fully understood, but there is increasing evidence that CS and chronic widespread musculoskeletal pain is associated with plasticity changes in of the central nervous system leading to hypersensitivity that can explain the clinical findings in chronic widespread LBP [133, 139, 141]. The main clinical manifestations are widespread lowered pain thresholds, exaggerated pain response to stimuli, and enlargement of pain referral areas. Most studies in the field have used clinical manifestations as the reference standard, meaning that the purpose of these studies were to identify the underlying physiology behind the presence of CS and widespread pain rather than a diagnostic validation of clinical findings.

In patients with chronic LBP it has been reported that 25–38% develop chronic widespread pain [164–166], and the condition is closely associated with systemic comorbidity and psychological disorders [167].

In our opinion, the suggested rule is useful for increasing the likelihood of identifying patients with CS in primary care. Central sensitization may coexist with other structure-specific syndromes in our diagnostic classification system because it is generally recognized that there is a structural pain generator behind initial nociception and peripheral sensitization involved [132]. However, we would not expect a patient with CS to fit any of the clinical patterns of specific pain producing structures in the classification system. In order to choose the best treatment strategy, the clinician has to make a decision as to which pain sources are the dominant in the individual patient with LBP [140, 163].

Reference standards

At the present time is seems obvious that there are no 'gold' standards, either in the form of clinical tests, high tech imaging or other procedures. What is available are *reference* standards that, while not perfect, are appropriate and quite adequate for the majority of patients, and for use as comparators with clinical tests in diagnostic accuracy studies. The diagnostic utility of discography and FJ or SIJ blocks is a matter of controversy. Some consensus reports do not support the use of these procedures due to insufficient evidence of validity [168], the main problem being the absence of gold standards for identifying a "true" pain source. In this review we have tried to reduce the possible false positive rate by using the strictest available criteria for the reference standards as a requirement for inclusion of studies.

What is apparent from our systematic review is that there generally is sufficient published data that can form a framework for an intelligent use of clinical examination procedures and more expensive and invasive diagnostic investigations when required. Diagnosis of the source and cause of presenting back pain remains a challenge, and only further high quality research will improve certainty for clinicians and patients alike.

It is true that for a large proportion of patients in the acute or subacute phase, an accurate patho-anatomic diagnosis is not required, even though possible with some degree of confidence. However for patients whose symptoms are not improving after several months, the need for a more precise diagnosis becomes increasingly valuable as a guide to more effective and targeted management. To this extent, the recommendations from this systematic review might be helpful, in that patient selection for expensive high tech imaging and minimally invasive diagnostic injection procedures is facilitated, with consequent better utilization of resources.

Implication for practice

Our recommendations are based on considerations of the consequences of false positives and false negatives. In most diagnoses, we put the most emphasis on tests with high specificity indicating few false positives and positive LRs to indicate the ratio of true positive tests results above the false positives. The consequence is that the clinician will be quite certain that a patient would actually have the disorder if the reference standard procedure were to be performed. Often, high specificity is a trade off at the expense of low sensitivity, meaning that a substantial proportion of patients with the disorders are not identified, and remain unclassified. However, the consequences in primary care are not serious inasmuch as the patient remains in the category of non-specific LBP. In daily clinical practice, referral to further diagnostics most often depends on assessment of red flags, severity of symptoms and functional limitations rather than diagnostic classification.

Only in cases where an undiagnosed spinal fracture is present, do primary treatment methods have potential to harm the patient if unidentified. Consequently, we have prioritized the recommendation of tests with a high sensitivity and low negative LRs in this diagnosis.

For the clinician, the diagnostic considerations do not stop here. The diagnostic certainty that a positive test will identify a pathological disorder is dependent on the prevalence of the disorder. Prevalence of categories like nerve root involvement, spinal stenosis, spondylolisthesis, and fracture are generally much lower in primary care settings than in secondary or tertiary settings of the vast majority of diagnostic studies. This means that the diagnostic accuracy of a positive test is likely much lower when the index tests are applied to primary care settings. For example, the pre-test probability of having a symptomatic spinal stenosis in primary care is estimated to be only 3% [168]. By use of the Cook rule, the posttest probability will rise to 7%. When improved walking tolerance with the spine in flexion or patient history report of relief by forward bending are added to the rule we would expect the post-test probability to rise further. By means of the LRs presented in this review, the clinician can use Fagan's nomogram [169] as a graphical tool for estimating how much the result on a diagnostic test changes the probability that a patient has the disorder in question.

In daily practice, it is unlikely that clinicians make conclusions based on a single finding. This practice is supported by our results that generally provide the most promising accuracy in diagnosis in which a composite of findings can be identified. Some studies do report diagnostic accuracy of test combinations and clusters, but this does not totally reflect the reasoning process of expert clinicians. Clinicians do not use individual tests or clusters of tests out of context from the total clinical picture. Sometimes pattern recognition is used, and sometimes a sequential, algorithmic or staged approach is used. Another way to utilize multiple test results is to consider the probability of specific disorders based on prevalence within a defined group or subgroup. Prevalence is equal to pre-test probability so the probability of any given disorder is equivalent to its prevalence in any given setting. The process of progressively reducing the size of the group labelled as 'non-specific', by abstracting out those cases with very high probability of a known condition, may be called 'Diagnosis by Subtraction'.

Diagnosis by subtraction

To illustrate, assume for this current purpose, that in a specific setting, the prevalence of 'centralizers' is 0.5 or 50%. The high specificity of this clinical finding to discogenic pain confirmed by discography indicates that these patients do not have 'non-specific' back pain but a 'specific' anatomical source of pain [33]. Whatever the prevalence of the remaining possible causes of pain in the whole group, it is twice as high in the 'non-centralizer' group. Thus the probability that a non-centralizer has of having, say sacroiliac joint pain or facet joint pain, is doubled. This review has shown that certain CDRs have high specificity for sacroiliac joint pain, spondylolisthesis, disc herniation with nerve root involvement, and spinal stenosis. If we sequentially subtract those cases satisfying the CDR's for these conditions, the prevalence / probability of other conditions being the cause of pain progressively rises as the size of the non-specific low back pain category reduces.

Limitations of this review

One of the main limitations in this review is that the search of the literature was not updated to year 2015 in all diagnostic categories. Due to limited resources, this has not been possible for the present authors. If an existing review fulfilled the criteria of being current, relevant, and of high-quality, then we chose to use our resources to conduct systematic searches within fields where recent reviews had not been published.

The vast majority of patients is most likely not representative of those that present for treatment in primary care. Almost all patients were preselected having a referral to specialist centers for specific diagnostic evaluation making them likely to have the target disorder in question.

Although some of the included reviews have used a QUADAS score of 10/14 as a marker for high versus low quality studies, we agree with the developers of the tool that no meaningful cut off exists [170].

It is our judgment that pooling of data was not feasible due to great variability across studies: The patient characteristics and prevalence of the target disorders varied considerably, the same reference standard was seldom used across studies, definition of a positive reference standard was not often specified, and execution of index tests was likely to vary among studies. Though it is tempting to pool data and perform a meta-analysis, we chose not to do this since in our opinion, pooling systematically homogenizes studies that are in fact acknowledged as heterogeneous. We chose to put emphasis on the results of those studies that had satisfactory quality assessments, and seemed to be closest in context to the environment this classification targets i.e. primary care.

Conclusions

In some diagnostic categories we have sufficient evidence to suggest a CDR. In others, we have only preliminary evidence that needs testing in future studies. The use of single clinical tests appears to be less useful than clusters of tests which is more closely in line with clinical decision making.

With respect to clinical diagnostic of symptomatic intervertebral disc, sacroiliac joint, spondylolisthesis, disc herniation with nerve root involvement, and spinal

Intervertebral disc
- Centralization of symptoms

Sacroiliac joint
- No centralization of symptoms
- Dominant pain in SIJ without tuber area
- 3 positive out of 5 physical examination findings: distraction, compression, thigh thrust, Gaenslen's test, sacral thrust

Disc herniation with nerve root involvement
- Straight leg raise test positive for referred leg pain
- 3 positive out of 4 history or physical examination findings: dermatomal pain location in concordance with a nerve root, and corresponding sensory deficits, reflex and motor weakness
- Supplementary physical examination finding: Crossed straight leg raise test positive

Spinal stenosis
- 3 positive out of 5 history findings: age more than 48 years, bilateral symptoms, leg pain more than back pain, pain during walking/standing, or pain relief upon sitting
- Supplementary physical examination finding: Improved walking tolerance with the spine in flexion or relief by forward bending

Spondylolisthesis
- Intervertebral slip by inspection or palpation
- Segmental hypermobility by use of manual passive physiological intervertebral motion test
- Supplementary physical examination finding in the elderly: Passive leg extension test positive

Fig. 1 Promising Clinical Diagnostic Rules based on best-evidence

stenosis, we were able to construct promising CDRs (see Fig. 1]. However, the accuracy of these findings in a primary care setting has yet to be confirmed.

Additional files

Additional file 1: Search strategy for disc, sacroiliac joint, and facet joint.

Additional file 2: Search strategy for spondylolisthesis.

Additional file 3: Search strategy for myofascial pain.

Additional file 4: Search strategy for peripheral nerve pain.

Additional file 5: Characteristics of the included studies.

Additional file 6: Quality assessment of included studies.

Additional file 7: Flow chart for selection of disc, sacroiliac joint and facet joint articles.

Additional file 8: Flow chart for selection of spondylolisthesis articles.

Additional file 9: Flow chart for selection of myofascial pain articles.

Additional file 10: Flow chart for selection of nerve pain articles.

Abbreviations
CDR: Clinical diagnostic rule; CS: Central sensitization; CT: X-ray computed tomography; FJ: Facet joint; ID: Lumbar intervertebral disc; LBP: Low back pain; LR: Likelihood ratio; MRI: Magnetic resonance imaging; NRI: Lumbar nerve root involvement; QUADAS: Quality Assessment of Diagnostic Accuracy Studies; ROM: Range of movement; SIJ: Sacroiliac joint; SLR: Straight leg raise; SS: Lumbar spinal stenosis; TrP: Myofascial trigger point

Acknowledgements
None.

Funding
No funding was received for the conduction of this review.

Authors' contributions
The authors have contributed in the following ways: TP provided concept/ research design, data collection, data analysis, and manuscript writing. ML provided concept/research design, analysis, and manuscript writing. CJ provided concept/research design and manuscript writing. All authors read and approved the final manuscript.

Competing interests
The authors declare that they have no competing interests.

Consent for publication
Not applicable.

Author details
[1]Back Center Copenhagen, Mimersgade 41, 2200 Copenhagen N, Denmark. [2]PhysioSouth Ltd, 7 Baltimore Green, Shirley, Christchurch 8061, New Zealand. [3]Southern Musculoskeletal Seminars, Christchurch, New Zealand. [4]Research Unit for Musculoskeletal Function and Physiotherapy, Department of Sports Science and Clinical Biomechanics, University of Southern Denmark, Odense, Denmark. [5]Department of Rehabilitation, University Hospital of Copenhagen, Herlev and Gentofte, Niels Andersen Vej 65, 2900 Hellerup, Denmark.

References

1. Foster NE, Dziedzic KS, van Der Windt DA, Fritz JM, Hay EM. Research priorities for non-pharmacological therapies for common musculoskeletal problems: nationally and internationally agreed recommendations. BMC Musculoskelet Disord. 2009;10:3.
2. Borkan JM, Koes B, Reis S, Cherkin DC. A report from the second international forum for primary care research on low back pain. Reexamining priorities. Spine. 1998;23(18):1992–6.
3. Kent P, Keating JL. Classification in nonspecific low back pain: what methods do primary care clinicians currently use? Spine. 2005;30(12):1433–40.
4. Hancock MJ, Maher CG, Laslett M, Hay E, Koes B. Discussion paper: what happened to the 'bio' in the bio-psycho-social model of low back pain? Eur Spine J. 2011;20(12):2105–10.
5. Jull G, Moore A. Hands on, hands off? The swings in musculoskeletal physiotherapy practice. Man Ther. 2012;17(3):199–200.
6. Ford JJ, Hahne AJ. Pathoanatomy and classification of low back disorders. Man Ther. 2013;18:165–8.
7. Pincus T, McCracken LM. Psychological factors and treatment opportunities in low back pain. Best Pract Res Clin Rheumatol. 2013;27(5):625–35.
8. Steenstra IA, Irvin E, Mahood Q, Hogg-Johnson S, Heymans MW. Systematic review of prognostic factors for workers' time away from work due to acute low back pain: an update of a systematic review. Toronto: Institute for Work & Health; 2011.
9. Delitto A, George SZ, Van Dillen LR, Whitman JM, Sowa G, Shekelle P, et al. Low back pain. J Orthop Sports Phys Ther. 2012;42(4):A1–57.
10. Ramond-Roquin A, Bouton C, Gobin-Tempereau AS, Airagnes G, Richard I, Roquelaure Y, et al. Interventions focusing on psychosocial risk factors for patients with non-chronic low back pain in primary care–a systematic review. Fam Pract. 2014;31(4):379–88.
11. Petersen T, Laslett M, Thorsen H, Manniche C, Ekdahl C, Jacobsen S. Diagnostic classification of non-specific low back pain. A new system integrating patho-anatomic and clinical categories. Physiother Theory Pract. 2003;19:213–37.
12. Petersen T, Olsen S, Laslett M, Thorsen H, Manniche C, Ekdahl C, et al. Inter-tester reliability of a new diagnostic classification system for patients with non-specific low back pain. Aust J Physiother. 2004;50:85–94.
13. Eirikstoft H, Kongsted A. Patient characteristics in low back pain subgroups based on an existing classification system. A descriptive cohort study in chiropractic practice. Man Ther. 2014;19(1):65–71.
14. Ford JJ, Hahne AJ, Surkitt LD, Chan AY, Richards MC, Slater SL, et al. Individualised physiotherapy as an adjunct to guideline-based advice for low back disorders in primary care: a randomised controlled trial. Br J Sports Med. 2015;50(4):237–45.
15. Karayannis NV, Jull GA, Hodges PW. Movement-based subgrouping in low back pain: synergy and divergence in approaches. Physiotherapy. 2015;102(2):159–69.
16. Main CJ, Foster N, Buchbinder R. How important are back pain beliefs and expectations for satisfactory recovery from back pain? Best Pract Res Clin Rheumatol. 2010;24(2):205–17.
17. Main CJ, Buchbinder R, Porcheret M, Foster N. Addressing patient beliefs and expectations in the consultation. Best Pract Res Clin Rheumatol. 2010; 24(2):219–25.
18. Berna C, Tracey I, Holmes EA. How a better understanding of spontaneous mental imagery linked to pain could enhance imagery-based therapy in chronic pain. J Exp Psychopathol. 2012;3:258–73.
19. Fardo F, Allen M, Jegindo EE, Angrilli A, Roepstorff A. Neurocognitive evidence for mental imagery-driven hypoalgesic and hyperalgesic pain regulation. Neuroimage. 2015;120:350–61.
20. Kamper SJ, Maher CG, Hancock MJ, Koes BW, Croft PR, Hay E. Treatment-based subgroups of low back pain: a guide to appraisal of research studies and a summary of current evidence. Best Pract Res Clin Rheumatol. 2010;24(2):181–91.
21. Airaksinen O, Brox JI, Cedraschi C, Hildebrandt J, Klaber-Moffett J, Kovacs F, et al. Chapter 4. European guidelines for the management of chronic nonspecific low back pain. Eur Spine J. 2006;15 Suppl 2:S192–300.
22. Kent P, Mjosund HL, Petersen DH. Does targeting manual therapy and/or exercise improve patient outcomes in nonspecific low back pain? A systematic review. BMC Med. 2010;8:22.
23. McGinn TG, Guyatt GH, Wyer PC, Naylor CD, Stiell IG, Richardson WS. Users' guides to the medical literature: XXII: how to use articles about clinical decision rules. Evidence-Based Medicine Working Group. JAMA. 2000;284(1):79–84.
24. Shamseer L, Moher D, Clarke M, Ghersi D, Liberati A, Petticrew M, et al. Preferred reporting items for systematic review and meta-analysis protocols (PRISMA-P) 2015: elaboration and explanation. BMJ. 2015;349:g7647.
25. Deeks JJ, Bossuyt PM, Gatsonis C. (editors). Cochrane handbook for diagnostic test accuracy reviews. The Cochrane Collaboration; 2009. http:// methods.cochrane.org/sdt/handbook-dta-reviews.
26. Reitsma JB, Rutjes AW, Whiting P, Vlassov VV, Leeflang MM, Deeks JJ. Chapter 9: Assessing methodological quality. In: Deeks JJ, Bossuyt PM, Gatsonis C, editors. Cochrane handbook for systematic reviews of diagnostic test accuracy version 1 0 0 The Cochrane Collaboration. 2009. Available from: http://methods.cochrane.org/sites/methods.cochrane.org.sdt/files/ public/uploads/ch09_Oct09.pdf.
27. Gopalakrishna G, Mustafa RA, Davenport C, Scholten RJ, Hyde C, Brozek J, et al. Applying Grading of Recommendations Assessment, Development and Evaluation (GRADE) to diagnostic tests was challenging but doable. J Clin Epidemiol. 2014;67(7):760–8.
28. Jaeschke R, Guyatt GH, Sackett DL. Users' guides to the medical literature. III. How to use an article about a diagnostic test. B. What are the results and will they help me in caring for my patients? The Evidence-Based Medicine Working Group. JAMA. 1994;271(9):703–7.
29. Slavin RE. Best evidence synthesis: an intelligent alternative to meta-analysis. J Clin Epidemiol. 1995;48(1):9–18.
30. Hancock MJ, Maher CG, Latimer J, Spindler MF, McAuley JH, Laslett M, et al. Systematic review of tests to identify the disc, SIJ or facet joint as the source of low back pain. Eur Spine J. 2007;10(16):1539–50.
31. Donelson R, Aprill CN, Medcalf R, Grant W. A prospective study of centralization of lumbar and referred pain. A predictor of symptomatic discs and anular competence. Spine. 1997;22(10):1115–22.
32. Young S, Aprill C, Laslett M. Correlation of clinical examination characteristics with three sources of chronic low back pain. Spine J. 2003;3(6):460–5.
33. Laslett M, Oberg B, Aprill CN, McDonald B. Centralization as a predictor of provocation discography results in chronic low back pain, and the influence of disability and distress on diagnostic power. Spine J. 2005;5(4):370–80.

34. Schwarzer AC, Aprill CN, Derby R, Fortin J, Kine G, Bogduk N. The prevalence and clinical features of internal disc disruption in patients with chronic low back pain. Spine. 1995;20(17):1878–83.

35. Manchikanti L, Pampati V, Fellows B, Ghafoor Baha A. The inability of the clinical picture to characterize pain from facet joints. Pain Physician. 2000;3(2):158–66.

36. Manchikanti L, Pampati V, Fellows B, Bakhit CE. Prevalence of lumbar facet joint pain in chronic low back pain. Pain Physician. 1999;2(3):59–64.

37. Revel M, Listrat VM, Chevalier XJ, Dougados M, N'guyen MP, Vallee C, et al. Facet joint block for low back pain: identifying predictors of a good response. Arch Phys Med Rehabil. 1992;73(9):824–8.

38. Revel M, Poiraudeau S, Auleley GR, Payan C, Denke A, Nguyen M, et al. Capacity of the clinical picture to characterize low back pain relieved by facet joint anesthesia. Proposed criteria to identify patients with painful facet joints. Spine. 1998;23(18):1972–7.

39. Laslett M, McDonald B, Aprill C, Tropp H, Oberg B. Clinical predictors of screening lumbar zygapophysial joint blocks: development of clinical prediction rules. Spine J. 2006;6:370–9.

40. Laslett M, Oberg B, Aprill CN, McDonald B. Zygapophysial joint blocks in chronic low back pain: a test of Revel's model as a screening test. BMC Musculoskelet Disord. 2004;5(1):43.

41. Manchikanti L, Manchikanti KN, Cash KA, Singh V, Giordano J. Age-related prevalence of facet-joint involvement in chronic neck and low back pain. Pain Physician. 2008;11(1):67–75.

42. Schwarzer AC, Derby R, Aprill CN, Fortin J, Kine G, Bogduk N. Pain from the lumbar zygapophysial joints: a test of two models. J Spinal Disord. 1994;7(4):331–6.

43. Fairbank JC, Park WM, McCall IW, O'Brien JP. Apophyseal injection of local anesthetic as a diagnostic aid in primary low-back pain syndromes. Spine. 1981;6(6):598–605.

44. Laslett M, Young S, Aprill C, McDonald B. Diagnosing painful sacroiliac joints. A validity study of a McKenzie evaluation and sacroiliac provocation tests. Aust J Physiother. 2003;49:89–97.

45. Van der Wurff P, Buijs EJ, Groen GJ. A multitest regimen of pain provocation tests as an aid to reduce unnecessary minimally invasive sacroiliac joint procedures. Arch Phys Med Rehabil. 2006;87(1):10–4.

46. Dreyfuss P, Michaelsen M, Pauza K, McLarty J, Bogduk N. The value of medical history and physical examination in diagnosing sacroiliac joint pain. Spine. 1996;21(22):2594–602.

47. Stanford G, Burnham RS. Is it useful to repeat sacroiliac joint provocative tests post-block? Pain Med. 2010;11(12):1774–6.

48. Ozgocmen S, Bozgeyik Z, Kalcik M, Yildirim A. The value of sacroiliac pain provocation tests in early active sacroiliitis. Clin Rheumatol. 2008;27(10):1275–82.

49. Van der Wurff P, Buijs EJ, Groen GJ. Intensity mapping of pain referral areas in sacroiliac joint pain patients. J Manipulative Physiol Ther. 2006;29(3):190–5.

50. Al Nezari NH, Schneiders AG, Hendrick PA. Neurological examination of the peripheral nervous system to diagnose lumbar spinal disc herniation with suspected radiculopathy: a systematic review and meta-analysis. Spine J. 2013;13(6):657–74.

51. Henrica De Vet, The Cochrane Collaboration Back Review Group. Personal communication. 2016.

52. Hancock MJ, Koes B, Ostelo R, Peul W. Diagnostic accuracy of the clinical examination in identifying the level of herniation in patients with sciatica. Spine (Phila Pa 1976). 2011;36(11):E712–9.

53. Vroomen PC, de Krom MC, Wilmink JT, Kester AD, Knottnerus JA. Diagnostic value of history and physical examination in patients suspected of lumbosacral nerve root compression. J Neurol Neurosurg Psychiatry. 2002;72(5):630–4.

54. Bertilson BC, Brosjo E, Billing H, Strender LE. Assessment of nerve involvement in the lumbar spine: agreement between magnetic resonance imaging, physical examination and pain drawing findings. BMC Musculoskelet Disord. 2010;11:202.

55. Kerr RS, Cadoux-Hudson TA, Adams CB. The value of accurate clinical assessment in the surgical management of the lumbar disc protrusion. J Neurol Neurosurg Psychiatry. 1988;51(2):169–73.

56. Suri P, Rainville J, Katz JN, Jouve C, Hartigan C, Limke J, et al. The Accuracy of the physical examination for the diagnosis of midlumbar and low lumbar nerve root impingement. Spine (Phila Pa 1976). 2011;36(1):63–73.

57. Gurdjian ES, Webster JE, Ostrowski AZ, Hardy WG, Lindner DW, Thomas LM. Herniated lumbar intervertebral discs – an analysis of 1176 operated cases. J Trauma. 1961;1:158–76.

58. Knutsson B. Comparative value of electromyographic, myelographic and clinical-neurological examinations in diagnosis of lumbar root compression syndrome. Acta Orthop Scand Suppl. 1961;49:1–135.

59. Stankovic R, Johnell O, Maly P, Willner S. Use of lumbar extension, slump test, physical and neurological examination in the evaluation of patients with suspected herniated nucleus pulposus. A prospective clinical study. Man Ther. 1999;4(1):25–32.

60. Vucetic N, Svensson O. Physical signs in lumbar disc hernia. Clin Orthop Relat Res. 1996;333:192–201.

61. Albeck MJ. A critical assessment of clinical diagnosis of disc herniation in patients with monoradicular sciatica. Acta Neurochir (Wien). 1996;138(1):40–4.

62. Spangfort EV. The lumbar disc herniation. A computer-aided analysis of 2,504 operations. Acta Orthop Scand Suppl. 1972;142:1–95.

63. Kosteljanetz M, Espersen JO, Halaburt H, Miletic T. Predictive value of clinical and surgical findings in patients with lumbago-sciatica. A prospective study (Part I). Acta Neurochir (Wien). 1984;73(1-2):67–76.

64. Hakelius A, Hindmarsh J. The significance of neurological signs and myelographic findings in the diagnosis of lumbar root compression. Acta Orthop Scand. 1972;43(4):239–46.

65. Weise MD, Garfin SR, Gelberman RH, Katz MM, Thorne RP. Lower-extremity sensibility testing in patients with herniated lumbar intervertebral discs. J Bone Joint Surg Am. 1985;67(8):1219–24.

66. van der Windt DA, Simons E, Riphagen II, Ammendolia C, Verhagen AP, Laslett M, et al. Physical examination for lumbar radiculopathy due to disc herniation in patients with low-back pain. Cochrane Database Syst Rev. 2010;2:CD007431.

67. Meylemans L, Vancraeynest T, Bruyninckx F, Rosselle N. [A comparative study of EMG and CAT scan in the lumbo-ischial syndrome. II: Pain in the lumbo-ischial syndrome and the diagnostic value of clinical examination, EMG and CAT scan. Acta Belg Med Phys. 1988;11(1):35–42.

68. Haldeman S, Shouka M, Robboy S. Computed tomography, electrodiagnostic and clinical findings in chronic workers' compensation patients with back and leg pain. Spine (Phila Pa 1976). 1988;13(3):345–50.

69. Poiraudeau S, Foltz V, Drape JL, Fermanian J, Lefevre-Colau MM, Mayoux-Benhamou MA, et al. Value of the bell test and the hyperextension test for diagnosis in sciatica associated with disc herniation: comparison with Lasegue's sign and the crossed Lasegue's sign. Rheumatology (Oxford). 2001;40(4):460–6.

70. Kosteljanetz M, Bang F, Schmidt Olsen S. The clinical significance of straight-leg raising (Lasegue's sign) in the diagnosis of prolapsed lumbar disc. Interobserver variation and correlation with surgical finding. Spine. 1988;13(4):393–5.

71. Demircan MN, Colak A, Kutlay M, Kibici K, Topuz K. Cramp finding: can it be used as a new diagnostic and prognostic factor in lumbar disc surgery? Eur Spine J. 2002;11(1):47–51.

72. Charnley J. Orthopaedic signs in the diagnosis of disc protrusion. With special reference to the straight-leg-raising test. Lancet. 1951;1(6648):186–92.

73. Majlesi J, Togay H, Unalan H, Toprak S. The sensitivity and specificity of the Slump and the Straight Leg Raising tests in patients with lumbar disc herniation. J Clin Rheumatol. 2008;14(2):87–91.

74. Vroomen PC, Van Hapert SJ, Van Acker RE, Beuls EA, Kessels AG, Wilmink JT. The clinical significance of gadolinium enhancement of lumbar disc herniations and nerve roots on preoperative MRI. Neuroradiology. 1998;40(12):800–6.

75. de Schepper EI, Overdevest GM, Suri P, Peul WC, Oei EH, Koes BW, et al. Diagnosis of lumbar spinal stenosis: an updated systematic review of the accuracy of diagnostic tests. Spine (Phila Pa 1976). 2013;38(8):E469–81.

76. Cook C, Brown C, Michael K, Isaacs R, Howers C, Richardson W, et al. The clinical value of a cluster of patient history and observational findings as a diagnostic support tool for lumbar stenosis. Physiother Res Int. 2011;16:170–8.

77. Konno S, Kikuchi S, Tanaka Y, Yamazaki K, Shimada Y, Takei H, et al. A diagnostic support tool for lumbar spinal stenosis: a self-administered self-reported history questionnaire. BMC Musculoskelet Disord. 2007;8:102.

78. Ljunggren AE. Discriminant validity of pain modalities and other sensory phenomena in patients with lumbar herniated intervertebral discs versus lumbar spinal stenosis. Neuro-Orthopedics. 1991;11(2):91–9.

79. Katz JN, Dalgas M, Stucki G, Katz NP, Bayley J, Fossel AH, et al. Degenerative lumbar spinal stenosis. Diagnostic value of the history and physical examination. Arthritis Rheum. 1995;38(9):1236–41.

80. Jensen OH, Schmidt-Olsen S. A new functional test in the diagnostic evaluation of neurogenic intermittent claudication. Clin Rheumatol. 1989;8(3):363–7.

81. Roach KE, Brown MD, Albin RD, Delaney KG, Lipprandi HM, Rangelli D. The sensitivity and specificity of pain response to activity and position in categorizing patients with low back pain. Phys Ther. 1997;77(7):730–8.

82. Sugioka T, Hayashino Y, Konno S, Kikuchi S, Fukuhara S. Predictive value of self-reported patient information for the identification of lumbar spinal stenosis. Fam Pract. 2008;25(4):237–44.

83. Fritz JM, Erhard RE, Delitto A, Welch WC, Nowakowski PE. Preliminary results of the use of a two-stage treadmill test as a clinical diagnostic tool in the differential diagnosis of lumbar spinal stenosis. J Spinal Disord. 1997;10(5):410–6.

84. Konno S, Hayashino Y, Fukuhara S, Kikuchi S, Kaneda K, Seichi A, et al. Development of a clinical diagnosis support tool to identify patients with lumbar spinal stenosis. Eur Spine J. 2007;16(11):1951–7.

85. Dong G, Porter RW. Walking and cycling tests in neurogenic and intermittent claudication. Spine. 1989;14(9):965–9.

86. Alqarni AM, Schneiders AG, Hendrick PA. Clinical tests to diagnose lumbar segmental instability: a systematic review. J Orthop Sports Phys Ther. 2011; 41(3):130–40.

87. Fritz JM, Piva SR, Childs JD. Accuracy of the clinical examination to predict radiographic instability of the lumbar spine. Eur Spine J. 2005;14(8):743–50.

88. Abbott JH, McCane B, Herbison P, Moginie G, Chapple C, Hogarty T. Lumbar segmental instability: a criterion-related validity study of manual therapy assessment. BMC Musculoskelet Disord. 2005;6:56.

89. Kasai Y, Morishita K, Kawakita E, Kondo T, Uchida A. A new evaluation method for lumbar spinal instability: passive lumbar extension test. Phys Ther. 2006;86(12):1661–7.

90. Kalpakcioglu B, Altinbilek T, Senel K. Determination of spondylolisthesis in low back pain by clinical evaluation. J Back Musculoskelet Rehabil. 2009;22(1):27–32.

91. Collaer JW, McKeough DM, Boissonnault WG. Lumbar isthmic spondylolisthesis detection with palpation: Interrater reliability and concurrent criterion-related validity. J Man Manipul Ther. 2006;14(4):22–9.

92. Ferrari S, Vanti C, Piccarreta R, Monticone M. Pain, disability, and diagnostic accuracy of clinical instability and endurance tests in subjects with lumbar spondylolisthesis. J Manipulative Physiol Ther. 2014;37(9):647–59.

93. Ahn K, Jhun HJ. New physical examination tests for lumbar spondylolisthesis and instability: low midline sill sign and interspinous gap change during lumbar flexion-extension motion. BMC Musculoskelet Disord. 2015;16(1):97.

94. Sundell CG, Jonsson H, Adin L, Larsen KH. Clinical examination, spondylolysis and adolescent athletes. Int J Sports Med. 2013;34(3):263–7.

95. Williams CM, Henschke N, Maher CG, van Tulder MW, Koes BW, Macaskill P, et al. Red flags to screen for vertebral fracture in patients presenting with low-back pain. Cochrane Database Syst Rev. 2013;1:CD008643.

96. Henschke N, Maher CG, Refshauge KM, Herbert RD, Cumming RG, Bleasel J, et al. Prevalence of and screening for serious spinal pathology in patients presenting to primary care settings with acute low back pain. Arthritis Rheum. 2009;60(10):3072–80.

97. van den Bosch MA, Hollingworth W, Kinmonth AL, Dixon AK. Evidence against the use of lumbar spine radiography for low back pain. Clin Radiol. 2004;59(1):69–76.

98. Gibson M, Zoltie N. Radiography for back pain presenting to accident and emergency departments. Arch Emerg Med. 1992;9(1):28–31.

99. Patrick JD, Doris PE, Mills ML, Friedman J, Johnston C. Lumbar spine x-rays: a multihospital study. Ann Emerg Med. 1983;12(2):84–7.

100. Deyo RA, Diehl AK. Lumbar spine films in primary care: current use and effects of selective ordering criteria. J Gen Intern Med. 1986;1(1):20–5.

101. Reinus WR, Strome G, Zwemer Jr FL. Use of lumbosacral spine radiographs in a level II emergency department. AJR Am J Roentgenol. 1998;170(2):443–7.

102. Roman M, Brown C, Richardson W, Isaacs R, Howes C, Cook C. The development of a clinical decision making algorithm for detection of osteoporotic vertebral compression fracture or wedge deformity. J Man Manip Ther. 2010;18(1):44–9.

103. Scavone JG, Latshaw RF, Rohrer GV. Use of lumbar spine films. Statistical evaluation at a university teaching hospital. JAMA. 1981;246(10):1105–8.

104. Tough EA, White AR, Richards S, Campbell J. Variability of criteria used to diagnose myofascial trigger point pain syndrome–evidence from a review of the literature. Clin J Pain. 2007;23(3):278–86.

105. Travell JG, Simons DG. Myofascial pain and dysfunction. The triggerpoint manual. Baltimore: Williams and Wilkins; 1982.

106. IASP. Myofascial pain. 2009. http://www.iasp-pain.org/files/Content/ ContentFolders/GlobalYearAgainstPain2/MusculoskeletalPainFactSheets/ MyofascialPain_Final.pdf.

107. Ge HY, Monterde S, Graven-Nielsen T, Arendt-Nielsen L. Latent myofascial trigger points are associated with an increased intramuscular electromyographic activity during synergistic muscle activation. J Pain. 2014; 15(2):181–7.

108. Wytrazek M, Huber J, Lisinski P. Changes in muscle activity determine progression of clinical symptoms in patients with chronic spine-related muscle pain. A complex clinical and neurophysiological approach. Funct Neurol. 2011;26(3):141–9.

109. Simons DG, Hong CZ, Simons LS. Endplate potentials are common to midfiber myofacial trigger points. Am J Phys Med Rehabil. 2002;81(3):212–22.

110. Couppé C, Midttun A, Hilden J, Jorgensen U, Oxholm P, Fuglsang-Frederiksen A. Spontaneous needle electromyographic activity in myofascial trigger points in the infraspinatus muscle: a blinded assessment. J Musculoskelet Pain. 2001;9(3):7–16.

111. Hubbard DR, Berkoff GM. Myofascial trigger points show spontaneous needle EMG activity. Spine. 1993;18(13):1803–7.

112. Ballyns JJ, Shah JP, Hammond J, Gebreab T, Gerber LH, Sikdar S. Objective sonographic measures for characterizing myofascial trigger points associated with cervical pain. J Ultrasound Med. 2011;30(10):1331–40.

113. Lewis C, Suovlis T, Sterling M. Sensory characteristics of tender points in the lower back. Man Ther. 2010;15:451–6.

114. Ge HY, Fernandez-de-las-Penas C, Madeleine P, Arendt-Nielsen L. Topographical mapping and mechanical pain sensitivity of myofascial trigger points in the infraspinatus muscle. Eur J Pain. 2008;12(7):859–65.

115. Myburgh C, Larsen AH, Hartvigsen J. A systematic, critical review of manual palpation for identifying myofascial trigger points: evidence and clinical significance. Arch Phys Med Rehabil. 2008;89(6):1169–76.

116. Lucas N, Macaskill P, Irwig L, Moran R, Bogduk N. Reliability of physical examination for diagnosis of myofascial trigger points: a systematic review of the literature. Clin J Pain. 2009;25(1):80–9.

117. Dixon JK, Keating JL. Variability in straight leg raise measurements. Physiother. 2000;86(7):361–70.

118. Shacklock M. Improving application of neurodynamic (neural tension) testing and treatments: a message to researchers and clinicians. Man Ther. 2005;10(3):175–9.

119. Boland RA, Adams RD. Effects of ankle dorsiflexion on range and reliability of straight leg raising. Aust J Physiother. 2000;46(3):191–200.

120. Gajdosik RL, LeVeau BF, Bohannon RW. Effects of ankle dorsiflexion on active and passive unilateral straight leg raising. Phys Ther. 1985;65(10): 1478–82.

121. Johnson EK, Chiarello CM. The slump test: the effects of head and lower extremity position on knee extension. J Orthop Sports Phys Ther. 1997;26(6): 310–7.

122. McHugh MP, Johnson CD, Morrison RH. The role of neural tension in hamstring flexibility. Scand J Med Sci Sports. 2012;22(2):164–9.

123. Davis DS, Anderson IB, Carson MG, Elkins CL, Stuckey LB. Upper limb neural tension and seated slump tests: the false positive rate among healthy young adults without cervical or lumbar symptoms. J Man Manip Ther. 2008;16(3):136–41.

124. Herrington L, Bendix K, Cornwell C, Fielden N, Hankey K. What is the normal response to structural differentiation within the slump and straight leg raise tests? Man Ther. 2008;13(4):289–94.

125. Lew PC, Briggs CA. Relationship between the cervical component of the slump test and change in hamstring muscle tension. Man Ther. 1997;2(2): 98–105.

126. Laessoe U, Voigt M. Modification of stretch tolerance in a stooping position. Scand J Med Sci Sports. 2004;14(4):239–44.

127. Coppieters MW, Kurz K, Mortensen TE, Richards NL, Skaret IA, McLaughlin LM, et al. The impact of neurodynamic testing on the perception of experimentally induced muscle pain. Man Ther. 2005;10(1):52–60.

128. Landis JR, Koch GG. The measurement of observer agreement for categorical data. Biometrics. 1977;33(1):159–74.

129. Walsh J, Hall T. Agreement and correlation between the straight leg raise and slump tests in subjects with leg pain. J Manipulative Physiol Ther. 2009; 32(3):184–92.

130. Philip K, Lew P, Matyas TA. The inter-therapist reliability of the slump test. Aust J Physiother. 1989;35:89–94.

131. IASP. Taxonomy. 2012. www.iasp-pain.org/Taxonomy.

132. Arendt-Nielsen L, Graven-Nielsen T. Translational musculoskeletal pain research. Best Pract Res Clin Rheumatol. 2011;25(2):209–26.

133. Pelletier R, Higgins J, Bourbonnais D. Is neuroplasticity in the central nervous system the missing link to our understanding of chronic musculoskeletal disorders? BMC Musculoskelet Disord. 2015;16:25.

134. Nijs J, Torres-Cueco R, van Wilgen CP, Girbes EL, Struyf F, Roussel N, et al. Applying modern pain neuroscience in clinical practice: criteria for the classification of central sensitization pain. Pain Physician. 2014;17(5):447–57.

135. Haanpaa M, Treede RD. Diagnosis and classification of neuropatic pain. Pain - clinical updates. 2010. http://iasp.files.cms-plus.com/Content/ContentFolders/Publications2/PainClinicalUpdates/Archives/PCU_18-7_final_1390260761555_9.pdf].

136. Haanpaa M, Attal N, Backonja M, Baron R, Bennett M, Bouhassira D, et al. NeuPSIG guidelines on neuropathic pain assessment. Pain. 2011;152(1):14–27.

137. Mayer TG, Neblett R, Cohen H, Howard KJ, Choi YH, Williams MJ, et al. The development and psychometric validation of the central sensitization inventory. Pain Pract. 2012;12(4):276–85.

138. Neblett R, Cohen H, Choi Y, Hartzell MM, Williams M, Mayer TG, et al. The Central Sensitization Inventory (CSI): establishing clinically significant values for identifying central sensitivity syndromes in an outpatient chronic pain sample. J Pain. 2013;14(5):438–45.

139. Woolf CJ. Central sensitization: Implications for the diagnosis and treatment of pain. Pain. 2011;152(3 suppl):S2–15.

140. Woolf CJ. What to call the amplification of nociceptive signals in the central nervous system that contribute to widespread pain? Pain. 2014;155(10):1911–2.

141. Arendt-Nielsen L, Skou ST, Nielsen TA, Petersen KK. Altered central sensitization and pain modulation in the CNS in chronic joint pain. Curr Osteoporos Rep. 2015;13(4):225–34.

142. Roussel NA, Nijs J, Meeus M, Mylius V, Fayt C, Oostendorp R. Central sensitization and altered central pain processing in chronic low back pain: fact or myth? Clin J Pain. 2013;29(7):625–38.

143. Hubscher M, Moloney N, Leaver A, Rebbeck T, McAuley JH, Refshauge KM. Relationship between quantitative sensory testing and pain or disability in people with spinal pain-a systematic review and meta-analysis. Pain. 2013;154(9):1497–504.

144. Smart KM, Curley A, Blake C, Staines A, Doody C. The reliability of clinical judgments and criteria associated with mechanisms-based classifications of pain in patients with low back pain disorders: a preliminary reliability study. J Man Manip Ther. 2010;18(2):102–10.

145. Smart KM, Blake C, Staines A, Doody C. The discriminative validity of "Nociceptive," "Peripheral Neuropathic," and "Central Sensitisation" as mechanisms-based classifications of musculoskeletal pain. Clin J Pain. 2011;27(8):655–63.

146. Rapala A, Rapala K, Lukawski S. Correlation between centralization or peripheralization of symptoms in low back pain and the results of magnetic resonance imaging. Ortop Traumatol Rehabil. 2006;8(5):531–6.

147. Albert HB, Hauge E, Manniche C. Centralization in patients with sciatica: are pain responses to repeated movement and positioning associated with outcome or types of disc lesions? Eur Spine J. 2012;21(4):630–6.

148. Falco FJ, Manchikanti L, Datta S, Sehgal N, Geffert S, Onyewu O, et al. An update of the systematic assessment of the diagnostic accuracy of lumbar facet joint nerve blocks. Pain Physician. 2012;15(6):E869–907.

149. Murakami E, Aizawa T, Noguchi K, Kanno H, Okuno H, Uozumi H. Diagram specific to sacroiliac joint pain site indicated by one-finger test. J Orthop Sci. 2008;13(6):492–7.

150. Wassenaar M, van Rijn RM, van Tulder MW, Verhagen AP, van Der Windt DA, Koes BW, et al. Magnetic resonance imaging for diagnosing lumbar spinal pathology in adult patients with low back pain or sciatica: a diagnostic systematic review. Eur Spine J. 2012;21(2):220–7.

151. Vucetic N, Astrand P, Guntner P, Svensson O. Diagnosis and prognosis in lumbar disc herniation. Clin Orthop Relat Res. 1999;361:116–22.

152. Simmonds AM, Rampersaud YR, Dvorak MF, Dea N, Melnyk AD, Fisher CG. Defining the inherent stability of degenerative spondylolisthesis: a systematic review. J Neurosurg Spine. 2015;23(2):178–89.

153. Standaert CJ, Herring SA. Spondylolysis: a critical review. Br J Sports Med. 2000;34(6):415–22.

154. Niggemann P, Kuchta J, Grosskurth D, Beyer HK, Hoeffer J, Delank KS. Spondylolysis and isthmic spondylolisthesis: impact of vertebral hypoplasia on the use of the Meyerding classification. Br J Radiol. 2012;85(1012):358–62.

155. Jarvik JG, Deyo RA. Diagnostic evaluation of low back pain with emphasis on imaging. Ann Intern Med. 2002;137(7):586–97.

156. Giamberardino MA, Affaitati G, Fabrizio A, Costantini R. Myofascial pain syndromes and their evaluation. Best Pract Res Clin Rheumatol. 2011;25(2):185–98.

157. Bennett R. Myofascial pain syndromes and their evaluation. Best Pract Res Clin Rheumatol. 2007;21(3):427–45.

158. Di Fabio RP. Neural mobilization: the impossible (editorial). J Orthop Sports Phys Ther. 2001;31:224–5.

159. Maitland GF. The slump test. Examination and treatment. Aust J Physiother. 1985;31(6):215–9.

160. Hall T, Zusman M, Elvey R. Adverse mechanical tension in the nervous system? Analysis of straight leg raise. Man Ther. 1998;3(3):140–6.

161. Nee RJ, Jull GA, Vicenzino B, Coppieters MW. The validity of upper-limb neurodynamic tests for detecting peripheral neuropathic pain. J Orthop Sports Phys Ther. 2012;42(5):413–24.

162. Nijs J, Apeldoorn A, Hallegraeff H, Clark J, Smeets R, Malfliet A, et al. Low back pain: guidelines for the clinical classification of predominant neuropathic, nociceptive, or central sensitization pain. Pain Physician. 2015; 18(3):E333–46.

163. Hansson P. Translational aspects of central sensitization induced by primary afferent activity - What is it and what is it not? Pain. 2014;155(10):1932–4.

164. Lapossy E, Maleitzke R, Hrycaj P, Mennet W, Muller W. The frequency of transition of chronic low back pain to fibromyalgia. Scand J Rheumatol. 1995;24(1):29–33.

165. Clauw DJ, Williams D, Lauerman W, Dahlman M, Aslami A, Nachemson AL, et al. Pain sensitivity as a correlate of clinical status in individuals with chronic low back pain. Spine. 1999;24(19):2035–41.

166. Mayer TG, Towns BL, Neblett R, Theodore BR, Gatchel RJ. Chronic widespread pain in patients with occupational spinal disorders: prevalence, psychiatric comorbidity, and association with outcomes. Spine (Phila Pa 1976). 2008;33(17):1889–97.

167. Phillips K, Clauw DJ. Central pain mechanisms in chronic pain states–maybe it is all in their head. Best Pract Res Clin Rheumatol. 2011;25(2):141–54.

168. Chou R, Loeser JD, Owens DK, Rosenquist RW, Atlas SJ, Baisden J, et al. Interventional therapies, surgery, and interdisciplinary rehabilitation for low back pain: an evidence-based clinical practice guideline from the American Pain Society. Spine. 2009;34(10):1066–77.

169. Schwarz A. Diagnostic test calculator. Free Software, available under the Clarified Artistic License. 2006. http://araw.mede.uic.edu/cgi-bin/testcalc.pl. Accessed 9 May 2017.

170. Whiting P, Harbord R, Kleijnen J. No role for quality scores in systematic reviews of diagnostic accuracy studies. BMC Med Res Methodol. 2005;5:19.

171. Manchikanti L, Benyamin RM, Singh V, Falco FJ, Hameed H, Derby R, et al. An update of the systematic appraisal of the accuracy and utility of lumbar discography in chronic low back pain. Pain Physician. 2013;16(2 Suppl): SE55–95.

172. Simopoulos TT, Manchikanti L, Singh V, Gupta S, Hameed H, Diwan S, et al. A systematic evaluation of prevalence and diagnostic accuracy of sacroiliac joint interventions. Pain Physician. 2012;15(3):E305–44.

173. Kreiner DS, Hwang SW, Easa JE, Resnick DK, Baisden JL, Bess S, et al. An evidence-based clinical guideline for the diagnosis and treatment of lumbar disc herniation with radiculopathy. Spine J. 2014;14(1):180–91.

174. Genevay S, Atlas SJ. Lumbar spinal stenosis. Best Pract Res Clin Rheumatol. 2010;24(2):253–65.

3

Correlation between lumbar dysfunction and fat infiltration in lumbar multifidus muscles in patients with low back pain

Markus Hildebrandt[1], Gabriela Fankhauser[2], André Meichtry[3] and Hannu Luomajoki[3*] (iD)

Abstract

Background: Lumbar multifidus muscles (LMM) are important for spinal motion and stability. Low back pain (LBP) is often associated with fat infiltration in LMM. An increasing fat infiltration of LMM may lead to lumbar dysfunction. The purpose of this study was to investigate whether there is a correlation between the severity of lumbar dysfunction and the severity of fat infiltration of LMM.

Methods: In a cross-sectional study, 42 patients with acute or chronic LBP were recruited. Their MRI findings were visually rated and graded using three criteria for fat accumulation in LMM: Grade 0 (0–10%), Grade 1 (10–50%) and Grade 2 (>50%). Lumbar sagittal range of motion, dynamic upright and seated posture control, sagittal movement control, body awareness and self-assessed functional disability were measured to determine the patients' low back dysfunction.

Results: The main result of this study was that increased severity of fat infiltration in the lumbar multifidus muscles correlated significantly with decreased range of motion of lumbar flexion ($p = 0.032$). No significant correlation was found between the severity of fat infiltration in LMM and impaired movement control, posture control, body awareness or self-assessed functional disability.

Conclusion: This is the first study investigating the relationship between the severity of fat infiltration in LMM and the severity of lumbar dysfunction. The results of this study will contribute to the understanding of the mechanisms leading to fat infiltration of LMM and its relation to spinal function. Further studies should investigate whether specific treatment strategies are effective in reducing or preventing fat infiltration of LMM.

Keywords: Low back pain, Multifidus muscle, Fat infiltration, Flexibility

Background

Low back pain (LBP) has a very high incidence rate with a lifetime prevalence of up to 84% [1]. Persisting pain for more than 12 weeks is defined as chronic low back pain (CLBP) [1]. Most LBP disorders are multifactorial in nature and there are diverse interpretations for the underlying pain mechanisms, even when specified radiological diagnosis are found. Eighty-five percent of CLBP disorders have no specific diagnosis or pathology and are therefore "nonspecific" [1]. A large group of these disorders are predominantly mechanically induced and lead to maladaptive processes that maintain the ongoing pain and can result in functional deficits [2]. There is evidence that persisting LBP influences lumbar motor control [3], alters brain function and structure [4], changes lumbar tactile acuity [5], decreases spinal mobility [6] and compromises postural control [7]. However, LBP does not only lead to dysfunction, it can also result in structural changes of the lumbar multifidi muscle (LMM) such as fat infiltration as a consequence of atrophy [8–10].

Lumbar multifidus muscles are important for providing segmental stability and they function as dynamic stabilizers of the lumbar spine. They reinforce lumbar lordosis during rotation [11] and antagonize lumbar flexion [41]. It is generally assumed that dysfunction of the back muscles results in pain inhibition, which can

* Correspondence: luom@zhaw.ch
[3]Institute of Physiotherapy, School of Health Professions, Zurich University of Applied Sciences, Technikumstrasse 71, 8401 Winterthur, Switzerland
Full list of author information is available at the end of the article

finally lead to fatty infiltration of the LMM [9, 12]. Additionally, metabolic [13] or neuropathic mechanisms [14] are possible causes for the appearance of muscle degeneration. The average fat content of LMM in healthy subjects is down to levels as low as 14.5%, whereas in subjects with CLBP, the fat content of LMM can average levels as high as 23.6% [15, 16]. Interestingly, there is no correlation between obesity and the presence of fat in LMM [16]. About 80% of people suffering from CLBP present LMM with increased fat infiltration between levels L2 to L5 [10, 16, 17]. Increased fat infiltration in association with pain, age or dysfunction has also been reported in other muscles [18–20]. Association between chronic neck pain, fatty infiltration of sub-occipital muscles [21] and dysfunction of standing balance [22] could be indicated. For the lower back, the relationship between sway-back posture and a greater fat deposition in LMM could be demonstrated [23]. However, further studies that investigate the association between fat infiltration and dysfunction of the lower back are missing.

The purpose of this study was to seek possible correlation between fat infiltration of LMM and specific lumbar dysfunction in patients suffering from LBP. Based on the fact that LMM are important for motion and stability of the spine, we hypothesized that fat infiltration of LMM could be associated with impaired movement and posture control.

Methods

This cross-sectional study was conducted in a private physiotherapy outpatient clinic in Bern, Switzerland, according to the Helsinki declaration of ethics in medical research. The duration of the study was 8 months (May-December 2013).

Participants

Forty-two patients with non-specific LBP and a referral for physiotherapy, who had a recent magnetic resonance imaging (MRI) of their lower spine, were consecutively recruited for this study from different healthcare centers. Patients were not allowed to be familiar with the measures used in this study and they should not have received manual therapy or lumbar stabilization programs prior to this study. Patient data for age, gender, body weight and duration of LBP (acute pain < 12 weeks, chronic pain > 12 weeks) were collected and the body mass index (BMI) for each patient was documented. Patients who were obese (BMI > 35) or not able to perform active lumbar flexion and extension due to pain inhibition were excluded from this study. Those who had prior back surgery, sacroiliac arthritis, acute lumbar trauma, neurological deficits, active malignancy, infectional diseases, and were under the age of 20 or over the age of 75 were excluded as well.

MRI evaluation

The patients' MR images were generated prior to this study for medical diagnostics and not for the purpose of this study. MR images were obtained with 1.5 T systems (GE Medical Systems, USA; Siemens Healthcare, Erlangen, Germany) and patients were positioned supine in the MRI device. Each MRI sample contained standard T1- and T2-weighted axial images of the lumbar spine. All images were stored as DICOM format for processing. Due to the clinical setting of this study, we had to accommodate the fact that MR images were produced in different radiology centers and MRI parameters were not standardized. Analyze software (OsiriX, Pixmeo SARL, Switzerland, Version 5.6) was used for image analysis. To determine fat infiltration of the lumbar multifidus muscles, all axial T1-weighted MR images were included in the analysis as such sequences provide excellent anatomical detail.

While many quantitative MRI-based methods like Dixon/IDEAL [24, 25] or proton-density fat-fraction [26] are more accurate to measure fat separation, we had to take the variable MRI parameters into account. Semi-quantitative assessment of fat infiltration of lumbar muscles have been reported to be valid and reproducible, and findings correlated with MR spectroscopic measurements [15]. There is also evidence that visual grading of fat infiltration in LMM, using MR images, is reliable [27, 28]. For that reason, a visual evaluation method was used for this study.

Images were analyzed slice per slice within the determined range between L3 and L5 (Fig. 1). In order to optimize image quality, grey scaling was used during analysis. The area demonstrating the highest quantity of fat infiltration in LMM (left and right side combined) was used for grading. To determine fat infiltration of LMM three criteria were used (Fig. 2): Grad 0 (0–10% fat), Grade 1 (10–50% fat) and Grade 2 (>50% fat) [16].

Grading for this study was performed by a doctor of chiropractic who is a clinician and instructor of radiological diagnostics at the national chiropractic academy with 25 years of experience. He was blinded to the patients functional assessments.

Measures

Lumbar dysfunction was specified as reduced spinal flexibility, impairment of movement and posture control, attenuation of body awareness and self-assessed functional disability. In order to assess the patients' extent of LBP and the functional abilities of the low back, a set of different tests were used. All tests were performed by the same investigator, a physical therapist with 20 years of experience in manual therapy. To minimize testing bias, procedures were standardized and trained prior to the study. Patients wore only underwear to allow the

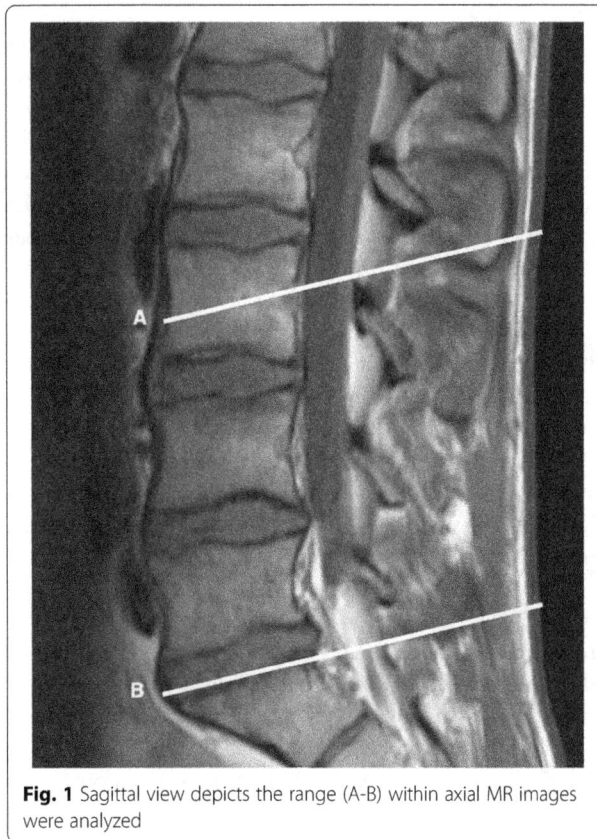

Fig. 1 Sagittal view depicts the range (A-B) within axial MR images were analyzed

observation of the entire body. The investigator was not aware of the patients' MRI findings.

Lumbar flexibility

Measurement of spinal flexibility was performed with the Spinal Mouse®, a hand-held computer-assisted device that can be used to measure the global and segmental range of motion of the spine [29]. The Spinal Mouse® has acceptable metrological properties to assess segmental and global lumbar flexibility during trunk flexion. However, its metrological properties are not acceptable to assess segmental mobility of L5-S1 alone [30] and the

segmental mobility of obese persons. Patients active range of motion of lumbar flexion (L1-S1), lumbar extension (L1-S1) and hip flexion were recorded in this study. Prior to the measurements, the landmarks of C7 and S3 were determined by palpation and were marked with a waterproof marker.

The device was then guided between the landmarks and along the midline of the spine to conduct the measurement.

Postural control

Postural control is based on the regulation of multisensory inputs and the reactions to stabilization. For this study, the upright Matthiass' arm-raising test [31] was used. This is a clinical test to detect posture changes under dynamic conditions. Patients had to hold two dumbbells with extended arms at shoulder height while posture was measured twice within an interval of 30 s with the Spinal Mouse® (Fig. 3). The overall weight of the dumbbells was calculated according to gender and bodyweight (women 5%, men 6.5% of bodyweight). Total and segmental evasive movements for the lumbar spine were calculated based on the differences between the two measurements.

Movement control

Movement control tests (MCT), a test battery consisting of six tests, are a reliable instrument for evaluating the ability to control flexion, extension and rotation of the lower back [3]. For practical reasons, MCT were modified for this study and only four tests were conducted to assess flexion and extension control (waiters bow, pelvic tilt, seated knee extension and prone active knee flexion). Patients received standardized instructions and each test was rated after three attempts. A correct movement (test negative) was rated with zero and an incorrect movement (test positive) was rated with one point. Total scores (max. four points) for all patients were calculated.

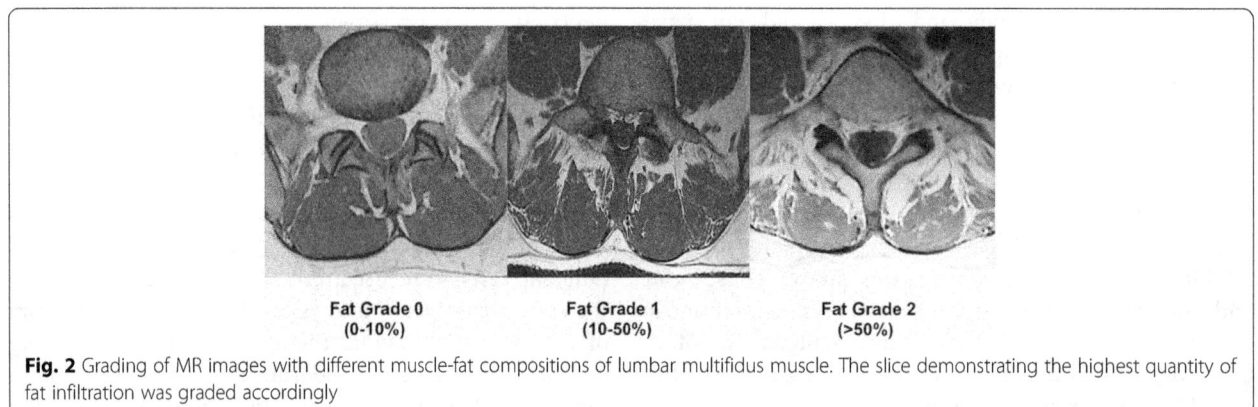

| Fat Grade 0 (0-10%) | Fat Grade 1 (10-50%) | Fat Grade 2 (>50%) |

Fig. 2 Grading of MR images with different muscle-fat compositions of lumbar multifidus muscle. The slice demonstrating the highest quantity of fat infiltration was graded accordingly

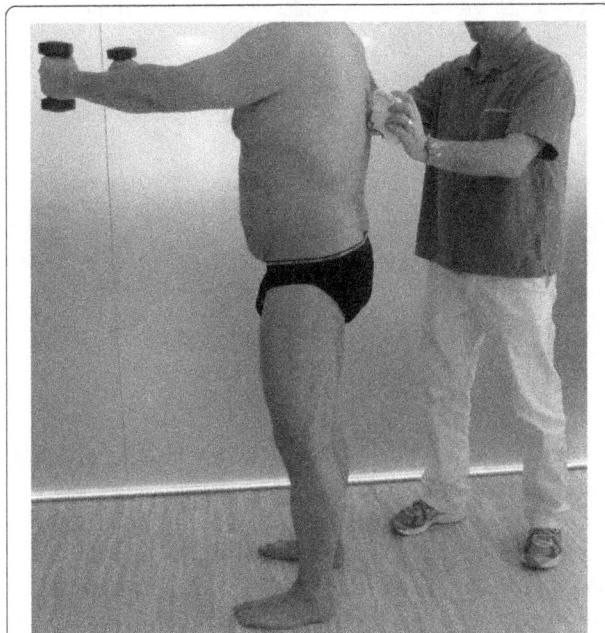

Fig. 3 Measurement of upright Matthiass' arm-raising test with the Spinal Mouse®. Segmental and total evasive movements for flexion or extension of the spine were calculated based on the difference between pre- and post-test posture

Body awareness

Impaired movement control of the lower back correlates positively with a disruption of the body image measured by two-point discrimination (TPD) of the back [5]. TPD threshold was measured using a plastic calliper ruler in the area between the first lumbar vertebra and the iliac crest. The threshold was defined as the distance between the calliper points at which the participants could decidedly detect two points instead of one. To find the TPD thresholds, descending runs with 10 mm increments starting from 8 cm as well as ascending calibrations with 5 mm increments were used. TPD was measured in prone position, left and right from the midline of the spine, horizontally and vertically. Mean values and standard deviations were calculated for horizontal and vertical thresholds.

Functional disability

To assess the implication of LBP on daily activities, the German version of the Oswestry Disability Index (ODI) questionnaire was used. The self-administered ODI is a valid instrument for measuring the degree of disability and for outcome measurement [32]. The German version of the ODI has been validated [33]. For this study the ODI was modified by using only nine sections, with a score ranging from 0 – 5 points per section. Total scores for all patients were calculated.

Statistical analysis

For each response, we fit a linear model to the data using fat, gender, age, duration of LBP and BMI as covariates. Our linear model for the j-th subject from group i was $Y_{ij} = \mu + \alpha_i + \text{covariates}_{ij} + \varepsilon_{ij}$, with μ as the intercept, α_i as the fat-effect of group i and the ε_{ij} as independent and normally distributed errors. We were interested in the covariate-adjusted effect of fat on the outcomes. Pairwise contrasts between the fat-groups were estimated from the estimated model. All simultaneous inference procedures controlled the family-wise error rate of $\alpha = 0.05$. Residual analysis was performed to check model assumptions, that is, independent and normally distributed errors. Breusch-Pagan tests were performed to test for homogeneous variances and Shapiro-Wilk tests for the normality assumption. For the association between fat content of LMM and age, status, gender and BMI, the Pearson correlation coefficient was calculated. A P value of less than .05 was considered to demonstrate a statistically significant difference.

The statistical analysis was performed with R, version 3.1.0 [34].

Results

A total of 42 patients, nineteen women (47.21 ± 13.15 years of age, 21–71 years) and 23 men (40.35 ± 10.21 years of age, 22–62 years) were tested. A detailed delineation of physical characteristics of the cohort is displayed in Table 1.

The results of main measurements are listed in Table 2.

69.1% of the patients reported chronic LBP and 30.9% reported acute LBP. Almost 85% of the patients showed fat infiltration in their LMM. Patients with chronic LBP were more likely to have fatty infiltration in LMM than patients with acute LBP ($p = 0.043$). Female patients demonstrated more fat infiltration in LMM than male patients ($p = 0.0019$), with a striking difference in fat grade 2. Whereas age correlated significantly with the presence of fat infiltration in LMM ($p = 0.025$), patients BMI did not interfere with fat infiltration in LMM.

Table 1 Physical characteristics in participating patients. Values for age and body mass index (BMI) represent mean and standard deviation

Fat Grade	Grade 0	Grade 1	Grade 2
Participants ($n = 42$)	$n = 6$	$n = 25$	$n = 11$
Gender (male, female)	6, 0	15, 10	2, 9
Duration of pain (acute, chronic)	4, 2	8, 17	1, 10
Age (years)	36 (10.49)	41.92 (11.60)	51 (10.50)
Body mass index (kg/m2)	25.24 (2.51)	23.53 (3.53)	22.49 (2.61)

Table 2 Descriptive data of main outcomes. Increased fat content of multifidus muscle correlates with decreased lumbar flexion ($p = 0.032$)

Fat Grade	Grade 0	Grade 1	Grade 2
Lumbar flexion (degrees)	24 (9.72)	22.56 (11.62)	11.55 (12.49)
Posture control (degrees)	−2.33 (1.37)	−1.08 (1.63)	−0.73 (0.90)
Movement control score (0–4)	2.17 (0.75)	1.68 (1.07)	1.18 (0.87)

Data represent mean and standard deviation. Negative values represent evasive movement in lumbar extension

Relationship between impairments and fat grade

Results showed that increased severity of fat infiltration in the lumbar multifidus muscles correlated with decreased range of motion of lumbar flexion ($p = 0.032$). Pairwise contrasts between the fat-groups indicated a significant difference ($p = 0.039$) between fat Grade 1 and fat Grade 2 (12.42°, 95% CI 0.513, 24.3) (Table 3).

However, none of the effect moderators (age, gender, duration of LBP, BMI) correlated with lumbar flexion (Table 4).

No significant correlation could be demonstrated between the severity of fat infiltration and movement control and there was no significant correlation found between fat infiltration and posture control (Fig. 4). But patients' posture control was affected by the duration of LBP. Patients with acute LBP demonstrated a significant ($p = 0.003$) greater lumbar evasive movement in extension than patients with chronic LBP. The ODI scores and the TPD values did not correlate with the severity of fat infiltration in lumbar multifidus muscles.

Discussion

The main result of our study was that increased severity of fat infiltration in the lumbar multifidus muscles correlated with decreased flexion range of motion of the lumbar spine. Although none of the effect moderators affected our main outcome, our study agreed with the existing evidence about the correlation between fat

Table 3 Table shows the estimated contrasts for lumbar flexion between the fat grades with the corresponding standard error (SE), degrees of freedom (df), t-statistic (t), the p-value (p) and the lower and upper bound of the 95% confidence interval (uCL and lCL)

Contrasts	Estimate	SE	df	lCL	uCL	t	p
Grade 0 - Grade 1	1.83	5.83	35	−18.35	22.0	0.315	0.947
Grade 0 - Grade 2	14.26	7.57	35	−11.93	40.4	1.885	0.158
Grade 1 - Grade 2	12.42	4.87	35	−4.42	29.3	2.553	0.039

The results are averaged over the levels of gender and status and taken at the mean of age and BMI. The p-values are adjusted for multiple testing. Results are averaged over the levels of: Gender, Status. Confidence level and P-value adjustments: tukey method for a family of 3 means.

Table 4 ANOVA table for the effect of fat grade and the covariates on lumbar flexion

Parameters	Df	SS	MS	F	P
Fat	2	1046	523	3.8	0.032
Age	1	72	72	0.52	0.474
Gender	1	54	54	0.39	0.535
Duration of pain	1	279	279	2.03	0.164
Body mass index	1	48	48	0.35	0.561
Residuals	35	4820	138		

Df Degrees of freedom; *SS* Sum of squares, *MS* Means squares, *F* F-statistics, *p* p-value

infiltration in LMM and age [35, 36], gender [17, 36], duration of pain [8] and BMI [15, 19].

In contrast to our hypothesis, we found no significant correlation between the severity of fat infiltration in LMM and impaired movement control or impaired posture control. Furthermore, correlation between fat infiltration of LMM and impaired body awareness or impaired self-assessed functional disability could not be demonstrated.

Decreased lumbar flexion

The relationship between spinal range of motion and disability in patients with low back pain has already been examined by various authors. Some found no significant correlation between lumbar flexion and reported disability [37, 38], while others reported decreased hip flexion and reduced spinal range of motion in all directions. The latter was found only in patients with LBP and limited straight leg raise [39]. The results of our study demonstrated that fat grade correlated with decrease of lumbar flexion only, whereas the amount of hip flexion increased, albeit not significantly. Therefore the increase of hip flexion might reflect a compensation for the loss of lumbar flexion. To explain the observed reduction in lumbar flexion, possible factors influencing spinal stability have to be highlighted. Shin et al. [40] demonstrated in their work that healthy subjects with the greatest lumbar flexibility had the highest activity levels of the LMM. Panjabi [41] described a model for spinal stability consisting of three subsystems (spinal column, spinal muscles and neural control unit) which together create optimal spinal flexibility and dynamic stability. As these systems are interdependent, one system could compensate for the deficits of another. If LBP occurs, inhibition of neural control is the consequence. Inhibition impedes alpha motor neuron activity in the anterior horn of the spinal cord and inhibits activity of LMM [12]. Thus, lumbar muscles cannot administrate their function anymore, which most likely debilitates postural control. Ongoing pain inhibition leads to alterations in neuro-

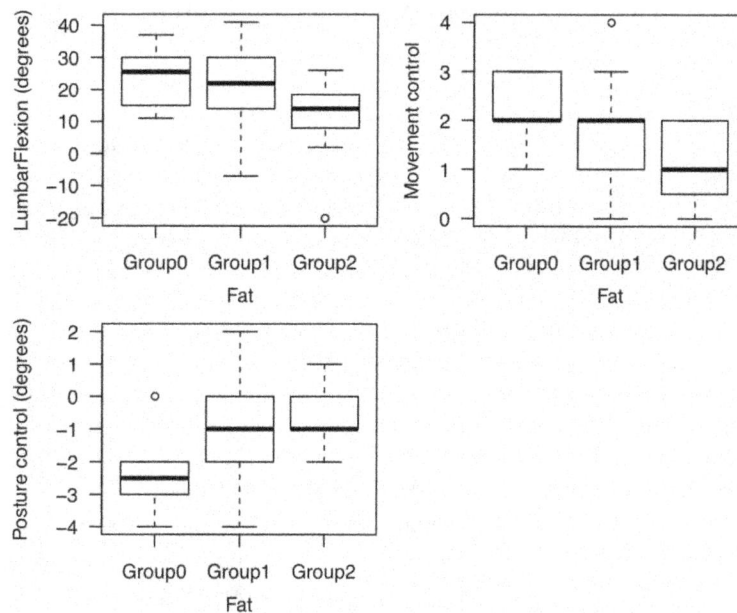

Fig. 4 Boxplots showing the association between the severity of fat infiltration (Grade 0, 1 and 2) and lumbar flexion, movement control and posture control. Only decreased lumbar flexion correlated significantly with increased severity of fat infiltration in multifidus muscles. No significant association was found between the severity of fat infiltration and impaired movement control or impaired posture control

muscular control, even after remission of LBP [10]. This mechanism becomes chronic and may result in atrophy of LMM. As important stabilizers, LMM act to maintain optimal joint forces, not only in the neutral zone of the spine, but also during prolonged flexion [42]. Therefore, atrophy in the muscular subsystem can lead to instability that must be compensated.

Superficial paraspinal and trunk muscles may have the ability to compensate for the deficit of LMM. Cholewicki et al. [43] investigated the stabilizing function of trunk flexor and extensor muscles in a neutral spine position. They demonstrated that active spinal stability was provided by flexor and extensor coactivation, but participants used different muscle recruitment strategies to achieve lumbar stability. The coactivation of local stabilizers such as LMM and M. tranversus abdominis increase intervertebral stiffness and allow superficial muscles to perform spinal movement. It has been hypothesized that recruitment strategies change in patients with LBP and global muscles try to compensate by global coactivation [44]. Although global coactivation increases stability, it also restricts spinal motion and function. Chan et al. [45] identified changed patterns of elasticity and cross-sectional area in LMM in relation to posture. In upright 25 and 45° forward stooping positions, the multifidus stiffness was higher in LBP patients than that in asymptomatic controls. There is also evidence that altered muscle activation strategies increase trunk stiffness in resting upright postures in recurrent LBP patients [6].

However defined, it cannot be determined whether reduced flexion range of motion of the lumbar spine is a cause or a result of fat infiltration of LMM. Referring to the results of our study, we hypothesize that once muscle activation strategies have changed, fatty infiltration of LMM proceeds. As a consequence, soft and ligamentous tissues that determine lumbar flexion are stiffening to compensate for the loss of dynamic stability. According to O'Sullivan [46], patients with LBP can be subgrouped into different movement dysfunction patterns. Patients with flexion patterns are probably the ones who have a dysfunction of their dorsal stabilizers. Potentially, fatty infiltrations of LMM is only present in the subgroup of patients with flexion patterns. The sample size of our study was too small to subgroup, but for future studies it would be worth trying to determine if there is a trend when subgrouping the patients. Lumbar pathology seen on MRI can play an important role in recurrence of LBP [47]. Whether decreased lumbar flexion and fat infiltration of LMM are risk factors for a recurrence of LBP remain unclear and has to be investigated.

Association between fat infiltration of LMM and movement control, postural control, body awareness and self-assessed functional disability

In contrast to our hypothesis we found no significant correlation between the grade of fat infiltration and impaired movement control or impaired postural control.

Likewise, there was no significant correlation found between LBP and impaired movement control and body awareness. This contradicts the findings of other authors [3, 48] but can be explained by the rather small sample size and the fact that patients in this study were not sub-grouped according to their LBP specificity. Interestingly, fat infiltration in LMM did not affect postural control, but patients with acute LBP demonstrated significantly higher impairment of posture control than patients with chronic LBP. These findings can be explained by using current evidence of the role of LMM in spinal stability and control. Multifidus muscles are predominantly occupied by muscle fiber type one [49] characterized by an extremly high cross-sectional area with very short muscle fibers that produce large forces over a narrow range of length [42]. The part that contributes the most to spinal stabilization is the deepest and also has a greater percentage of type 1 muscle fibers than the superficial part [50]. Ongoing loss of neural influence and mechanical loading leads to the atrophy of muscle fiber type I [51] whereas age-dependent atrophy of skeletal muscles affects predominately type two fibers [35]. The appearance of acute LBP changes corticomotor excitability [52] and first inhibits the deepest part of LMM which accordingly debilitates postural control more than movement control. This might explain our finding that patients with acute LBP demonstrated significantly higher impairment of posture control than patients with chronic LBP. Nevertheless, a correlation between duration of acute or chronic LBP and decreased lumbar flexion could not be demonstrated. In summary, our results revealed that fat infiltration of LMM has little impact on the measured functions of the lower back muscles.

Limitations
The results presented in this study should be considered cautiously because of the small sample size and the possible methodological bias of a single-center study with only one tester and one reviewer. Unfortunately, we had to accommodate the fact that patients for this study were referred from different healthcare centers and therefore patients' MRI were generated in different radiology centers. Differing MRI parameters and visual analysis are limiting factors for grading the amount of fat infiltration in LMM and the authors are aware of the possible inaccuracy of the MRI methodology. Standardized MRI protocols and quantitative MRI-based methods should be used in future studies. Likewise, the selection of patients should be refined in order to harmonize the physical characteristics of the cohort. For financial reasons, a control group with no fat infiltration of LMM and without LBP could not be included. The duration of LBP was measured, but the reoccurrence-rate of LBP was not evaluated. Although lumbar flexion was measured with a reliable instrument, other limiting factors for lumbar flexion (fear avoidance, straight leg raise etc.)

were not evaluated in this study and should be considered in continuing investigations.

Conclusion
Fat infiltration in LMM can be found both in acute or chronic LBP patients and in healthy subjects and therefore is not a pain-specific peculiarity. The presented study is the first that investigated the relationship between the severity of fat infiltration in LMM and the severity of lumbar dysfunction. The main result of this study was, that increased severity of fat infiltration in LMM correlated significantly with decreased range of motion of lumbar flexion. Neither the duration of pain, nor age, gender or BMI had an effect on this correlation. Moreover, the severity of fat infiltration in LMM did not correlate with altered movement control, posture control, body awareness and self-assessed functional disability. In summary, this cross-sectional study revealed that fat infiltration of LMM impaires more the flexibility of the lower spine than it affects active functions of the lower back muscles. Whether reduced flexion range of motion of the lumbar spine is a cause or a result of fat infiltration of LMM could not be identified with this study. And it is still not clear if fat infiltration of LMM is a prognostic factor and if patients with LBP and fat infiltration of LMM have to be subgrouped and need special treatment strategies. And last but not least, it has to be investigated whether asymptomatic subjects with decreased lumbar flexion also demonstrate increased fat infiltration of LMM. Further research is necessary to provide evidence whether specific strategies are effective for the treatment of LBP and for the prevention of progressive fat infiltration of LMM.

Abbreviations
BMI: Body-Mass-Index; CLBP: Chronic Low Back Pain; LBP: Low Back Pain; LMM: Lumbar Multifidus Muscles; MCT: Movement Control Tests; ODI: Oswestry Disability Index; TPD: Two Point Discrimination

Acknowledgements
The authors would like to acknowledge Dr. Alfred Schlup for rating the MRI scans and the idiag AG of Switzerland for placing a Spinal Mouse® at our disposal at no charge. Further we would like to acknowledge the input from reviewers who contributed to an improved manuscript.

Funding
This study was unfunded.

Authors' contributions
MH originated the idea of the study. MH, GF and HL designed the trial protocol. MH and GF conducted all measurements for this study. AM provided statistical support. All authors read and approved the final manuscript.

Competing interests

The authors declare that they have no competing interests.

Consent for publication

Patients gave written consent for publication of their anonymized data.

Author details

[1]Physio Hildebrandt, Sickingerstrasse 4, 3014 Bern, Switzerland. [2]Hauptstrasse 26, 3254 Messen, Switzerland. [3]Institute of Physiotherapy, School of Health Professions, Zurich University of Applied Sciences, Technikumstrasse 71, 8401 Winterthur, Switzerland.

References

1. Airaksinen O, Brox JI, Cedraschi C, Hildebrandt J, Klaber-Moffett J, Kovacs F, et al. Chapter 4. European guidelines for the management of chronic nonspecific low back pain. Eur Spine J. 2006;15:192–300.

2. O'Sullivan PB, Burnett A, Floyd AN, Gadsdon K, Logiudice J, Miller D, et al. Lumbar repositioning deficit in a specific low back pain population. Spine. 2003;28:1074–9.

3. Luomajoki H, Kool J, de Bruin ED, Airaksinen O. Movement control tests of the low back; evaluation of the difference between patients with low back pain and healthy controls. BMC Musculoskelet Disord. 2008;9(1):170.

4. Wand BM, Parkitny L, O'Connell NE, Luomajoki H, McAuley JH, Thacker M, et al. Cortical changes in chronic low back pain: current state of the art and implications for clinical practice. Man Ther. 2011;16(1):15–20.

5. Luomajoki H, Moseley GL. Tactile acuity and lumbopelvic motor control in patients with back pain and healthy controls. Br J Sports Med. 2011;45(5): 437–40.

6. Hodges P, van den Hoorn W, Dawson A, Cholewicki J. Changes in the mechanical properties of the trunk in low back pain may be associated with recurrence. J Biomech. 2009;42:61–6.

7. Mok NW, Brauer SG, Hodges PW. Failure to use movement in postural strategies leads to increased spinal displacement in low back pain. Spine. 2007;32(19):E537–543.

8. Hides J, Gilmore C, Stanton W, Bohlscheid E. Multifidus size and symmetry among chronic LBP and healthy asymptomatic subjects. Man Ther. 2008;13: 43–9.

9. Freeman MD, Woodham MA, Woodham AW. The role of the lumbar multifidus in chronic Low back pain: a review. PM & R. 2010;2:142–6.

10. D'hooge R, Cagnie B, Crombez G, Vanderstraeten G, Dolphens M, Danneels L. Increased intramuscular fatty infiltration without differences in lumbar muscle cross-sectional area during remission of unilateral recurrent low back pain. Man Ther. 2012;17(6):584–8.

11. Bogduk N. Clinical Anatomy of the Lumbar Spine and Sacrum, Fourth edition. Philadelphia: Elsevier; 2005. ISBN 0-443-10119-1.

12. Danneels LA, Vanderstraeten GG, Cambier DC, Witvrouw EE, De Cuyper HJ, Danneels L. CT imaging of trunk muscles in chronic low back pain patients and healthy control subjects. Eur Spine J. 2000;9(4):266–72.

13. Schakman O, Kalista S, Barbé C, Loumaye A, Thissen JP. Glucocorticoid-induced skeletal muscle atrophy. Int J Biochem Cell Biol. 2013;45:2163–72.

14. Nishida Y, Saito Y, Yokota T, Kanda T, Mizusawa H. Skeletal muscle MRI in complex regional pain syndrome. Intern Med. 2009;48(4):209–12.

15. Mengiardi B, Schmid MR, Boos N, Pfirrmann CWA, Brunner F, Elfering A, et al. Fat content of lumbar paraspinal muscles in patients with chronic Low back pain and in asymptomatic volunteers: quantification with MR Spectroscopy1. Radiology. 2006;240(3):786–92.

16. Kjaer P, Bendix T, Sorensen JS, Korsholm L, Leboeuf-Yde C. Are MRI-defined fat infiltrations in the multifidus muscles associated with low back pain? BMC Med. 2007;5:2.

17. Kader DF, Wardlaw D, Smith FW. Correlation between the MRI changes in the lumbar multifidus muscles and Leg pain. Clin Radiol. 2000;55(2):145–9.

18. Elliott J, Sterling M, Noteboom JT, Treleaven J, Galloway G, Jull G. The clinical presentation of chronic whiplash and the relationship to findings of MRI fatty infiltrates in the cervical extensor musculature: a preliminary investigation. Eur Spine J. 2009;18:1371–8.

19. Marcus RL, Addison O, Kidde JP, Dibble LE, Lastayo PC. Skeletal muscle fat infiltration: impact of age, inactivity, and exercise. J Nutr Health Aging. 2010; 14(5):362–6.

20. Nardo L, Karampinos DC, Lansdown DA, Carballido-Gamio J, Lee S, Maroldi R, et al. Quantitative assessment of fat infiltration in the rotator cuff muscles using water-fat MRI. J Magn Reson Imaging. 2013; doi:10.1002/jmri.24278.

21. Andary MT, Hallgren RC, Greenman PE, Rechtien JJ. Neurogenic atrophy of suboccipital muscles after a cervical injury: a case study. Am J Phys Med Rehabil. 1998;77(6):545–9.

22. McPartland JM, Brodeur RR, Hallgren RC. Chronic neck pain, standing balance, and suboccipital muscle atrophy-a pilot study. J Manipulative Physiol Ther. 1997;20:24–9.

23. Pezolato A, de Vasconcelos EE, Defino HLA, Nogueira-Barbosa MH. Fat infiltration in the lumbar multifidus and erector spinae muscles in subjects with sway- back posture. Eur Spine J. 2012;21(11):2158–64.

24. Dixon W. Simple proton spectroscopic imaging. Radiology. 1984;153:189–94.

25. Gerdes CM, Kijowski R, Reeder SB. IDEAL imaging of the musculoskeletal system: robust water fat separation for uniform fat suppression, marrow evaluation, and cartilage imaging. Am J Roentgenol. 2007;189(5):284–91.

26. Reeder S, Hu H, Sirlin C. Proton density fat-fraction: A standardized mr-based biomarker of tissue fat concentration. JMRI. 2012;36(5):1011–14.

27. Solgaard Sorensen J, Kjaer P, Jensen ST, Andersen P. Low-field magnetic resonance imaging of the lumbar spine: reliability of qualitative evaluation of disc and muscle parameters. Acta Radiol. 2006;47(9):947–53.

28. Battaglia PJ, Maeda Y, Welk A, Hough B, Kettner N. Reliability of the Goutallier classification in quantifying muscle fatty degeneration in the lumbar multifidus using magnetic resonance imaging. J Manipulative Physiol Ther. 2014;37(3):190–7.

29. Mannion AF, Knecht K, Balaban G, Dvorak J, Grob D. A new skin-surface device for measuring the curvature and global and segmental ranges of motion of the spine: reliability of measurements and comparison with data reviewed from the literature. Eur Spine J. 2004;13(2):122–36.

30. Guermazi M, Ghroubi S, Kassis M, Jaziri O, Keskes H, Kessomtini W, et al. Validity and reliability of spinal mouse to assess lumbar flexion. Ann Readapt Med Phys. 2006;49(4):172–7.

31. Mahlknecht JF. The prevalence of postural disorders in children and adolescents: a cross sectional study. Z Für Orthop Unfallchirurgie. 2007; 145(3):338–42.

32. Fairbank JC, Pynsent PB. The oswestry disability index. Spine. 2000;25(22): 2940–52.

33. Osthus H, Cziske R, Jacobi E. Cross-cultural adaptation of a German version of the oswestry disability index and evaluation of its measurement properties. Spine. 2006;31:E448–53.

34. R Development Core Team. R: A language and environment for statistical computing. 2011. Vienna: R Foundation for Statistical Computing. ISBN 3-900051-07-0, URL https://www.r-project.org.

35. Lexell J. Human aging, muscle mass, and fiber type composition. J Gerontol A Biol Sci Med Sci. 1995;50:11–6.

36. Crawford RJ, Filli L, Elliott JM, Nanz D, Fischer MA, Marcon M, Ulbrich EJ. Age- and level-dependence of fatty infiltration in lumbar paravertebral muscles of healthy volunteers. AJNR Am J Neuroradiol. 2016;37(4):742–8.

37. Grönblad M, Hurri H, Kouri JP. Relationships between spinal mobility, physical performance tests, pain intensity and disability assessments in chronic low back pain patients. Scand J Rehabil Med. 1997;29:17–24.

38. Sullivan MS, Shoaf LD, Riddle DL. The relationship of lumbar flexion to disability in patients with low back pain. Phys Ther. 2000;80(3):240–50.

39. Wong TKT, Lee RYW. Effects of low back pain on the relationship between the movements of the lumbar spine and hip. Hum Mov Sci. 2004;23(1):21–34.

40. Shin G, Shu Y, Li Z, Jiang Z, Mirka G. Influence of knee angle and individual flexibility on the flexion-relaxation response of the low back musculature. J Electromyogr Kinesiol. 2004;14(4):485–94.

41. Panjabi MM. Clinical spinal instability and low back pain. J Electromyogr Kinesiol. 2003;13(4):371–9.

42. Ward SR, Kim CW, Eng CM, Gottschalk 4th LJ, Tomiya A, Garfin SR, et al. Architectural analysis and intraoperative measurements demonstrate the unique design of the multifidus muscle for lumbar spine stability. J Bone Joint Surg Am. 2009;91(1):176–85.

43. Cholewicki J, Panjabi M, Khachatryan A. Stabilizing function of trunk flexor-extensor muscles around a neutral spine posture. Spine. 1997;22:2207–12.

44. Barr KP, Griggs M, Cadby T. Lumbar stabilization: core concepts and current literature, Part 1. Am J Phys Med Rehabil. 2005;84(6):473–80.

45. Chan S-T, Fung P-K, Ng N-Y, Ngan T-L, Chong M-Y, Tang C-N, et al. Dynamic changes of elasticity, cross-sectional area, and fat infiltration of multifidus at different postures in men with chronic low back pain. Spine J. 2012;12(5):381–8.

46. O'Sullivan P. Diagnosis and classification of chronic low back pain disorders: maladaptive movement and motor control impairments as underlying mechanism. Man Ther. 2005;10(4):242–55.

47. Hancock MJ, Maher CM, Petocz P, Lin CW, Steffens D, Luque-Suarez A, Magnussen JS. Risk factors for a recurrence of low back pain. Spine J. 2015; 15(11):2360–8.

48. Saner J, Kool J, de Bie R, Sieben J, Luomajoki H. Movement control exercise versus general exercise to reduce disability in patients with low back pain and movement control impairment. A randomised controlled trial. BMC Musculoskelet Disord. 2011;12:207.

49. Demoulin C, Crielaard J-M, Vanderthommen M. Spinal muscle evaluation in healthy individuals and low-back-pain patients: a literature review. Joint Bone Spine. 2007;74:9–13.

50. MacDonald DA, Lorimer Moseley G, Hodges PW. The lumbar multifidus: does the evidence support clinical beliefs? Man Ther. 2006;11(4):254–63.

51. Ciciliot S, Rossi AC, Dyar KA, Blaauw B, Schiaffino S. Muscle type and fiber type specificity in muscle wasting. Int J Biochem Cell Biol. 2013;45(10):2191–9.

52. Tsao H, Tucker KJ, Hodges PW. Changes in excitability of corticomotor inputs to the trunk muscles during experimentally-induced acute low back pain. Neuroscience. 2011;181:127–33.

4

An update on the prevalence of low back pain in Africa

Linzette Deidrè Morris[1,2*], Kurt John Daniels[1], Bhaswati Ganguli[3] and Quinette Abegail Louw[1]

Abstract

Background: Low back pain (LBP) remains a common health problem and one of the most prevalent musculoskeletal conditions found among developed and developing nations. The following paper reports on an updated search of the current literature into the prevalence of LBP among African nations and highlights the specific challenges faced in retrieving epidemiological information in Africa.

Methods: A comprehensive search of all accessible bibliographic databases was conducted. Population-based studies into the prevalence of LBP among children/adolescents and adults living in Africa were included. Methodological quality of included studies was appraised using an adapted tool. Meta-analyses, subgroup analyses, sensitivity analyses and publication bias were also conducted.

Results: Sixty-five studies were included in this review. The majority of the studies were conducted in Nigeria ($n = 31;47\%$) and South Africa ($n = 16;25\%$). Forty-three included studies (66.2%) were found to be of higher methodological quality. The pooled lifetime, annual and point prevalence of LBP in Africa was 47% (95% CI 37;58); 57% (95% CI 51;63) and 39% (95% CI 30;47), respectively.

Conclusion: This review found that the lifetime, annual and point prevalence of LBP among African nations was considerably higher than or comparable to global LBP prevalence estimates reported. Due to the poor methodological quality found among many of the included studies, the over-representation of affluent countries and the difficulty in sourcing and retrieving potential African studies, it is recommended that future African LBP researchers conduct methodologically robust studies and report their findings in accessible resources.

Keywords: Low back pain, Africa, Prevalence, Epidemiology, Systematic review, Meta-analysis

Background

Low back pain (LBP) is arguably the most prevalent musculoskeletal condition found among both developed and developing nations [1–4]. Broadly defined as pain or discomfort in the lumbar region of the spine [1, 2]; LBP is the leading cause of activity limitation, results in significant losses in productivity at work and incurs billions of dollars in medical expenditure annually [1, 3, 4]. The prevalence of LBP worldwide is estimated to be between 30 and 80% among the general population and has been found to increase with age [5]. In addition, a higher prevalence of LBP has been associated with a lower socioeconomic status and lower education levels [5, 6]. According to the Global Burden of Disease (GBD) 2010 study, LBP is currently the sixth highest burden on a list of 291 conditions and is the cause of more years lived with disability (YLDs) globally than any other disease [4]. Affecting just about anyone, of any gender, race or socioeconomic background [6], LBP has a substantial impact on the overall and financial well-being of an

* Correspondence: ldmorris@sun.ac.za
[1]Division of Physiotherapy, Department of Health and Rehabilitation Sciences, Faculty of Medicine and Health Sciences, Stellenbosch University, PO BOX 241, Cape Town 8000, South Africa
[2]Division of Epidemiology and Biostatistics, Faculty of Medicine and Health Sciences, Stellenbosch University, Tygerberg, South Africa
Full list of author information is available at the end of the article

individual and society [5, 7]. Therefore, it was postulated that the burden of LBP would be greater in lower and middle income countries (LMICs) like those situated in Africa [7, 9]. A systematic review published in 2007 revealed that the prevalence of LBP in Africa was comparable to that of developing nations, and was rising [10].

Despite the GBD 2010 and World Health Organization (WHO) reports [4, 8, 9], and coupled with the high prevalence of LBP in Africa [10]; LBP and other musculoskeletal conditions remain less prioritized in LMICs, due to more pressing health issues like HIV/AIDS [3]. This is most likely due to the fact that although LBP causes significant disability and related health costs, it is not life-threatening [4, 11]. LBP however remains a global health concern and an immense burden for LMICs, such as those in Africa where health budgets are already restricted and channelled to other higher priority conditions [1, 2, 5, 7]. Of concern is that due to various epidemiologic challenges faced in various LMICs in Africa and the subsequent lack of accurate data, the true burden of LBP is still not well understood or known. In the 7 years since the previous review was published, a large number of studies have emerged. The following paper therefore reports on an updated search of the current literature into the prevalence of LBP among African nations (children, adolescents, adults; males and females). It was hoped that a better understanding of the current burden of LBP in African LMICs would be established. Furthermore, this paper also highlights the specific challenges faced in retrieving epidemiological information in Africa and on conducting meta-analyses of LBP data, as well as the methodological shortcomings of published African studies.

Methods

The MOOSE (Meta-analysis Of Observational Studies in Epidemiology) were used [12]. The protocol for this updated review was registered on PROSPERO prior to commencement (protocol registration number: CRD42014010417) [13].

Studies had to primarily report on the prevalence of LBP among nations situated on the African continent were included. Studies could report on the prevalence of musculoskeletal conditions as a whole, yet had to provide subgroup data for LBP prevalence. Studies could report on the following recall periods for LBP prevalence, namely: point, annual or lifetime prevalence. Subjects included in the studies could be any race, gender and age. Studies could be published in English, Afrikaans or French, since these are three of the most common languages in which scholarly communication in Africa is conducted [14]. French studies were translated by a French-speaking African native. To validate the translations, we cross-checked the French translations with the English abstract of the article (which is typically available online) to check for any marked discrepancies and reverse translations were done to ensure validity of translations. Dissertations, conference proceedings, commentaries/letters and other grey literature were excluded from this review.

A comprehensive update of the previous search [10] was conducted in the following bibliographic databases via the Stellenbosch University's library website: *Ebsco-Host (including CiNAHL, Africa-Wide Information, Health Source: Nursing/Academic edition, SPORTDiscus) , Medline, ScienceDirect, Scopus, PEDro, PubMed, SA ePublications, Cochrane Library, ProQuest Medical Library, African Journals Online (AJOL)* and *Web of Science*. The main search terms were: *low back pain, Africa* and *prevalence*. The original search strategy was revised where necessary and excluded *management* and *rehabilitation*. The full search strategy is available on request from the corresponding author. Secondary searching (PEARLing) was conducted (PEARLing is a search method whereby the reference lists of all included and excluded studies are searched for other studies which may not have been identified during the database search). Manual searching was not conducted due to the difficulty in replicating this method. The search was commenced and conducted between June 2014 and October 2014, and an updated search was conducted in March 2015 and July 2016. A final search was conducted in April 2017, prior to submission. Articles published and indexed from inception of the databases to the end of the search period were included.

The titles and abstracts of all potentially relevant population-based studies were screened by two reviewers independently. Methodological appraisal of included studies was conducted using the same critical appraisal tool as in the original review [10, 15]. The tool was however further adapted for use in this review (Table 1), by reducing the previous items 7, 8 and 9 to one item (7a- c), as all these items pertained to the validation of the data collection tool used in the study. For the purposes of this review, all items in the appraisal tool were equally weighed and the total score for the tool was 10. No subminimum criteria were applied.

Appraisal of studies was conducted independently by two reviewers. Studies scoring 60% or less on the appraisal tool were deemed as low quality studies and were excluded from the meta-analyses. The 60% cut-off was deemed appropriate based on the fact that no subminimum criteria were applied due to the heterogeneous nature of LBP data and that the average methodological score of all studies was 66%. It was therefore decided that all studies which were below the average score were relatively lower in methodological quality compared to the rest of the included studies.

Table 1 Methodological appraisal tool for LBP prevalence studies (adapted) [15]

Criteria	Yes/No	Comments
Is the final sample representative of the target population?		
1. At least 1 of the following must apply in the study: an entire target population, randomly selected sample or sample stated to represent the target population.		
2. At least 1 of the following: reasons for non-response described, non-responders described, comparison of responders and non-responders, or comparison of sample and target population.		
3. Response rate, and if applicable, drop-out rate reported		
Quality of data		
4. Were the data primary data of LBP, or was it taken from a survey not specifically designed for that purpose?		
5. Were the data collected from each subject directly or were they collected from a proxy?		
6. Was the same mode of data collection used for all subjects?		
7. At least 1 of the following in case of: a) Questionnaire: a validated questionnaire or at least tested for reproducibility? b) Interview: interview validated, tested for reproducibility, or adequately described and standardized? c) Examination: examination validated, tested for reproducibility, adequately described and standardized?		
Definition of LBP		
8. Was there a precise anatomic delineation of the lumbar area or reference to an easily obtainable article that contains such specification?		
9. Was there further useful specification of the definition of LBP, or question(s) put to study subjects quoted such as frequency, duration, or intensity, and character of the pain. Or was there reference to an easily obtainable article that contains such specification?		
10. Were the recall periods clearly stated: e.g. 1 week, 1 month, lifetime?		
Total score (10)		

Data were extracted using specifically-designed extraction sheets and were entered into Microsoft (MS) Excel spreadsheets [16]. The following data were extracted from included studies: *author name(s), year of publication, country of publication, study design, data collection tool/ outcome measure tool(s), population, study setting (including if rural or urban setting), sample size, age group/age (range and/or mean ± standard deviation), gender, data collection period, LBP definition, LBP recall period, reliability/validity of measurement tools, response rates and LBP prevalence rates (point, annual and lifetime).*

From the data extracted, the pooled point, annual and lifetime prevalence (summary estimates) of LBP among African nations, as well as the 95% confidence intervals (CI), were calculated for conducting meta-analyses of observational data. A random effects model to adjust for heterogeneity was used since LBP data inherently varies between studies due to differences in risk factors and characteristics between populations. Sub-group analyses were conducted for age group (adults and children/adolescents), country status (low income, low middle income and upper middle income), gender (male and female) and setting (community, industry, hospital, professional and school). Sensitivity analyses were conducted to assess if the inclusion of the lower methodological quality studies would change the results of the analyses. Publication bias was also assessed using Duval and Tweedie's Trim and Fill method [81].

Results

The results of the comprehensive updated search of literature into the prevalence of LBP in Africa are depicted in Fig. 1. A total of 65 studies were included in this review (of which 40 were published after the original review was conducted) [17–70, 81–91]. A list of the excluded studies and the reasons for their exclusion is available from the corresponding author.

General description of included studies

More than 72.3% of the included studies were conducted in lower income and lower middle income countries [17, 21, 22, 25–29, 31–34, 36, 37, 40–44, 46–48, 50–53, 57–60, 63–67, 69, 83–91]. The majority of the studies were conducted in Nigeria, which is a lower middle income country ($n = 31$; 47.7%) [22, 25, 27, 29, 32, 33, 36, 41, 44, 46–48, 50, 52, 53, 57–60, 64–66, 81–83, 86–91] and South Africa, which is an upper middle income country ($n = 16$; 24.6%) [19, 20, 23, 24, 30, 35, 38, 39, 45, 49, 54–56, 61, 62, 70]. Three of the included studies were published in the French language [18, 26, 51], the rest were published in English. Fifteen (27.8%) of the 54 independent African countries (countries as recognised by the United Nations) are represented in this review. Forty-five studies included both male and female participants (75%) [17, 18, 20–22, 27–37, 40, 46, 48–53, 55, 57–59, 61, 62, 67–70, 81, 82, 84–86, 89, 90]. Fourteen of the included studies included children and/or adolescents between the ages 11 and 19 years (21.5%) [17–19, 31, 34, 35, 41, 44, 53, 56, 59, 67, 69, 85]. The response rates were reported by 72. 3% of the studies ($n = 47$) [19–25, 27, 28, 30–41, 46–50, 52–54, 59, 61–64, 66–70, 82, 85–91] and ranged from 11 to 100%. Forty-two of the studies were conducted in an urban setting (64.6%), while nine studies (13.8%) where

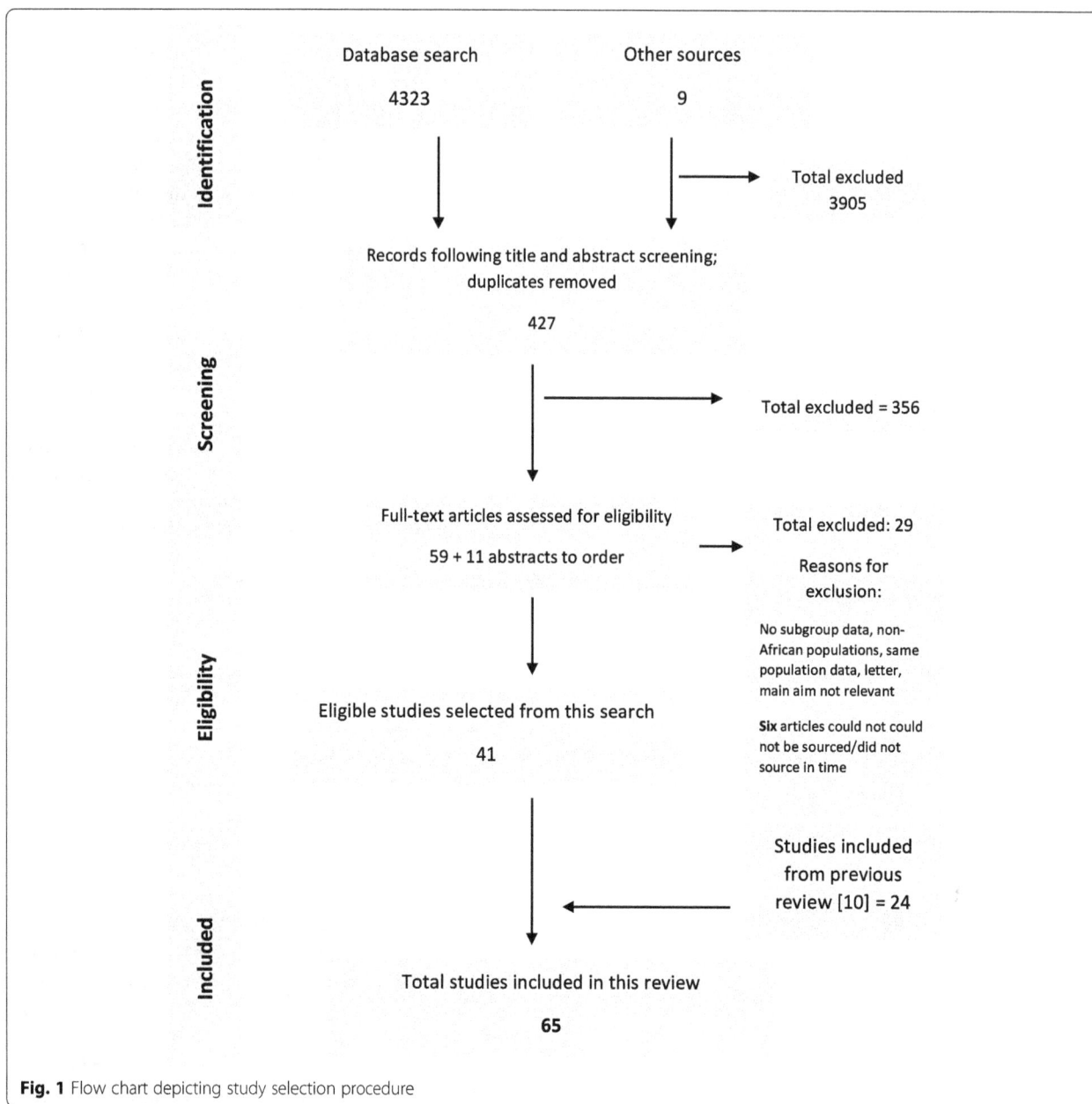

Fig. 1 Flow chart depicting study selection procedure

conducted in a rural setting. The rest of the studies ($n = 14$; 21.5%) were conducted in a setting which incorporated both rural and urban communities.

The most common study design was cross-sectional ($n = 60$; 92.3%). Two studies used a prospective study design [17, 42] and three used a retrospective study design [21, 26, 84]. Most of the included studies used questionnaires. Three studies reviewed medical records [21, 26, 84], and eight studies included a physical examination [17, 40, 42–45, 47, 58]. Twelve studies conducted interviews [17, 20, 40–44, 54, 55, 57, 58, 60]. It was unclear in three of the studies which sampling method was used [19, 50, 59]. Nine studies did not explicitly provide a clear recall period (point, lifetime or annual) for LBP (15%) [17, 41,

42, 44, 45, 49, 70, 71, 84]. Two studies used the index pregnancy (up to 40 weeks) as the recall period [60, 83].

The most common population studied was health professionals and hospital staff ($n = 17$; 26.2%) [22, 28, 30, 37, 45, 46, 48–52, 55, 61–63, 82, 91]. Health professions studies included physiotherapists, general surgeons, dentists, nurses, general surgeons and oral hygienists. Workers were studied in 21 of the eligible studies (32.3%) [20, 24, 26, 27, 32, 33, 36, 38, 39, 43, 44, 47, 54, 57, 64–66, 81, 87–90] and included the following sectors: commercial, industry, transport and farming. Computer-users were only studied in one included study [36] and two studies included sports players [19, 56]. The sports players studied were cricketers. One study reported on LBP prevalence among school teachers [68]. An overview summary of the descriptive data extracted from the included studies is provided in Table 2.

Methodological quality of included studies

Twenty-two (33.8%) of the included studies scored 60% or less on the specified critical appraisal tool and were therefore excluded from further analysis [17, 19, 21, 23, 26, 36, 38, 42, 44–46, 49–51, 55, 56, 58, 64, 83, 84, 86, 90]. Sixty-five percent (n = 42) of the included studies reported on the validity and/or reliability of their data collection tools (questionnaire, interview or examination) [31, 32, 34, 35, 39, 41–48, 50, 52–70, 81, 83, 85–91]. Only 24 of the included studies (36.9%) provided a case definition for LBP [18, 24, 25, 30–32, 34, 35, 37, 40, 41, 48, 52, 57, 65–69, 81, 83–85, 91]. Table 3 illustrates the methodological appraisal of the included studies.

Lifetime, annual and point prevalence of LBP among African nations

Lifetime, annual and point prevalence data of LBP among African nations were calculated to provide a summary estimate. Lifetime prevalence pertains to the experience of LBP at any point in the individual's lifetime; annual prevalence pertains to the experience of LBP at any point in the past 6–12 months; and point prevalence pertains to the experience of LBP at the time of the study's data collection. For these purposes, only African studies reporting a recall period of lifetime, annual or point prevalence for LBP, were included for analyses.

- *Lifetime prevalence of LBP in Africa*

Sixteen studies reported on the lifetime prevalence of LBP in Africa [18, 26, 30, 31, 34, 35, 37, 39, 64, 67, 70, 85, 86, 91]. The lifetime prevalence for LBP in Africa was estimated at 47% (95% CI 37;58). The summary analyses for lifetime prevalence of LBP among Africans is depicted in Fig. 2.

Sensitivity and subgroup analyses were conducted to ensure that the exclusion of the poorer methodological quality studies would not have influenced the results significantly if included. Figure 3 illustrates the sensitivity and subgroup analyses conducted for lifetime LBP prevalence among Africans. A significant difference between the summary estimates calculated with only the higher quality studies or only the lower quality studies, compared to all studies (combined) was found.

- *Annual prevalence of LBP in Africa*

Thirty-four studies reported on the annual prevalence of LBP in Africa [22, 25, 27–29, 32–34, 37, 39, 43, 46–54, 56, 57, 59, 61, 62, 65, 66, 68, 81, 82, 85–89]. The annual prevalence of LBP in Africa was estimated at 57% (95% CI 51;63).

The summary analyses for annual prevalence of LBP among Africans is depicted in Fig. 4.

Figure 5 illustrates the sensitivity and subgroup analyses for annual LBP prevalence among African nations. No significant differences between the summary estimates calculated with only the higher quality studies or only the lower quality studies, compared to all studies (combined) were found.

- *Point prevalence of LBP in Africa*

Twenty-three studies reported on point prevalence of LBP in Africa [17, 19–21, 23, 33, 39–42, 45, 54, 55, 58, 59, 63, 67, 69, 84–86, 91]. The point prevalence of LBP in Africa was estimated at 39% (95% CI 30;47). The summary analyses for point prevalence of LBP among Africans is depicted in Fig. 6.

Figure 7 illustrates the subgroup and sensitivity analyses for point LBP prevalence among Africans. No significant differences between the summary estimates calculated with only the higher quality studies or only the lower quality studies, compared to all studies (combined) were found.

Publication bias

Duval and Tweedie's "Trim and Fill" method was used to assess publication bias [80]. Under the random effects model the point estimate and 95% confidence interval for the combined studies is 0.49 (95% CI 0.39, 0.57). Using Trim and Fill the imputed point estimate is 0.31 (95% CI 0.24, 0.39). The method suggests that a total of 13 studies may be missing from this review.

Discussion

This paper provides an updated synthesis of the literature into the prevalence of LBP among African populations. The current review indicates that although a number of years have passed after our initial review [10], LBP remains a health concern in Africa.

Meta-analyses of the observational data collected from the eligible studies provides a summary estimate of the lifetime, annual and point prevalence. Lifetime, annual and point prevalence of LBP among African populations was found to be higher than recently reported estimates for global LBP prevalence [2, 4, 5]. The global prevalence of LBP reported by Hoy et al. in 2012 was calculated from a total of 165 studies conducted in 54 countries around the globe (developed and developing countries), over a period of 29 years [2]. In our review, the point prevalence of LBP among Africans was estimated at 39% (95% CI 30;47), which is considerably higher than the global LBP prevalence estimate (18.3%) reported by Hoy et al. [2]. Similarly, the annual prevalence for LBP among Africans (57%; 95% CI 51;63) found in our review was substantially higher than the global annual LBP

Table 2 General description of included studies (n = 65)

Study ID	Year	Country	Population description	Study setting	Design/tool	Sampling method	Age (years)	Gender	n	RR
Mulimba [17]	1990	Nairobi	Private patients	Private clinic	P; I/E	population	11–75	F/M	2201	NP
Bezzaoucha [18]	1992	Algiers	General population	Community	C; Q	population	15 and over	F/M	6956	NP
Harris [19]	1993	South Africa	Cricketers	Cricket clubs/schools	C; Q	unclear	15–35	M	110	90
Schierhout et al. [20]	1993	South Africa	Factory workers	Factories	C; I	block random	18 and older	F/M	155	100
Mijiyawa et al. [21]	2000	Togo	OPD patients	Rheumatology clinic	R; MR	population	17–94	F/M	9065	100
Omokhodion et al. [22]	2000	Nigeria	Hospital staff	Hospital	C; Q	population	20–60	F/M	74	93
Worku [23]	2000	Lesotho	Mothers	Community	C; Q	stratification	18 and older	F	4001	100
Wallner-Schlotfeldt et al. [24]	2000	South Africa	Material handlers	Industry	C; Q	population	23–59	M	126	68
Omokhodion et al. [25]	2002	Nigeria	General population	Community	C; Q	stratification	20–85	F/M	900	100
Mbaye et al. [26]	2002	Senegal	Public transport employees	Industry	R; MR	population	18–55	M	1500	NP
Omokhodion et al. [27]	2003	Nigeria	Civil service workers	Corporate	C; Q	stratification	20–60	F/M	840	66
Igumbor et al. [28]	2003	Zimbabwe	Physiotherapists	Physiotherapy practices	C; Q	population	23–76	F/M	107	72
Omokhodion et al. [29]	2004	Nigeria	General population	Community	C; Q	stratification	20–82	F/M	474	NP
Govender [30]	2004	South Africa	Nurses	Hospital	C; Q	random	20–62	F/M	320	68
Prista et al. [31]	2004	Mozambique	School children	Schools	C; Q	stratification	11–16	F/M	204	85
Fabunmi et al. [32]	2005	Nigeria	Peasant farmers	Farm settlement	C; Q	multi-stage	18 and older	F/M	500	100
Sanya et al. [33]	2005	Nigeria	Industrial workers	Industry	C; Q	population	20–60	F/M	604	53
Bejia et al. [34]	2005	Tunisia	School children	Schools	C; Q	random	11–19	F/M	622	98
Jordaan et al. [35]	2005	South Africa	Adolescents	Schools	C; I	stratified cluster	13–18	F/M	1004	89
Adedoyin et al. [36]	2005	Nigeria	Computer users	University campus	C; Q	convenience	29 ± 2.5	F/M	1041	93
Bejia et al. [37]	2005	Tunisia	Hospital staff	Hospital	C; Q	random	18–60	F/M	350	100
Van Vuuren et al. [38]	2005	South Africa	Steel plant workers	Industry	C; Q	population	31.76 ± 7.80	M	366	96
Van Vuuren et al. [39]	2005	South Africa	Manganese plant workers	Industry	C; Q	convenience	35.2 ± 9.29	M	109	100
Galukande et al. [40]	2005	Uganda	OPD patients	OPD Clinic	C; Q/E	population	19–86	F/M	1033	100
Ayanniyi et al. [41]	2006	Nigeria	Pregnant females	Antenatal clinics	C; I	consecutive	12–45 (26.95 ± 5.37)	F	2187	88
Hill et al. [42]	2007	Ghana	Community women	Hospital	P; I/E	convenience	18 and older	F	1328	NP
Bio et al. [43]	2007	Ghana	Gold miners	Gold mines	C; I/E	simple random	27–53/(40 ± 5.6)	M	280	NP
Balogun and Owoaje [44]	2007	Nigeria	Female traders	Trade market	C; I/E	population	16–80/(37.3 ± 12.8)	F	281	NP
Naidoo and Coopoo [45]	2007	South Africa	Nurses	Public hospitals	C; Q/E	volunteered	37	F	107	NP
Odebiyi et al. [87]	2007	Nigeria	Commercial/private drivers	Industry	C; Q	unclear	30 and older	M	500	100
Adegoke et al. [46]	2008	Nigeria	Physiotherapists	2°and 3° hospitals	C; Q	population	22–57 (33.7 ± 6.8)	F/M	126	58
Akinbo et al. [47]	2008	Nigeria	Commercial drivers/cyclists	Commercial driver garages	C; Q/E	random	37.1 ± 10.5 / 31.13 ± 8.13	M	599	75
Sikiru and Shmaila [48]	2009	Nigeria/Ethiopia	Nurses	Specialized hospitals	C; Q	population	33.69 ± 8.83	F/M	508	82/83

Table 2 General description of included studies (n = 65) (Continued)

Study ID	Year	Country	Population description	Study setting	Design/tool	Sampling method	Age (years)	Gender	n	RR
Booysens et al. [49]	2009	South Africa	Oral hygienists	Dental practices	C; Q	population	20 and older	F/M	362	38
Isa et al. [81]	2009	Nigeria	Commercial motorcyclists	Industry	C; Q	convenience	21–50	F/M	600	NP
Tinubu et al. [50]	2010	Nigeria	Nurses	Private / public hospitals	C; Q	unclear	22–58(36.4 ± 7.75)	F/M	118	80
Ouédraogo et al. [51]	2010	Burkina Faso	Hospital workers	Tertiary hospital	C; Q	consecutive	22–58 (38 ± 8.25)	F/M	436	NP
Sikiru and Hanifa [52]	2010	Nigeria	Nurses	Specialized hospitals	C; Q	volunteered	25–55 (39.20 ± 9.09)	F/M	408	82
Abiodun- Solanke et al. [82]	2010	Nigeria	Dentists/ dental auxiliaries	Dental hospitals	C;Q	cluster random	21–60	F/M	210	77.3
Ayanniyi et al. [53]	2011	Nigeria	Adolescents (school children)	Schools	C; Q	cluster random	10–19 (15.0 ± 1.7)	F/M	3185	72
Saidu et al. [64]	2011	Nigeria	Factory workers	Factories	C; Q	convenience	21–58	F/M	420	84
Himalowa and Frantz [54]	2012	South Africa	Manual construction workers	Construction sites	C; I	population	17–65 (31.9 ± 10.7)	M	212	100
Desai et al. [55]	2012	South Africa	General surgeons	University	C; I	population	33.57 ± 6.48	F/M	76	NP
Noorbhai et al. [56]	2012	South Africa	Adolescent cricket players	Top cricketing schools	C; Q	purposive	14–17 (15.1 ± 1)	M	234	NP
Birabi et al. [57]	2012	Nigeria	Peasant farmers	Farm settlement	C; I	cluster random	18–58(36.71 ± 8.98)	F/M	310	NP
Ogunbode et al. [58]	2013	Nigeria	Adult patients	Family practice clinic	C; I/E	population	18–85 (42.5 ± 15.5)	F/M	485	NP
Oyeyemi et al. [83]	2013	Nigeria	Pregnant females	Teaching Hospital	C;Q	convenience	25.61 ± 5.02	F	310	NP
Akinpelu et al. [59]	2013	Nigeria	Adolescent students	Community	C; Q	unclear	12–17	F/M	900	90
Jimoh et al. [60]	2013	Nigeria	Pregnant females	Antenatal care clinics	C; I	population	29.93 ± 4.80	F	200	NP
Madiba et al. [61]	2013	South Africa	Nurses	Tertiary hospital	C; Q	purposive	29–65	F/M	125	74
Tella et al. [65]	2013	Nigeria	Peasant farmers	Farms	C; Q	convenience	unclear	F/M	604	NP
Rufa'i et al. [66]	2013	Nigeria	Professional drivers	Motor parks	C;Q	convenience	19–64	M	200	86.3
Botha et al. [62]	2014	South Africa	Dentists	Dental practices	C; Q	convenience	45 ± 13	F/M	338	11
El-Soud et al. [63]	2014	Egypt	Nurses	Tertiary hospitals	C; Q	Population	18 and older	F/M	150	100
Chiwaridzo et al. [67]	2014	Zimbabwe	Adolescents	Government schools	C; Q	cluster random	13–19	F/M	544	97.8
Erick and Smith [68]	2014	Botswana	School teachers	Schools	C; Q	cluster random	38.5 ± 8.62	F/M	1747	56.3
Mwaka et al. [69]	2014	Uganda	Pupils	Schools	C; Q	cluster random	Mean 13.6	F/M	532	67.9
Major-Helstoot et al. [70]	2014	South Africa	General population	Communities	C; Q	cluster random	44.8 ± 13.95	F/M	489	97
Akodu et al. [88]	2014	Nigeria	Traffic wardens	Traffic centres	C; Q	unclear	38.22 ± 2.98	F/M	187	82
Triki et al. [84]	2015	Tunisia	Children/adolescents	Sports education institute	R; MR	population	18.5–24.5	F/M	5958	NP
Adegoke et al. [85]	2015	Nigeria	Children/adolescents	School	C; Q	cluster random	10–19	F/M	571	83.97
Vincent-Onabajo et al. [86]	2016	Nigeria	University students	University	C; Q	purposive	20–47	F/M	207	71
Akodu et al. [89]	2016	Nigeria	Filling stations workers	Industry	C; Q	unclear	20–64	F/M	241	95
Odebiyi et al. [90]	2016	Nigeria	Call centre workers	Industry	C; Q	Random	20–49	F/M	120	93.5
Belay et al. [91]	2016	Ethiopia	Nurses	Profession	C; Q	Random	20–60	F	179	91.9

Key: *M* male, *F* female, *SD* standard deviation, *C* cross-sectional, *P* prospective, *R* retrospective, *RR* response rate, *NP* not provided, *I* interview, *E* examination, *Q* questionnaire, *MR* medical records

Table 3 Methodological appraisal of included studies (n = 65)

Criterion study ID	1	2	3	4	5	6	7	8	9	10	%	MA
Mulimba [17]	+	−	−	+	+	+	−	−	−	−	40	No
Bezzaoucha [18]	+	−	+	+	+	+	−	+	−	+	70	Yes
Harris [19]	−	−	+	+	+	+	−	−	+	+	60	No
Schierhout et al. [20]	+	+	+	+	+	+	−	−	−	+	70	Yes
Mijiyawa et al. [21]	−	−	−	+	−	+	−	−	−	+	30	No
Omokhodion et al. [22]	+	−	+	+	+	+	−	−	+	+	70	Yes
Worku [23]	+	−	+	+	−	+	−	−	+	+	60	No
Wallner-Schlotfeldt et al. [24]	−	+	+	+	+	+	−	+	+	+	80	Yes
Omokhodion et al. [25]	+	+	+	+	+	+	−	+	+	+	90	Yes
Mbaye et al. [26]	−	−	+	+	+	+	−	−	+	+	60	No
Omokhodion et al. [27]	+	+	+	+	+	+	−	−	−	+	70	Yes
Igumbor et al. [28]	+	+	+	+	+	+	−	−	+	+	80	Yes
Omokhodion et al. [29]	+	+	+	+	+	+	−	−	+	+	80	Yes
Govender [30]	+	+	+	+	+	+	−	+	+	+	90	Yes
Prista et al. [31]	+	−	+	+	+	+	+	+	+	+	90	Yes
Fabunmi et al. [32]	+	−	−	+	+	+	+	+	+	+	80	Yes
Sanya et al. [33]	+	−	+	+	+	+	−	−	+	+	70	Yes
Bejia et al. [34]	+	+	+	+	+	+	+	+	+	+	100	Yes
Jordaan et al. [35]	+	+	+	+	+	+	+	+	+	+	100	Yes
Adedoyin et al. [36]	−	+	+	−	+	+	−	−	+	+	60	No
Bejia et al. [37]	+	+	+	+	+	+	−	+	+	+	90	Yes
Van Vuuren et al. [38]	−	−	+	+	+	+	−	−	+	+	60	No
Van Vuuren et al. [39]	+	+	+	+	+	+	+	−	+	+	90	Yes
Galukande et al. [40]	−	+	+	+	+	+	−	+	+	+	80	Yes
Ayanniyi et al. [41]	+	+	+	−	+	+	+	+	+	−	80	Yes
Hill et al. [42]	+	+	−	−	+	+	+	−	−	−	50	No
Bio et al. [43]	+	+	−	+	+	+	+	−	+	+	80	Yes
Balogun and Owoaje [44]	+	−	−	−	+	+	+	−	−	−	40	No
Naidoo and Coopoo [45]	−	+	+	+	+	+	+	−	−	−	60	No
Odebiyi et al. [87]	−	−	+	+	+	+	+	−	+	+	70	Yes
Adegoke et al. [46]	+	−	+	−	+	+	+	−	−	+	50	No
Akinbo et al. [47]	+	+	−	−	+	+	+	−	+	+	70	Yes
Sikiru and Shmaila [48]	+	−	+	+	+	+	+	+	+	+	90	Yes
Booysens et al. [49]	+	−	+	−	+	+	−	−	+	−	50	No
Isa et al. [82]	+	−	−	+	−	+	+	+	+	+	70	Yes
Tinubu et al. [50]	−	−	+	−	+	+	+	−	−	+	50	No
Ouédraogo et al. [51]	−	−	−	+	+	+	−	−	−	+	40	No
Sikiru and Hanifa [52]	−	−	−	+	+	+	+	+	+	+	70	Yes
Abiodun-Solanke et al. [83]	+	+	−	−	+	+	−	−	+	+	60	Yes
Ayanniyi et al. [53]	+	−	+	−	+	+	+	−	+	+	70	Yes
Saidu et al. [64]	−	−	+	−	+	+	+	−	+	−	50	No
Himalowa and Frantz [54]	+	+	+	+	+	+	+	−	−	+	80	Yes
Desai et al. [55]	−	−	−	−	+	+	+	−	+	+	50	No
Noorbhai et al. [56]	+	−	−	−	+	+	+	−	+	+	60	No

Table 3 Methodological appraisal of included studies ($n = 65$) *(Continued)*

Criterion study ID	1	2	3	4	5	6	7	8	9	10	%	MA
Birabi et al. [57]	+	−	−	+	+	+	+	+	+	+	80	Yes
Ogunbode et al. [58]	+	−	−	+	+	+	+	−	−	+	60	No
Oyeyemi et al. [84]	−	−	−	−	+	+	+	+	+	+	60	Yes
Akinpelu et al. [59]	−	−	+	+	+	+	+	−	+	+	70	Yes
Jimoh et al. [60]	+	+	−	+	+	+	+	−	+	+	80	Yes
Madiba et al. [61]	+	−	+	−	+	+	+	−	+	+	70	Yes
Tella et al. [65]	−	−	−	+	+	+	+	+	+	+	70	Yes
Rufa'i et al. [66]	−	+	+	+	+	+	+	+	−	+	80	Yes
Botha et al. [62]	+	−	+	−	+	+	+	−	+	+	70	Yes
El-Soud et al. [63]	+	+	+	+	+	+	+	−	+	−	80	Yes
Chiwaridzo et al. [67]	+	+	+	+	+	+	+	+	+	+	100	Yes
Erick and Smith [68]	+	+	+	+	+	+	+	+	+	+	100	Yes
Mwaka et al. [69]	+	−	+	−	+	+	+	+	+	−	70	Yes
Major-Helstoot et al. [70]	+	+	+	+	+	+	+	−	−	+	80	Yes
Akodu et al. [88]	−	−	+	+	+	+	+	−	+	+	70	Yes
Triki et al. [84]	+	−	−	+	+	+	−	+	−	−	50	No
Adegoke et al. [85]	+	−	+	+	+	+	+	+	+	+	90	Yes
Vincent-Onabajo et al. [86]	−	−	+	+	+	+	+	−	+	+	60	Yes
Akodu et al. [89]	−	−	+	+	+	+	+	−	+	+	70	Yes
Odebiyi et al. [90]	+	−	+	−	+	+	+	−	−	+	60	Yes
Belay et al. [91]	+	−	+	+	+	+	+	+	+	+	90	Yes

Key: + criteria fulfilled; − criteria not fulfilled; *MA* Methodologically acceptable

prevalence (38.5%) reported by Hoy et al. [2]. The lifetime prevalence for LBP among Africans (47%; 95% CI 37;58) was also found to be considerably higher than the estimates (38.9%) reported by Hoy et al. [2]. The summary estimates found in this review were compared specifically to North American and Western European countries. It was found that the point LBP prevalence among Africans was substantially higher than estimates provided for Canada (28.7%), Denmark (12–13.7%) and Sweden (23.2%), and was comparable to Germany (39.2) and Belgium (33%) [5]. One year LBP prevalence among Africans was considerably higher than Spain (20%), and on par with Denmark (56%) and Ukraine (50.3%) [5]. The findings of this review therefore reiterates the fact that LBP is a burden and is therefore a public health concern among developing nations in Africa [4, 7, 8]. Despite the high burden, LBP remains a lower priority compared to epidemics such as HIV/AIDS in Africa [3]. African healthcare budgets and systems may be generally ill-prepared to deal with the management of LBP which could partly explain the high LBP prevalence among African populations [4, 9, 10, 71]. The successful development and implementation of strategies and policies to address the burden of LBP in poorer countries or countries with emerging economies, like those in Africa, is therefore warranted [9].

The lifetime, annual and point prevalence of LBP was estimated to be higher among African adults compared to African children and adolescents. This finding confirms that similarly to developed nations, the prevalence of LBP among Africans increases with age [1, 2, 6]. These summary estimates for annual and lifetime LBP prevalence among African children and adolescents were however found to be higher than estimates reported for the United Kingdom (15.6–24%), Finland (9.7%), and Iran (15%), and comparable to Iceland (34%) and Denmark (32.4%) [5], although point prevalence was found to be lower or on par (11%). Of concern is that the early onset of LBP in childhood or adolescents is a risk factor for developing chronic LBP later in life [53, 72], and once the younger generation become the working class, the ongoing pain and related disability will ultimately affect work productivity and the economy of a country [1, 3, 53]. Therefore, in developing countries or countries with emerging economies like African countries, where budgets are already stringent [10], it would make sense to implement effective prevention strategies to the risk of developing LBP in childhood and/or adolescence,

Author(s) and Year	Cases	Sample Size	Lifetime prevalence [95% CI]	Population	Country
Bezzaoucha, 1992	632	6956	0.09 [0.08 , 0.10]	General population	Algiers
Mbaye et al, 2002	236	1500	0.16 [0.14 , 0.18]	Public transport	Senegal
Govender, 2004	102	218	0.47 [0.40 , 0.53]	Nurses	South Africa
Prista et al , 2004	58	204	0.28 [0.22 , 0.35]	School children	Mozambique
Bejia et al , 2005	177	622	0.28 [0.25 , 0.32]	School children	Tunisia
Jordaan et al, 2005	528	1004	0.53 [0.50 , 0.56]	Adolescents	South Africa
Bejia et al , 2005	202	350	0.58 [0.53 , 0.63]	Hospital staff	Tunisia
Van Vuuren et al , 2005	234	366	0.64 [0.59 , 0.69]	Steel plant	South Africa
Van Vuuren et al , 2005	78	109	0.72 [0.63 , 0.80]	Manganese plant	South Africa
Saidu et al, 2011	360	420	0.86 [0.82 , 0.89]	Factory workers	Nigeria
Chiwardizo et al, 2014	228	532	0.43 [0.39 , 0.47]	Adolescents	Nigeria
Major–Helstoot et al , 2014	358	489	0.73 [0.69 , 0.77]	General population	South Africa
Adegoke et al, 2015	331	571	0.58 [0.54 , 0.62]	Children/adolescents	Nigeria
Vincent–Onajabo et al , 2016	94	207	0.45 [0.39 , 0.52]	University students	Nigeria
Odebiyi et al , 2016	120	374	0.32 [0.27 , 0.37]	Call centre workers	Nigeria
Belay et al, 2016	181	395	0.46 [0.41 , 0.51]	Nurses	Ethiopia
RE Model			0.47 [0.37 , 0.58]		

Fig. 2 Summary analysis for lifetime prevalence of LBP among African populations

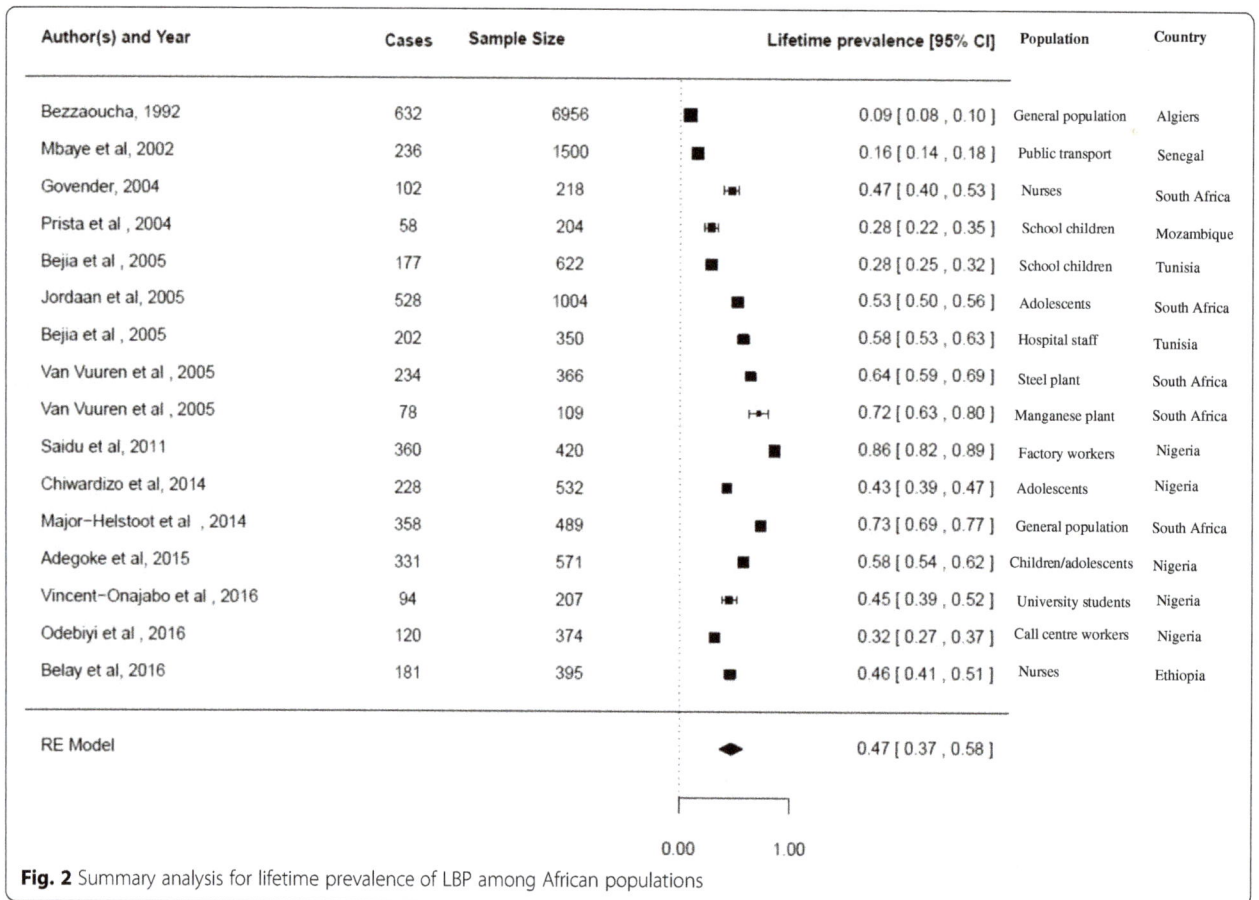

in anticipation of the future economically drain LBP may place on the individual, the industry and the state [53]. Future studies should therefore investigate the factors which lead to the early onset of LBP among African children and adolescents and develop prevention strategies which are effective, feasible and accessible to all people living in rural and urban areas of Africa.

The findings of this review also clearly show a notable difference in point and annual LBP prevalence of close to 20% between African males and females, with males reporting a higher prevalence. These results indicate a reverse gender pattern compared to global trends which generally indicate that females experience a higher prevalence [92]. What is interesting

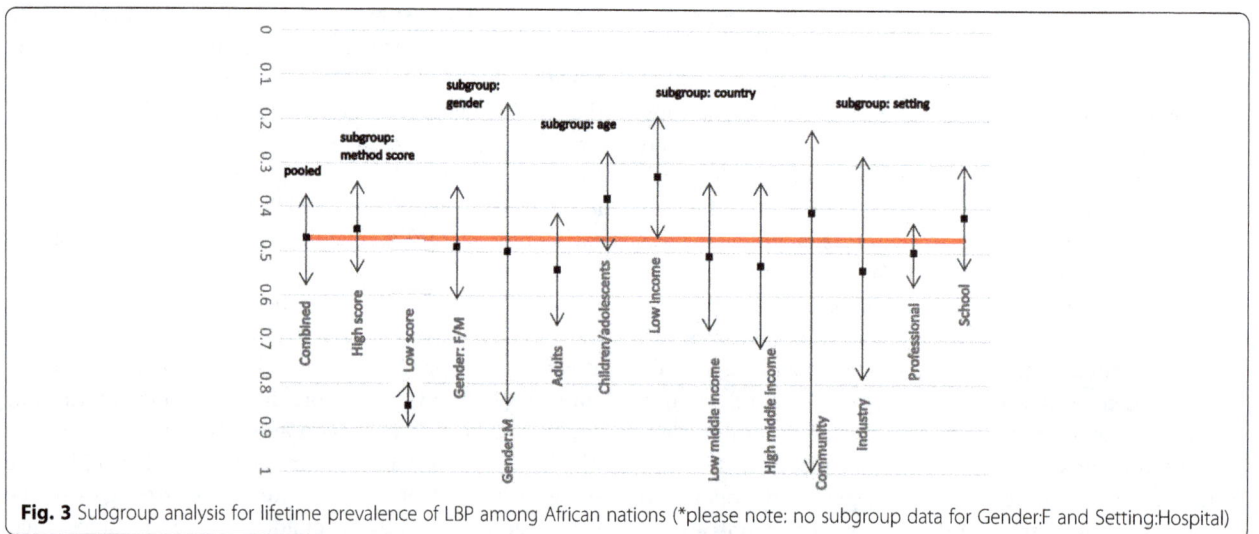

Fig. 3 Subgroup analysis for lifetime prevalence of LBP among African nations (*please note: no subgroup data for Gender:F and Setting:Hospital)

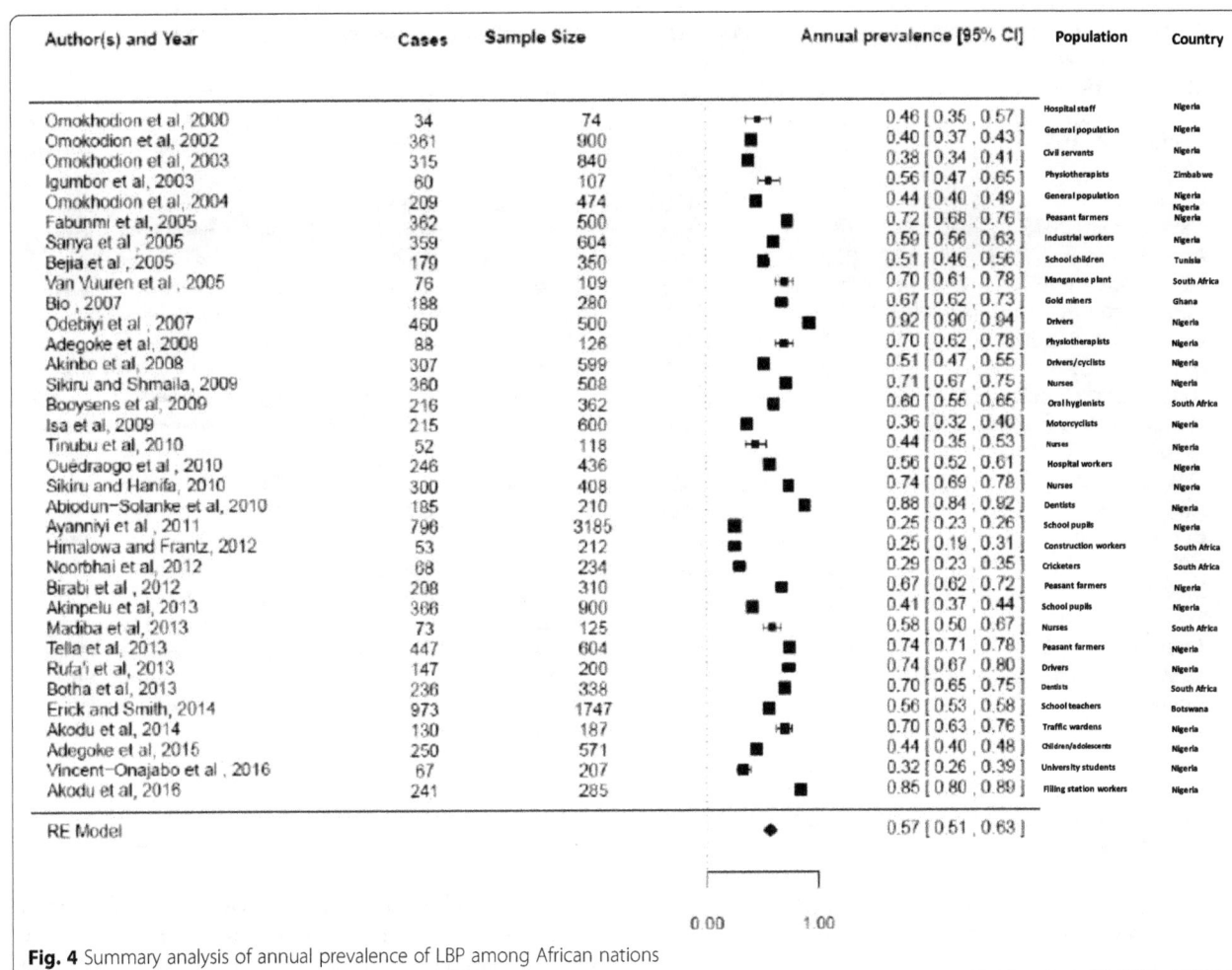

Author(s) and Year	Cases	Sample Size	Annual prevalence [95% CI]	Population	Country
Omokhodion et al, 2000	34	74	0.46 [0.35 , 0.57]	Hospital staff	Nigeria
Omokodion et al, 2002	361	900	0.40 [0.37 , 0.43]	General population	Nigeria
Omokodion et al, 2003	315	840	0.38 [0.34 , 0.41]	Civil servants	Nigeria
Igumbor et al, 2003	60	107	0.56 [0.47 , 0.65]	Physiotherapists	Zimbabwe
Omokhodion et al, 2004	209	474	0.44 [0.40 , 0.49]	General population	Nigeria
Fabunmi et al, 2005	362	500	0.72 [0.68 , 0.76]	Peasant farmers	Nigeria
Sanya et al, 2005	359	604	0.59 [0.56 , 0.63]	Industrial workers	Nigeria
Bejia et al, 2005	179	350	0.51 [0.46 , 0.56]	School children	Tunisia
Van Vuuren et al, 2005	76	109	0.70 [0.61 , 0.78]	Manganese plant	South Africa
Bio, 2007	188	280	0.67 [0.62 , 0.73]	Gold miners	Ghana
Odebiyi et al, 2007	460	500	0.92 [0.90 , 0.94]	Drivers	Nigeria
Adegoke et al, 2008	88	126	0.70 [0.62 , 0.78]	Physiotherapists	Nigeria
Akinbo et al, 2008	307	599	0.51 [0.47 , 0.55]	Drivers/cyclists	Nigeria
Sikiru and Shmaila, 2009	360	508	0.71 [0.67 , 0.75]	Nurses	Nigeria
Booysens et al, 2009	216	362	0.60 [0.55 , 0.65]	Oral hygienists	South Africa
Isa et al, 2009	215	600	0.36 [0.32 , 0.40]	Motorcyclists	Nigeria
Tinubu et al, 2010	52	118	0.44 [0.35 , 0.53]	Nurses	Nigeria
Ouédraogo et al, 2010	246	436	0.56 [0.52 , 0.61]	Hospital workers	Nigeria
Sikiru and Hanifa, 2010	300	408	0.74 [0.69 , 0.78]	Nurses	Nigeria
Abiodun-Solanke et al, 2010	185	210	0.88 [0.84 , 0.92]	Dentists	Nigeria
Ayanniyi et al, 2011	796	3185	0.25 [0.23 , 0.26]	School pupils	Nigeria
Himalowa and Frantz, 2012	53	212	0.25 [0.19 , 0.31]	Construction workers	South Africa
Noorbhai et al, 2012	68	234	0.29 [0.23 , 0.35]	Cricketers	South Africa
Birabi et al, 2012	208	310	0.67 [0.62 , 0.72]	Peasant farmers	Nigeria
Akinpelu et al, 2013	366	900	0.41 [0.37 , 0.44]	School pupils	Nigeria
Madiba et al, 2013	73	125	0.58 [0.50 , 0.67]	Nurses	South Africa
Tella et al, 2013	447	604	0.74 [0.71 , 0.78]	Peasant farmers	Nigeria
Rufa'i et al, 2013	147	200	0.74 [0.67 , 0.80]	Drivers	Nigeria
Botha et al, 2013	236	338	0.70 [0.65 , 0.75]	Dentists	South Africa
Erick and Smith, 2014	973	1747	0.56 [0.53 , 0.58]	School teachers	Botswana
Akodu et al, 2014	130	187	0.70 [0.63 , 0.76]	Traffic wardens	Nigeria
Adegoke et al, 2015	250	571	0.44 [0.40 , 0.48]	Children/adolescents	Nigeria
Vincent-Onajabo et al, 2016	67	207	0.32 [0.26 , 0.39]	University students	Nigeria
Akodu et al, 2016	241	285	0.85 [0.80 , 0.89]	Filling station workers	Nigeria
RE Model			0.57 [0.51 , 0.63]		

0.00   1.00

Fig. 4 Summary analysis of annual prevalence of LBP among African nations

about this finding is that within most African cultures, African males actually tend to under-report health issues as it is perceived to reduce their masculinity [93]. A higher prevalence for African females would therefore have been expected. However, this said, these findings may also be linked to the fact that half of the studies on industry included mostly males or males only, whereas the workers included in the professional subgroup included more females. Since industry-related jobs include more intense physical labour, an over-representation of males may have therefore resulted.

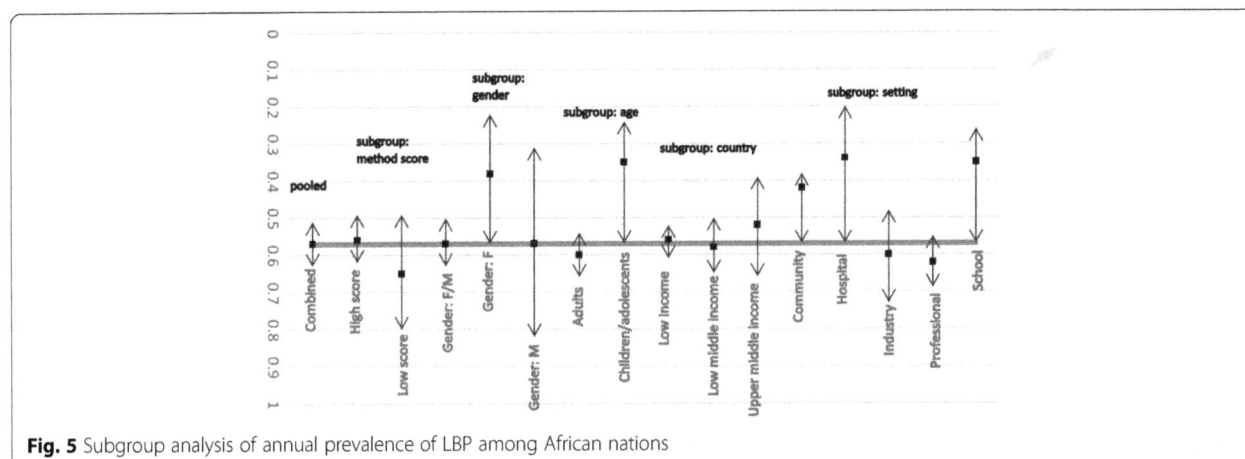

Fig. 5 Subgroup analysis of annual prevalence of LBP among African nations

Author(s) and Year	Cases	Sample Size		Point prevalence [95% CI]	Population	Country
Mulimba, 1990	227	2201		0.10 [0.09 , 0.12]	Private patients	Nairobi
Harris, 1993	68	110		0.62 [0.53 , 0.71]	Cricketers	South Africa
Schierhout, 1993	40	155		0.26 [0.19 , 0.33]	Factory workers	South Africa
Mijiyawa, 2000	3204	9065		0.35 [0.34 , 0.36]	OPD patients	Togo
Worku, 2000	2340	4001		0.58 [0.57 , 0.60]	Mothers	Lesotho
Sanya et al , 2005	361	604		0.60 [0.56 , 0.64]	Industrial workers	Nigeria
Adedoyin et al , 2005	770	1041		0.74 [0.71 , 0.77]	Computer users	Nigeria
Galukande et al, 2005	204	1033		0.20 [0.17 , 0.22]	OPD patients	Uganda
Van Vuuren et al , 2005	41	109		0.38 [0.29 , 0.47]	Industrial workers	South Africa
Ayanniyi et al, 2006	763	2187		0.35 [0.33 , 0.37]	Pregnant females	South Africa
Hill et al , 2007	258	1328		0.19 [0.17 , 0.22]	Community women	Ghana
Naidoo and Coopoo, 2007	43	107		0.40 [0.31 , 0.49]	Nurses	South Africa
Himalowa and Frantz, 2012	146	212		0.69 [0.63 , 0.75]	Construction workers	South Africa
Desai et al, 2012	46	76		0.61 [0.50 , 0.72]	General surgeons	South Africa
Ogunbode et al , 2013	227	485		0.47 [0.42 , 0.51]	Adult patients	Nigeria
Akinpelu et al, 2013	116	900		0.13 [0.11 , 0.15]	Adolescent students	Nigeria
El-Soud et al, 2014	119	150		0.79 [0.73 , 0.86]	Nurses	Nigeria
Chiwardizo et al, 2014	49	532		0.09 [0.07 , 0.12]	Adolescents	Zimbabwe
Mwaka et al, 2014	201	532		0.38 [0.34 , 0.42]	Pupils	Uganda
Triki et al , 2015	882	5958		0.15 [0.14 , 0.16]	Children/adolescents	Tunisia
Adegoke et al, 2015	146	571		0.26 [0.22 , 0.29]	Children/adolescents	Nigeria
Vincent-Onajabo et al , 2016	24	207		0.12 [0.07 , 0.16]	Call centre workers	Nigeria
Belay et al, 2016	179	395		0.45 [0.40 , 0.50]	Nurses	Egypt
RE Model				0.39 [0.30 , 0.47]		

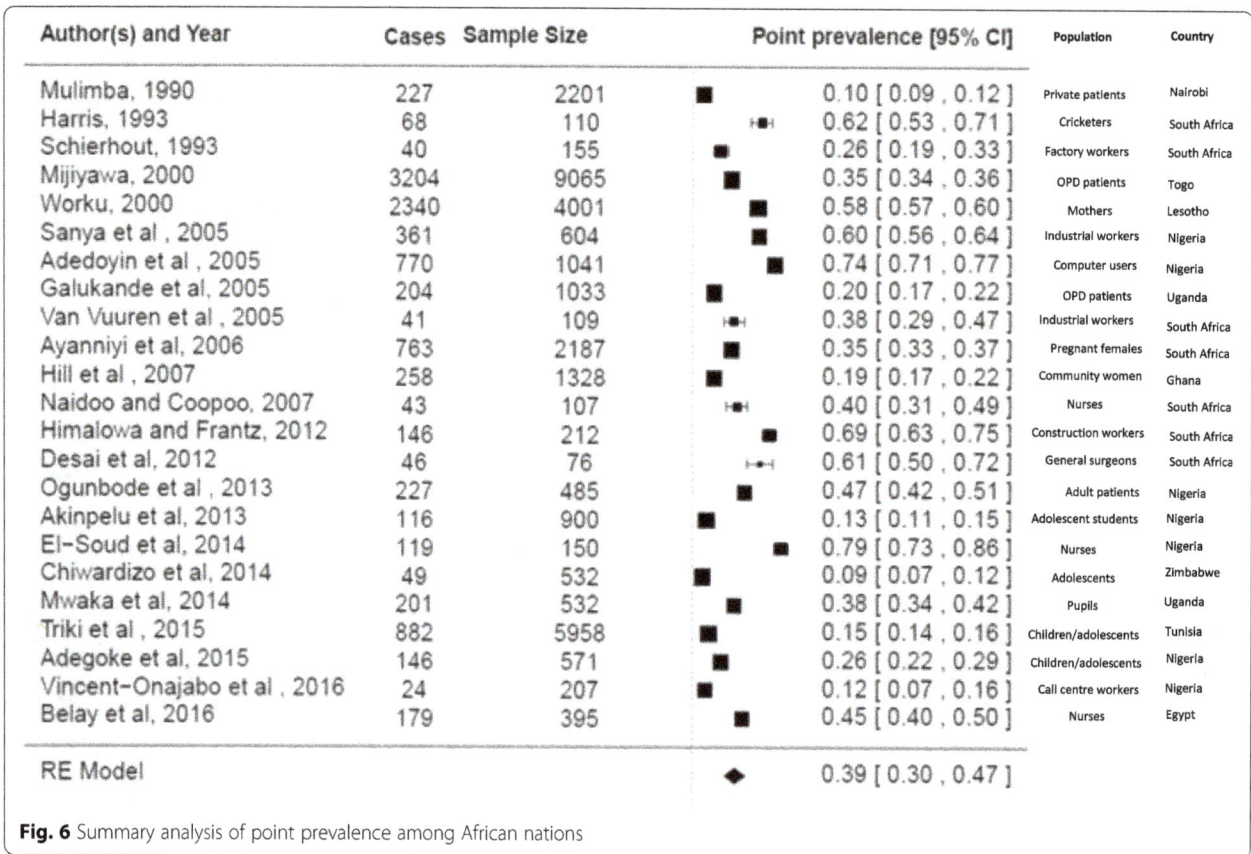

Fig. 6 Summary analysis of point prevalence among African nations

Epidemiologic and methodological challenges in conducting LBP prevalence reviews among African populations

The review process highlighted a number of challenges related to conducting, sourcing and pooling relevant epidemiologic data in Africa. One of the first methodological challenges when conducting such a review, was the uncertainty of whether all relevant data were included in the review. This is because a number of African research studies may not have been published in journals which are indexed in accessible and commonly-used international databases [73, 74]. Many African LBP studies are published in local journals or as a postgraduate thesis, and not all African universities may have information technology systems which allow online access to their postgraduate theses [74]. Data may therefore only be available in the local university libraries. Furthermore, African LBP researchers may not have the

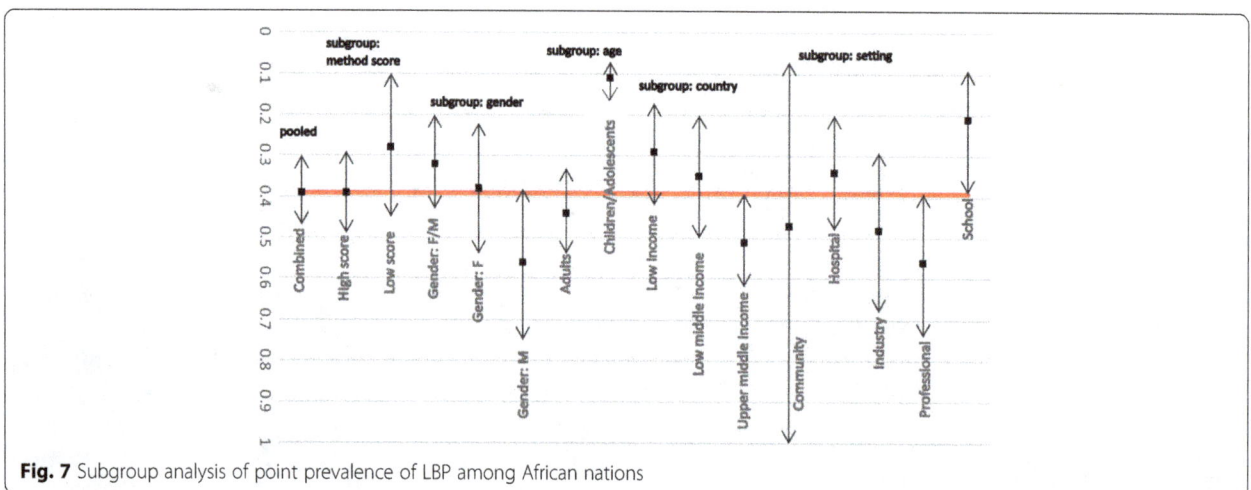

Fig. 7 Subgroup analysis of point prevalence of LBP among African nations

opportunity to publish in open access journals due to the associated high publication costs [73–75], which leads to difficulty in publishing, as well as accessing and retrieving such publications. The inclusion of all relevant African literature on LBP prevalence can therefore not be guaranteed.

Another challenge in conducting this review is the fact that Africa is riddled by huge economic inequality between countries. We found that most studies were conducted in Nigeria and South Africa, which have the strongest economies in Africa and are currently ranked first and third, respectively in terms of Gross Domestic Product [75]. In these relatively more affluent countries, factors such as economic growth and urbanisation have already followed patterns noted in the developed world and this could have an effect on LBP occurrence and reporting [75]. While research fields such as HIV/AIDS and TB in Africa are well funded by international bodies, this is not the case with LBP research [3]. LBP research in poorer African countries is consequently not possible or encouraged due to prioritisation of research funding towards other pressing health issues. The economic inequality between African countries could therefore have biased our review findings to more affluent countries.

The poor methodological quality of included studies posed another challenge in conducting this review since just over 60% of the studies could be used in the analyses. Of concern was that most of the shortcomings in the methods reported by the poor quality studies could have been avoided. Similarly, to the previous review [10], and other reviews [2], the poor quality studies in this review generally did not provide a definition of LBP, lacked adequate representation of the population, did not provide response rates or drop-out rates, and neglected to use reliable and/valid instruments (be it a questionnaire, interview, or examination) for collection of data. According to Dionne et al., it is highly recommended that epidemiologic studies should at least provide the case definition used in establishing the prevalence of LBP in a specified population [76]. In addition, this case definition for LBP should be standardized to ensure that greater comparisons between countries (developed or developing) can be made [76, 77], for a greater understanding of LBP to be gained [2]. The validity and reliability of instruments should also be established prior to their administration in a specific population to ensure accurate estimates of prevalence [78]. One important area to address is the development of a valid and reliable LBP measurement instrument which should ideally take context and culture into account. Furthermore, improved collaboration between researchers in different African countries, will facilitate standardization of measuring LBP among Africans to assist with comparisons across countries as well as meta-analytical approaches. It is

therefore recommended that future studies prioritize conducting studies with improved methodological quality, provide and use a standardized case definition of LBP, and report essential information, which will lead to accurate assessment, interpretation, translation and comparison of results across studies [79].

Lastly, although measures were taken to ensure that the heterogeneity among studies was considered during meta-analyses, the summary estimates provided in this review should still be viewed with caution [2]. Heterogeneity in observational studies is however expected [76, 77, 79], since populations, and even cultural groups within a specific population, inherently differ [94]. More specifically, heterogeneity of LBP data remains considerable across studies due to the lack of a standardized or universal case definition for LBP [76, 77]. For this reason, the pooling and comparison of LBP data based on different definitions is a challenge on its own, regardless of population and other study characteristic variability [77].

Conclusion

Since the original review was published in 2007, a number of epidemiologic studies into the prevalence of LBP in Africa have emerged. This review found that the lifetime, annual and point prevalence of LBP among African nations, was higher than the global LBP prevalence reported. Prevention strategies addressing the early onset of LBP among the youth would most likely be the answer to addressing the burden of LBP on future economies in Africa. Caution must however be taken when interpreting the summary estimates provided in this current review, since high heterogeneity, which is expected, was displayed among the included studies. Furthermore, due to the poor methodological quality found among many of the included studies, the over-representation of more affluent African countries and the difficulty in sourcing and retrieving potential African studies, it is recommended that future African LBP researchers conduct methodologically robust studies and report their findings in accessible resources.

Abbreviations

CI: Confidence interval; GBD: Global burden of disease; LBP: Low back pain; LMICs: Lower and middle income countries; WHO: World Health Organization; YLDs: Years lived with disability

Acknowledgements

The authors would like to acknowledge the staff at the Stellenbosch University Medical and Health Sciences Library for their assistance in retrieving the articles; Prof. Karen Grimmer for assistance in the conceptualization of the idea for the initial review published in 2007 [10], as well as Dr. Faheema Kimmie-Dhansay for assistance in part of the analyses.

Authors' contributions

LM: Conceptualization of review update idea and developed the protocol, conducted the update of the search, conducted appraisal of studies, extracted the data, assisted with analyses of the data, wrote the manuscript.

QL: conceptualization of main review idea, supervised the process, assisted with analyses of the data, contributed to writing the manuscript.
KD: independently conducted search, appraisal and extraction of data, assisted with analyses of data, contributed to the writing of the manuscript.
BG: conducted the analyses, produced the graphics and contributed to the interpretation and writing of the statistical sections of this manuscript. All authors read and approved the final manuscript.

Competing interests
The authors declare that they have no competing interest.

Author details
[1]Division of Physiotherapy, Department of Health and Rehabilitation Sciences, Faculty of Medicine and Health Sciences, Stellenbosch University, PO BOX 241, Cape Town 8000, South Africa. [2]Division of Epidemiology and Biostatistics, Faculty of Medicine and Health Sciences, Stellenbosch University, Tygerberg, South Africa. [3]Department of Statistics, University of Calcutta, Kolkata, India.

References
1.   Manchikanti L. Epidemiology of low back pain. Pain Physician. 2000;3(2):167–92.
2.   Hoy D, Bain C, Williams G, March L, Brooks P, Blyth F, et al. A systematic review of the global prevalence of low back pain. Arthritis Rheum. 2012;64(6):2028–37.
3.   Froud R, Patterson S, Eldridge S, Seale C, Pincus T, Rajendran D, et al. A systematic review and meta-synthesis of the impact of low back pain on people's lives. BMC Musculoskelet Disord. 2014;15:50.
4.   Hoy D, Smith E, Cross M, Sanchez-Riera L, Buchbinder R, Blyth F, et al. The global burden of musculoskeletal conditions for 2010: estimates from the global burden of disease 2010 study. Ann Rheum Dis. 2014;73:968–74.
5.   Hoy D, Brooks P, Blyth F, Buchbinder R. The epidemiology of low back pain. Best Pract Res Clin Rheumatol. 2010;24(6):769–81.
6.   Majid K, Truumees E. Epidemiology and natural history of low back pain. Semin Spine Surg. 2008;20:87–92.
7.   Woolf AD, Erwin J, March L. The need to address the burden of musculoskeletal conditions. Best Pract Res Clin Rheumatol. 2012;26(2):183–224.
8.   March L. The global burden of musculoskeletal conditions – why is it important? Best Pract Res Clin Rheumatol. 2011;24(6):721.
9.   Woolf AD, Kristina A. Prevention of musculoskeletal conditions in the developing world. Best Pract Res Clin Rheumatol. 2008;22(4):759–72.
10. Louw QA, Morris LD, Grimmer-Somers K. The prevalence of low back pain in Africa: a systematic review. BMC Musculoskel Disord. 2007;8:105.
11. Hoy D, March L, Brooks P, Woolf A, Blyth F, Vos T, et al. Measuring the global burden of low back pain. Best Pract Res Clin Rheumatol. 2010;24(2): 155–65.
12. Guidelines for reporting of Meta-analysis Of Observational Studies in Epidemiology. https://www.elsevier.com/__data/promis_misc/ISSM_MOOSE_Checklist.pdf. Accessed 11 May 2018.
13. Prospero website. Available: http://www.crd.york.ac.uk/PROSPERO/display_record.php?ID=CRD42014010417. Accessed May 2018.
14. Ondari-Okemwa E. Scholarly publishing in sub-Saharan Africa in the twenty-first century: challenges and opportunities. First Monday. 2007;12:10.
15. Walker B. The prevalence of low back pain: a systematic review of the literature from 1966 to 1998. J Spinal Dis. 2000;13(3):205–17.
16. Microsoft Excel. Microsoft 2010 software. Microsoft Corporation Redmond, Washington.
17. Mulimba J. The problems of low back pain in Africa. East Afr Med J. 1990;67(4):250–3.
18. Bezzaoucha A. Descriptive epidemiology of low-back pain in Algiers. Rev Rhum Mal Ostéoartic. 1992;59(2):121–4.
19. Harris I. Prevalence of low back pain in cricketers-an undergraduate epidemiological study. Physiotherapy. 1993;49:65–6.
20. Schierhout G, Myers J, Bridger R. Musculoskeletal pain and workplace ergonomic stressors in manufacturing industry in South Africa. Int J Ind Ergon. 1993;12:3–11.
21. Mijiyawa M, Oniankitan O, Kolani B, Koriko T. Low back pain in hospital outpatients in Lome(Togo). Joint Bone Spine. 2000;67:533–8.
22. Omokhodion F, Umar U, Ogunnowo B. Prevalence of low back pain among staff in a rural hospital in Nigeria. Occup Med. 2000;50:107–10.
23. Worku Z. Prevalence of low back pain in Lesotho mothers. JMPT. 2000;23:147–54.
24. Wallner-Schlotfeldt PJ, Stewart A. The predisposing factors to low back pain in workers. SAJP. 2000;56:33–8.
25. Omokodion F. Low back pain in a rural community in south West Nigeria. West Afr J Med. 2002;2:87–90.
26. Mbaye I, Fall M, Wone I, Dione P, Ouattara B, Sow M. Chronic low back pain in a Senegalese pubic transport's company. Dakar Med. 2002;47(2):176–8.
27. Omokodion F, Sanya A. Risk factors for low back pain among office workers in Ibadan, Southwest Nigeria Short report. Occ Med. 2003;53:287–9.
28. Igumbor E, Useh U, Madzivire D. An epidemiological study of work-related low back pain among physiotherapists in Zimbabwe. SAJP. 2003;59:7–14.
29. Omokodion F. Low back pain in an urban population in Southwest Nigeria. Trop Dr. 2004;34:17–20.
30. Govender S. Low back pain in the nursing profession-a pilot study. SAOJ. 2004:7–13.
31. Prista A, Balague F, Nordin M, Skovron M. Low back pain in Mozambican adolescents. Eur Spine J. 2004;13:341–5.
32. Fabunmi A, ABa S, Odunaiya N. Prevalence of low back pain among peasant farmers in a rural community in south-West Nigeria. Afr J Med Med Sci. 2005;34(3):259–162.
33. Sanya A, Ogwumike O. Low back pain prevalence amongst industrial workers in the private sector in Oyo state, Nigeria. Afr J Med Med Sci. 2005;34:245–9.
34. Bejia I, Abid N, Salem K, Letaief M, Younes M, Touzi M, et al. Low back pain in a cohort of 622 Tunisian schoolchildren and adolescents: an epidemiological study. Eur Spine J. 2005;14:331–336 (a).
35. Jordaan R, Kruger M, Stewart A, Becker P. The association between low back pain, gender and age in adolescents. SAJP. 2005;61:15–20.
36. Adedoyin R, Idowu B, Adagunodo R, Ooyomi A, Idowu P. Musculoskeletal pain associated with the use of computer systems in Nigeria. Technol Health Care. 2005;13:125–30.
37. Bejia I, Younes M, Jamila H, Khalfallah T, Salem K, Touzi M, et al. Prevalence and factors associated with low back pain among hospital staff. Joint Bone Spine. 2005;72:254–259 (b).
38. Van Vuuren B, Becker P, Van Heerden H, Zinzen E, Meeusen R. Lower back problems and occupational risk factors in a south African steel industry. Am J Ind Med. 2005;47:45–457.
39. Van Vuuren B, Zinzen E, Van Heerden H, Becker P, Meeusen R. Psychosocial factors related to lower back problems in a south African manganese industry. J Occup Rehabil. 2005;15:215–25.
40. Galukande M, Muwazi S, Mugisa D. Aetiology of low back pain in Mulago hospital, Uganda. Afr Health Sci. 2005;5:164–7.
41. Ayanniyi O, Sanya A, Ogunlade S, Oni-Orisan M. Prevalence and pattern of back pain among pregnant women attending ante-natal clinics in selected health care facilities. Afr J Biomed Res. 2006;9:149–56.
42. Hill A, Darko R, Seffah J, Adanu R, Anarfi J, Duda R. Health of urban Ghanaian women as identified by the Women's health study of Accra. Int J Gynaecol Obstet. 2007;99:150–6.
43. Bio F, Sadhra S, Jackson C, Burge P. Low back pain in underground gold miners in Ghana. Ghana Med J. 2007;41(1):21–5.
44. Balogun M, Owoaje E. Work conditions and health problems of female traders in Ibadan Nigeria. Afr J Med Med Sci. 2007;36(1):57–63.
45. Naidoo R, Coopoo Y. The health and fitness profiles of nurses in KwaZulu-Natal. Curationis. 2007;30(2):66–73.
46. Adegoke B, Akodu A, Oyeyemi A. Work-related musculoskeletal disorders among Nigerian physiotherapists. BMC Musculoskel Disord. 2008;9:112.
47. Akinbo S, Odebiyi D, Osasan A. Characteristics of back pain among commercial drivers and motorcyclists in Lagos, Nigeria. West Afr J Med. 2008;27(2):85–9.
48. Sikiru L, Shmaila H. Prevalence and risk factors of low back pain among nurses in Africa: Nigerian and Ethiopian specialized hospitals survey study. East Afr J Pub Health. 2009;6(1):22–6.
49. Booyens S, van Wyk P, Postma T. Musculoskeletal disorders amongst practising south African oral hygienists. SADJ. 2009;64(9):400–3.

50. Tinubu B, Mbada C, Oyeyemi A, Fabunmi A. Work-related musculoskeletal disorders among nurses in Ibadan, south-West Nigeria: a cross-sectional survey. BMC Musculoskel Disord. 2010;11:12.

51. Ouédraogo D, Ouédraogo V, Ouedraogo L, Kinda M, Tiéno H, Zoungrana E, et al. Prevalence and risk factors associated with low back pain among hospital staff in Ouagadougou (Burkina Faso). Med Trop. 2010;70:277–80.

52. Sikiru L, Hanifa S. Prevalence and risk factors of low back pain among nurses in a typical Nigerian hospital. Afr Health Sci. 2010;10(1):26–30.

53. Ayanniyi O, Mbada C, Muolokwu C. Prevalence and profile of back pain in Nigerian adolescents. Med Princ Pract. 2011;20:368–73.

54. Himalowa S, Frantz J. The effect of occupationally-related low back pain on functional activities among male manual workers in a construction company in cape town, South Africa. Occup Healt SA. 2012;18(5):28–32.

55. Desai F, Ellapen T, van Heerden H. The point prevalence of work-related musculoskeletal pain among general surgeons in KwaZulu-Natal, South Africa. Ergonomics SA. 2012;24(2):18–30.

56. Noorbhai M, Essack F, Thwala S, Ellapen T, van Heerden J. Prevalence of cricket-related musculoskeletal pain among adolescent cricketers in KwaZulu-Natal. SAJSM. 2012;24(1):3–9.

57. Birabi B, Dienye P, Ndukwu G. Prevalence of low back pain among peasant farmers in a rural community in south South Nigeria. Rural Remote Health. 2012;12:1920.

58. Ogunbode A, Adebusoye L, Alonge T, Ogunbode A. Prevalence of low back pain and associated risk factors amongst adult patients presenting to a Nigerian family practice clinic, a hospital-based study. Afr J Prim Health Care. 2012;5(1):1–8.

59. Akinpelu A, Oyewole O, Hammed G, Gbiri C. Prevalence of low back pain among adolescent students in a Nigerian Urban Community. AJPARS. 2013;5(1&2):29–34.

60. Jimoh A, Omokanye L, Salaudeen A, Saidu R, Saka M, Akinwale A. Prevalence of low back pain among pregnant women in Ilorin, Nigeria. Med Pract Rev. 2013;4(4):23–6.

61. Madiba S, Hoque M, Rakgase R. Musculoskeletal disorders among nurses in high acuity areas in a tertiary hospital in South Africa. Occup Healt SA. 2013;19(1):20–3.

62. Botha P, Chikte U, Barrie R, Esterhuizen T. Self-reported musculoskeletal pain among dentists in South Africa: a 12-month prevalence study. SADJ. 2014;69(5):208–13.

63. El-Soud A, El-Najjar A, EL-Fattah N and Hassan A. Prevalence of low back pain in working nurses in Zagazig University hospitals: and epidemiological study. Egyptian Rheumatology and Rehabilitation. 2014;41:109–15.

64. Sa'idu I, Utti V, Jaiyesimi A, Rufa'i A, Maduagwu S, Onuwe H, et al. Prevalence of musculoskeletal injuries among factory workers in Kano metropolis, Nigeria. Int J Occup Saf Ergon. 2011;17:99–102.

65. Tella B, Akinbo S, Asafa S, Gbiri C. Prevalence and impacts of low back pain among peasant farmers in south-West Nigeria. Int J Occup Med Environ Health. 2013;26:621–7.

66. Rufa'i A, Sa'idu I, Ahmad R, Elmi O, Aliyu S, Jarere A, et al. Prevalence and risk factors for low back pain among professional drivers in Kano. Nigeria: Archives of Environmental and Occupational Health; 2013. [Epub ahead of print].

67. Chiwaridzo M, Naidoo N. Prevalence and associated characteristics of recurrent non-specific low back pain in Zimbabwean adolescents: a cross-sectional study. BMC Musculoskelet Disord. 2014;15:381.

68. Erick P, Smith D. Low back pain among school teachers in Botswana, prevalence and risk factors. BMC Musculoskelet Disord. 2014;15:359.

69. Mwaka E, Munabi I, Buwembo W, Kukkiriza J, Ochieng J. Musculoskeletal pain and school bag use: a cross-sectional study among Ugandan pupils. BMC Research Notes. 2014;7:222.

70. Major-Helstoot M, Crous L, Grimmer-Somers K, Louw Q. Management of LBP at primary care level in South Africa: up to standards? Afr Health Sci. 2014;14:698–706.

71. Mousavi S, Akbari M, Mehdian H, Mobini B, Montazeri A, Akbarnia B, et al. Low back pain in Iran: a growing need to adapt and implement evidence-based practice in developing countries. Spine (Phila Pa 1976). 2011;36(10):E638–46.

72. Calvo-Muñoz I, Gómez-Conesa A, Sánchez-Meca J. Prevalence of low back pain in children and adolescents: a meta-analysis. BMC Pediatr. 2013;13:14.

73. Sawyerr A. African universities and the challenge of research capacity development. JHEA/RESA. 2004;2:211–40.

74. Ngobeni S. Scholarly publishing: the challenges facing the African university press. ASC working paper 100 2012.

75. Mutula S. Challenges of doing research in sub-Saharan African universities: digital scholarship opportunities. Inkanyiso: Journal of Humanities and Social Sciences. 2009;1:1.

76. Dionne C, Dunn K, Croft P, Nachemson A, Buchbinder R, Walker B, et al. A consensus approach toward the standardization of back pain definitions for use in prevalence studies. Spine (Phila Pa 1976). 2008;33:95–103.

77. Videman T, Batti MC. Commentary: back pain epidemiology — the challenge of case definition and developing new ideas. Spine. 2012;12:71–2.

78. Stroup D, Berlin J, Morton S, Olkin I, Williamson G, Rennie D, et al. Meta-analysis of observational studies in epidemiology: a proposal for reporting. JAMA. 2000;283(15):2008–12.

79. Beaton D, Bombardier C, Guillemin F, Ferraz M. Guidelines for the process of cross-cultural adaptation of self-report measures. Spine. 2000;25:3186–91.

80. Duval S, Tweedie R. Trim and fill: a simple funnel-plot-based method of testing and adjusting for publication bias in meta-analysis. Biometrics. 2000;56(2):455–63.

81. Isa U, Saminu A, Rufai Y. Prevalence of low back pain complaints among commercial motorcyclists in Kano, Northwest Nigeria. Nigerian Medical Practitioner. 2009;56:19–23.

82. Abiodun-Solanke I, Agbaje J, Ajayi D, Arotiba J. Prevalence of neck and back pain among dentists and dental auxillaries in south western Nigeria. Afr J Med Med Sci. 2010;39:137–42.

83. Oyeyemi A, Rafa'I A, Lawan A. Low back pain incidence, anthropometric characteristics and activities of daily living in pregnant women in a teaching hospital center antenatal clinic. Trop J Obstet Gynaecol. 2013;30:29–37.

84. Triki M, Koubaa A, Masmoudi L, Fellman N, Tabka Z. Prevalence and risk factors of low back pain among undergraduate students of a sports and physical education institute in Tunisia. Libyan J Med. 2015;10:26802.

85. Adegoke B, Odole A, Adeyinka A. Adolescent low back pain among secondary school students in Ibadan, Nigeria. Afr Health Sci. 2015;15:429–37.

86. Vincent-Onabajo G, Nweze E, Kachalla G, Ali M, Usman A, Alhaji M, Umeonwuka C. Prevalence of Low Back Pain among Undergraduate Physiotherapy Students in Nigeria. Pain Res Treat. 2016;123038:4.

87. Odebiyi D, Ogwezi D, Adegoke B. The prevalence of low back pain in commercial motor drivers and private automobile drivers. Nig J Med Rehabil. 2007;21(1 & 2):21-4.

88. Akodu A, Taiwo A, Jimoh O. Prevalence of low back pain among traffic wardens in Lagos state. Nigeria AJPARS. 2014;6(1 & 2):37–41.

89. Akodu A, Okafor U, Adebayo A. Prevalence of low back pain among filling stations attendants in Lagos, Southwest Nigeria Afr J Biomed Res. 2016;19: 109–15.

90. Odebiyi D, Akanle O, Akinbo S, Balogun S. Prevalence and impact of work-related musculoskeletal disorders on job performance of call center operators in Nigeria. Int J Occup Environ Med. 2016;7:98–106.

91. Belay M, Worku A, Gebrie S, Wamisho B. Epidemiology of Low Back Pain among Nurses Working in Public Hospitals of Addis Ababa, Ethiopia East & Central African Journal of Surgery. 2016;21(1):113-31.

92. Wáng Y, Wáng J, Káplár X. Increased low back pain prevalence in females than in males after menopause age: evidences based on synthetic literature review. Quantitative Imaging in Medicine and Surgery. 2016;692:199–206.

93. Thorpe R, Wilson-frederick S, Whitfield K. Health behaviors and all-cause mortality in African-American men. Am J Mens Health. 2013;7(40):8S–18S.

94. Le Gal M, Mainguy Y, Le Lay K, Nadjar A, Allain D, Galissié M. Linguistic validation of six patient-reported outcomes instruments into 12 languages for patients with fibromyalgia. Joint Bone Spine. 2010;77:165–70.

5

A multimedia campaign to improve back beliefs in patients with non-specific low back pain: a process evaluation

Arnela Suman[1] [iD], Frederieke G. Schaafsma[1,2]*, Jiman Bamarni[3], Maurits W. van Tulder[4] and Johannes R. Anema[1,2]

Abstract

Background: Low back pain (LBP) is one of the most prevalent and costly disorders worldwide. To reduce its burden in the Netherlands, implementation of a multidisciplinary guideline for LBP was supported by a multifaceted eHealth campaign for patients with LBP. The current study aims 1) to evaluate whether the implementation strategy was performed as planned; 2) to assess the feasibility, barriers and facilitators of the patient based eHealth campaign; 3) to gain insight into the satisfaction and experiences of patients with various ethnic backgrounds with the implementation strategy and to make a comparison between them; and 4) to explore the association between exposure to and satisfaction with the implementation strategy.

Methods: This process evaluation was performed using the Linnan and Steckler framework, and used a mixed methods approach for data collection and analysis. The relationship between satisfaction of patients and exposure to the strategy was statistically examined. Semi-structured interviews were analysed using qualitative data analysis methods.

Results: Two hundred and fourteen patients participated in the quantitative, and 44 in the qualitative analysis. Most were female and had a high level of education. Many patients did not use the campaign at all or only once, and those that did rated it as reasonable. Patient satisfaction with the campaign increased significantly with an increase in its use. Qualitative analysis showed that four main themes played a role in campaign rating and use: satisfaction with intervention components, perceived benefits of the intervention, usage of the intervention, and satisfaction with the medium used.

Conclusion: This process evaluation showed that the eHealth campaign was used only by a small proportion of patients with non-specific LBP. It seemed that the campaign was offered to the patients too late, that the lay-out of the campaign did not meet patient needs, and that healthcare providers rarely discussed the campaign with their patients, while involvement of those providers seemed to improve trustworthiness of the campaign and increase its usage. It is important to invest effort into healthcare providers to motivate patients to use eHealth intervention and to tailor strategies better to the needs of users.

Keywords: Implementation, Guidelines as topic, Process Assessment (Health Care), Multimedia, eHealth, Low back pain, Attitude to Health, Patient Satisfaction

* Correspondence: f.schaafsma@vumc.nl
[1]Amsterdam Public Health research institute, Department of Public and Occupational Health, VU University Medical Centre, PO Box 70571007 MB Amsterdam, The Netherlands
[2]Department of Public and Occupational Health, Research Centre for Insurance Medicine, Collaboration between AMC-UMCG-UWV-VUmc, VU University medical centre, PO Box 70671007 MB Amsterdam, The Netherlands
Full list of author information is available at the end of the article

Background

Low back pain (LBP) is the leading cause of disability worldwide [1], and one of the most common conditions for which people in industrialised countries seek medical care [2]. While LBP represents an important economic burden on societies [3], in 85 to 95% of patients with LBP the pain cannot be attributed to a specific cause and is thus referred to as non-specific [4, 5]. Psychosocial risk factors, including stress, anxiety, depression, and pain coping strategies have been shown to play a substantial role in the aetiology and prognosis of non-specific LBP [4, 5]. A biopsychosocial approach for the treatment of LBP has been increasingly adopted [6]. This approach often exists of multidisciplinary programmes that encompass a combination of physical, psychological, educational, and work-related components for treatment [6]. A recent Cochrane review has shown that this approach to LBP rehabilitation is more effective than usual care and physical treatment in decreasing pain and disability, and improving work outcomes [6]. However, despite the widespread efforts to reduce the burden of LBP, it remains a highly prevalent and costly disorder.

In an attempt to reduce the burden of LBP in the Netherlands, in 2010 the 'Multidisciplinary guideline for nonspecific low back pain' was developed [7]. This guideline was implemented using a patient and professional multifaceted implementation strategy that is evaluated in a randomised controlled trial (RCT). Implementing guidelines into clinical practice can be challenging, with many factors influencing the uptake of these guidelines by health care professionals (HCPs) [8]. In order to better understand why implementation efforts do or do not result in sustainable changes, it is important that trials implementing guidelines also evaluate the implementation process [9]. Process evaluations can explain differences between observed and expected results, and can shed a light on the underlying mechanisms responsible for the observed effects [10]. These evaluations can thus be useful in improving existing strategies for the implementation of interventions, and they can be useful for the development of future implementation strategies [10, 11]. The current paper describes the process evaluation of the implementation strategy targeted at patients. A process evaluation of the HCP based strategy is reported elsewhere [12].

The goals of the current study were: 1) to evaluate whether the implementation strategy was performed as planned; 2) to assess the feasibility, barriers and facilitators of the patient based eHealth campaign; 3) to gain insight into the satisfaction and experiences of patients with various ethnic backgrounds with the implementation strategy and to make a comparison between them; and 4) to explore the association between exposure to and satisfaction with the strategy.

Methods

This process evaluation was performed alongside a stepped-wedge RCT to test the cost-effectiveness of a multifaceted implementation strategy for the Dutch multidisciplinary guideline for nonspecific LBP. Details of the procedures and methods of the RCT, as well as details on the medical ethical review for this study have been reported elsewhere [13]. In this trial, multidisciplinary collaboration between HCPs was promoted by means of continuing medical education (CME) training sessions for health care professionals combined with a multimedia strategy for these HCPs. For patients with LBP, an interactive multifaceted eHealth strategy was developed.

Study population

The study population for this process evaluation consisted primarily of LBP patients that participated in the trial. These patients were recruited through their participating HCPs. Patients in the trial allocated to the intervention group were invited to participate in this process evaluation by means of a quantitative evaluation questionnaire. Patients that completed the questionnaire were asked if they were also willing to participate in a qualitative evaluation of the intervention, and if so, these patients were personally contacted by telephone and e-mail. Furthermore, patients from the intervention group were invited to participate in the qualitative analysis by means of a call in monthly newsletters, and through calls via social media. The majority of the trial patients were native Dutch or western immigrants. Because 35% of Amsterdam citizens consists of non-western ethnic minorities of which the majority is of Turkish, Moroccan or Surinamese origin [14], extra effort was put into recruiting Turkish, Moroccan, and Surinamese LBP patients for this process evaluation to gain insight into their experiences and satisfactions as well. These patients did not participate in the trial but received access to parts of the intervention for the sole purpose of evaluating these parts of the process. These patients were recruited in several ways, including a personal invitation to evaluate the intervention by their HCP; via posters and take-away brochures in HCP practices and university buildings, and via posters in various meeting places in the city.

Multifaceted implementation strategy

The multifaceted implementation strategy for patients consisted of a multimedia eHealth campaign that comprised of several components, described in more detail below.

Interactive website

An interactive website that included extensive written information about acute and chronic LBP was developed. The website provided information about the aetiology of LBP, the expected prognosis, and tips and tricks on how to self-manage LBP. Twelve short video-messages in which HCPs such as surgeons, doctors and therapists, and patients with LBP share their insights and advice on LBP and staying active, continuing or returning to work, and coping with LBP were also developed for this campaign. The video-messages were uploaded one by one on the website every 1 to 2 months. Furthermore, the website contained several physical therapy exercises in video and diagram format, and other downloadable documents such as information leaflets and self-help toolkits. Links to other informative websites and applications, video material, and reading material were also provided on the website. In order to prevent contamination by exposing patients from the control group to the intervention strategy, the website was protected by login. Eligible patients received login credentials after they had completed a baseline questionnaire at their inclusion in the study. The website was modified in such a way that only administrators could generate these login credentials. This was an extra effort to prevent undesirable exposure of the website to the control group.

Social media

The website contained a forum on which patients could chat with each other or with members of the research team, where they could ask questions, or share information. Also, a Facebook page and a Twitter account were opened to regularly post updates or interesting information about the study or about LBP in general. Except for the forum, which was part of the protected website, the social media options were open to anyone who had an account and wished to follow the research pages.

Monthly newsletters

Monthly newsletters were sent to the patients. The newsletters included updates on the study, news, reminders about new content on the website (e.g. new video-messages), tips and tricks for self-management of LBP, frequently asked questions, anecdotal items, and reminders to fill in follow-up questionnaires.

Translations

In order to involve the two largest local ethnic minority groups (e.g. Turkish and Moroccan immigrants) in the study, several items of the strategy were translated into Turkish and Arab languages. These included instructions and explanations of the follow-up questionnaires, instructions and an explanation of the main page of the website, and re-voiced copies of the video-messages.

Data collection and analysis

This process evaluation was based on components developed by the Linnan and Steckler framework [11]. Using a mixed methods approach, quantitative and qualitative methods were applied to collect data on the components: recruitment, reach, dose delivered, dose received, satisfaction and barriers and facilitators (Table 1).

Quantitative data collection

All patients that participated in the trial were sent an electronic evaluation questionnaire in the months January and February 2016. The questionnaire was designed to measure their usage of and satisfaction with the intervention. Table 2 shows the evaluation questionnaire items. Using regression modelling in IBM SPSS Statistics 22.0, the association between satisfaction with the intervention (outcome variable) and exposure to the intervention (i.e. usage of the website) was explored. To measure intervention use objectively, login data of the website and amount of followers on social media were registered.

Dose delivered

The dose delivered refers to the extent to which the strategy was delivered by the intervention providers according to protocol for the various implementation strategy components. Points were assigned to strategy components if they were delivered as planned, and the sum of component scores was used to calculate the overall dose delivered. Only the provision of video-messages and newsletters was protocolled, whereas the social media component was set up to provide ad hoc messages.

Video-messages During 12 months, one video-message per one to two months was to be uploaded on the website. For each video-message that was timely delivered 1 point was scored, thus amounting to a maximum total of 12 points that could be scored for this component.

Monthly Newsletters During 24 months, one newsletter was to be sent out to participating patients. For each newsletter that was timely delivered 1 point was scored, thus amounting to a maximum total of 24 points that could be scored for this component.

Qualitative data analysis

To gain more in-depth knowledge about the satisfaction and experiences of patients with the intervention, and to get insight into barriers and facilitators for the use of this intervention by patients, semi-structured, qualitative interviews were conducted among a subset of participating patients. Sampling of patients was guided by the willingness of the patients to participate in an interview, and interviews were conducted until redundancy was reached [15].

The topic lists for the interviews addressed the same items as the evaluation questionnaire, and was designed to elicit opinions about the various intervention components and the manner in which they were offered.

Table 1 Process evaluation components

Component	Definition	Data collection method
1. Recruitment	Procedures used to recruit patients	Description and minutes of recruitment procedure
2. Reach	Number of patients participating in the study as proportion of patients invited; and number of patients participating in the process evaluation as proportion of patients participating in the study	Minutes of research organisation
3. Dose delivered	Extent to which the protocol for implementation strategy was delivered by the intervention providers as planned	Minutes of research organisation
4. Dose received	Extent to which intervention was used by patients	Evaluation questionnaire Login registration data website Followers data social media
5. Satisfaction	Experiences of patients with intervention Patients' overall satisfaction with intervention	Evaluation questionnaire Qualitative interviews
6. Barriers and facilitators	Barriers and facilitators for intervention use by patients	Qualitative interviews

Interviews were recorded and transcribed verbatim immediately after they had taken place. All interviews were analysed using a constant comparison approach in three subsequent steps. The first step was the fragmentation of transcripts into short, descriptive summaries (open coding). Subsequently, the fragments that were closely related to each other were grouped to create provisional themes (axial coding). In the third and last step, connection between the provisional themes was made to structure the data into meaningful entities [16]. To enhance the quality of analyses, one researcher coded all interviews, and two other researchers coded a random sample of interviews. Any disagreements in coding were resolved by consensus. The patients participating in this study were divided into four ethnic groups, and the satisfaction and experiences with the implementation strategy were compared between those groups.

Results

Three hundred and 31 patients with LBP received the multifaceted intervention of this implementation study. A total of 214 (64.7%) patients completed the quantitative evaluation questionnaire for the current process evaluation, and 44 patients participated in the qualitative evaluation of the intervention.

Table 2 Items of evaluation questionnaire

Items	
1. How often did you visit the website? [a]	11. Did you find the links useful? [c]
2. Did your HCP recommend this website to you? [b]	12. How often did you use the exercises provided? [f]
3. Did your HCP discuss this website with you? [b]	13. Did you find the exercises useful? [c]
4. Did you experience any added value from the website in addition to the treatment you received from your HCP? [c]	14. Were the advices applicable to you? [c]
5. Was the information on the website clear to you? [c]	15. Did you find the monthly newsletter useful? [c]
6. Did you find the website useful? [c]	16. Did you use social media for this study, if yes, which one(s)? [g]
7. How many video-messages have you watched? [d]	17. Did the website contribute to your recovery? [b]
8. Did you find the video-messages useful? [c]	18. If the website contributed to your recovery, which component(s) was/were the most helpful to you? [h]
9. On a scale from 0 (lowest) to 10 (highest), how would you rate your appreciation of the video-messages? [e]	19. Would you recommend this website to others with back pain? [b]
10. How often did you use the links provided? [f]	20. On a scale from 0 (lowest) to 10 (highest), how would you rate your appreciation of the website? [e]

[a] Never/Once/At least once per month/At least once, not every month
[b] Yes/No
[c] No/A little/Yes
[d] None/One/Some (2–12)/All (12)
[e] 0–10
[f] Never/Once/More than once
[g] Forum/Facebook/Twitter
[h] Information/Videos/Links/Exercises/Social media

Quantitative results
Recruitment and reach
A total of 5203 patients with LBP were invited by their HCP to participate in the trial. Of these patients, 890 (17.1%) agreed to participate in the trial and 753 (14.5%) actually participated, 286 patients (5.5%) declined participation, and 4005 patients (77.0%) did not respond at all. Three hundred and 31 (44.0%) of the participating patients were randomised to the intervention group and thus received the intervention, and were invited to participate in this process evaluation. Two hundred and 14 (64.7%) patients from the intervention group filled in the evaluation questionnaire. Table 3 shows the characteristics of these patients. Demographic characteristics of patients that did not respond to the evaluation questionnaire ($n = 117$) were evaluated to compare with demographic characteristics of the responders. Non-responders were on average 51.9 years old (SD 14.4), mostly female ($n = 73$), native Dutch ($n = 94$), and had a background in higher ($n = 57$) or vocational educational ($n = 31$).

Dose delivered
Eleven out of 12 video-messages were uploaded according to protocol, thus receiving 11 points for this component of the dose delivered. Out of 24 monthly newsletters, 17 newsletters were sent according to protocol, and 7 newsletters were not. Thus, the newsletters scored 17 points, making the total dose delivered points amount to 28 out of 36 points (77.8% overall dose delivered).

Dose received and Satisfaction
Eleven (5.2%) patients stated that the website was recommended by their HCP, and 4 (1.9%) patients stated that they discussed the content of the website with their HCP. The Facebook page had 9 followers, and the Twitter account had 14 followers. Two patients stated that they used Facebook, and 1 patient stated using the forum. None of the patients indicated using Twitter. The monthly newsletters were considered a little useful by 137 (66.2%) patients, and not useful to 70 (33.8%) patients. The website login log showed that a total of 302 logins were registered, belonging to 170 unique patients (55% of intervention group). One hundred patients (71.4%) stated that they would recommend the website to others, and the mean satisfaction with the website was 6.7. Table 4 shows other results of the evaluation questionnaire. The majority of patients only visited the website once or not at all. More than half of the patients (53%) did not watch any of the videos. Patients who watched the videos seemed to appreciate the video-messages to an ample degree (graded 6.9 out of 10 points), but the majority felt little added value of the website to their recovery.

Statistical analysis showed that patients who had not visited the website at all or only visited it once, rated the intervention with 6.4 points on average. Increasing the number of visits to monthly visits, or regular visits that were not per se monthly, resulted in an increase of average rating of 0.8 points, and the increase was statistically significant for patients that regularly visited the website. Table 5 shows the results of this linear regression analysis.

Qualitative results (satisfaction, barriers and facilitators)
Forty-four semi-structured, qualitative interviews were conducted among patients with LBP, of which 19 participated in the entire study, and 25 only participated in this process evaluation. Fifteen patients were of Dutch or other western origin (mean age 57), 9 were of Moroccan origin (mean age 44.3), 10 were of

Table 3 Characteristics of patients that completed evaluation questionnaire ($n = 214$)

Mean age (SD)	56 (13.5)		Occupational status (%)	
Gender (%)	Male	Female	Student	7 (3.3)
	101 (47.6)	111 (52.4)	Employed	94 (44.3)
			Self-Employed	33 (15.6)
Back pain (%)[a]	124 (57.9)		Unemployed	36 (17)
Mean Disability Score (SD)[b]	4 (4)		Retired	42 (19.8)
Disability pension (%)	11 (5.2)			
			Volunteer work	26 (12.3)
Level of education (%)				
None/Elementary	6 (2.8)		Ethnicity	
High School	14 (6.6)		Native Dutch	198 (93.4)
Vocational	55 (25.9)		Western ethnic minority	8 (3.8)
Higher	137 (64.6)		Non-western ethnic minority	6 (2.8)

[a]N patients that reported having LBP at start of the study
[b]As measured with Roland Morris Disability Questionnaire [41], scale range 0–24

Table 4 Results of evaluation questionnaire (*n* = 214)

Website visits n (%)		Website clear n (%)	
Never	66 (31.3)	No	2 (1.4)
Once	91 (42.9)	Little	15 (10.5)
At least once per month	14 (6.6)	Yes	126 (88.1)
At least once, not every month	41 (19.3)		
Website useful n (%)		Added value of website n (%)	
No	11 (7.7)	No	44 (30.8)
Little	56 (39.2)	Little	61 (42.7)
Yes	76 (53.2)	Yes	38 (26.6)
Videos viewed n (%)		Videos useful n (%)	
None	76 (53.1)	No	12 (18.5)
One	26 (18.2)	Little	53 (81.5)
Some (2–12)	39 (27.3)	Yes	0 (00.0)
All	2 (1.4)	Mean appreciation videos (SD)	6.9 (1.3)
Links viewed n (%)		Links useful n (%)	
Never	75 (53.2)	No	5 (7.5)
Once	44 (31.2)	Little	61 (92.4)
More than once	22 (15.6)	Yes	0 (00.0)
Exercises viewed n (%)		Exercises useful n (%)	
Never	63 (44.7)	No	12 (15.4)
Once	31 (22)	Little	66 (84.6)
More than once	47 (33.3)	Yes	0 (00.0)
Contribution to recovery n (%)	22 (15.6)	Advice applicable	
Information	11	No	36 (25.5)
Videos	4	Little	63 (44.7)
Links	2	Yes	42 (29.8)
Exercises	19		
Social media	2		

Surinamese or Indonesian origin (mean age 34.6), and 10 were of Turkish or Iraqi origin (mean age 37.6). The overall mean age of the patients was 45 years, 25 were female and 18 were male. The majority of patients (*n* = 25) had a high educational level, followed by 15 patients with vocational education, and 4 patients with elementary education. The characteristics

Table 5 Results of linear regression analysis on intervention rating

Group	B	Sig. (*p* = .05)	95% CI
Website visited 0 or 1 times (*n* = 157, 74.2%)	6.4	-	6.1–6.7
Website visited monthly (*n* = 14, 6.6%)	7.2	>0.100	6.0–8.3
Website visited regularly (*n* = 41, 19.3%)	7.2	<0.001	6.3–8.0

of these 44 patients are shown in Table 6. Data of the interviews were analysed and categorised into four themes, discussed by theme below.

Satisfaction with intervention components

The information on the website was appreciated by most of the patients. The website was considered to be clear and understandable, although somewhat basic. Patients indicated that the amount of information on the website was satisfactory, and most patients felt that their expectations were met by the website. Some patients even felt that there was too much (especially written) information on the website. The content of the website was perceived to be interesting and helpful by most patients, although they indicated that the website would have been more

Table 6 Characteristics of patients that participated in the qualitative evaluation

ID	Age	Gender	Ethnicity	Educational level	Study participant	ID	Age	Gender	Ethnicity	Educational level	Study participant
1	30	F	Polish	Higher	√	23	29	F	Iraqi	Higher	-
2	55	M	Moroccan	Elementary	√	24	42	F	Moroccan	Vocational	-
3	63	M	Moroccan	Vocational	√	25	26	M	Moroccan	Vocational	-
4	55	F	Peruvian	Elementary	√	26	18	F	Turkish	Vocational	-
5	50	M	Surinamese	Higher	√	27	41	F	Indonesian	Higher	-
6	38	F	Surinamese	Vocational	√	28	27	F	Surinamese	Vocational	-
7	42	M	British	Vocational	√	29	44	F	Moroccan	Higher	-
8	65	M	Moroccan	Higher	√	30	32	F	Turkish	Higher	-
9	66	M	Dutch	Higher	√	31	25	F	Surinamese	Vocational	-
10	28	F	German	Higher	√	32	76	M	Dutch	Higher	√
11	73	F	Dutch	Higher	√	33	60	F	Dutch	Higher	√
12	59	M	Turkish	Higher	-	34	65	M	Dutch	Higher	√
13	46	M	Moroccan	Elementary	-	35	74	F	Swiss	Higher	√
14	38	M	Dutch	Higher	-	36	56	F	Dutch	Vocational	√
15	45	F	Iraqi	Vocational	-	37	58	F	Swiss	Higher	√
16	34	F	Surinamese	Vocational	-	38	64	M	Dutch	Higher	√
17	26	F	Moroccan	Higher	-	39	70	M	Dutch	Higher	√
18	55	F	Turkish	Vocational	-	40	26	F	Turkish	Higher	-
19	32	M	Moroccan	Higher	-	41	42	F	Turkish	Elementary	-
20	56	M	Surinamese	Vocational	-	42	48	M	Surinamese	Vocational	-
21	22	M	Turkish	Higher	-	43	34	F	Surinamese	Higher	-
22	18	F	Turkish	Vocational	-	44	23	F	Surinamese	Higher	-

useful to them if had they received access at the start of their first episode of LBP, when they did not have much information about and experience with LBP yet. One patient mentioned that this was a reason to drop out of the study by stating: *"... I thought: Been there, done that. And that's where I quit." (Patient 6).*

Although for many patients the exercises provided on the website were not new (having received them from healthcare providers on earlier occasions), the exercises were perceived to be the most helpful and interesting of all components by most patients. The ability to look up the exercises at any time of the day, to always have instructions at hand, and to be reminded to exercise were deemed positive effects of providing exercises on the website. Some patients mentioned they would have appreciated additional and more specific instructions regarding the exercises, such as an overview of when and which effects on the LBP should be expected when certain exercises are performed, and how often and how intensive the exercises should be performed. For example, one participant would have liked to know *"...Which muscle groups you train when you perform certain exercises, and why this is good for your back." (Patient 20).*

Most patients did not look at the provided links to other websites and additional information. The most frequently provided explanation for this was the perceived unnecessity of those links: patients felt that they had learned enough from the website alone, or they already had all the information they wanted before they visited the website. Patients that had already recovered from LBP felt no need for (additional) information. Patients indicated that they already knew enough about LBP and they stated that they preferred all available information in one place, so that looking up information is more convenient and less time-consuming. As one patient stated regarding the convenience of having all information in one place: *"You should be careful with providing too many links, for one could not see the forest for the trees anymore." (Patient 43).*

Patients were satisfied with the option to download material from the website to their computer, mainly because they could print this information and then have it available off-line and in other formats. This was beneficial for patients if they were not able to use their computer for a prolonged period of time, as one patient illustrated: *"I just print it. Reading on the computer is a bit difficult for me sometimes, because I have a cataract." (Patient 8).* Patients mostly downloaded and printed the exercises from the website, although the download materials were overall not often used.

The newsletters' most common effect was reminding patients to visit the website, or to (re)start following advice they read on the website or received from their healthcare provider. One patient said: *"It is a nice reminder for me to take a look at the website again. And I like reading updates about the study." (Patient 35).* Also, the newsletters triggered patients to think about their LBP and their current state of health, and the patients appreciated reading about new information, insights, and updates from the research team. Since the patients received the newsletters directly to their e-mail, most could open the letter on their mobile device and thus read it at their convenience. This direct and approachable way of communicating information was appreciated by most patients, as *Patient 24* illustrated by saying: *"You get the newsletter in your mailbox and you can download and read it immediately. It's no trouble at all. And I think it is interesting to read about what is going on."* However, some patients indicated that they would have preferred another frequency of the newsletters (i.e. either more often or less often), and that they would appreciate more information about international research on LBP, for example on the aetiology and possible treatment options of LBP.

Many patients did not watch (all of) the provided video-messages due to time constraints, too much information on the website or technical issues with the website. Those that did watch the video-messages considered them informative, clear, and concise. The videos were considered easily accessible, and those patients appreciated the fact that the information was provided in a concise and present-day manner. They most often watched the videos in which a healthcare professional was interviewed; the videos with LBP patients were less often watched. The patients that watched the videos considered them to be informative, because they recognized their complaints in the stories told, and this made them more confident that their LBP is normal, and that medical interventions were not necessary. Even some patients that did not recognize their complaints in the video-messages considered the videos to be informative, because the stories reassured them and made them think more positively about their LBP and recovery. The patients mentioned that the experiences of other patients with LBP motivated them to actively work on their LBP, and gave them hope that recovery from their LBP is possible, as one participant stated: *"It is good to hear from someone that has gone through this in his life, and who really has gotten better. It gives you more willpower to do it yourself as well." (Patient 26).*

The majority of patients did not notice the option to connect to the research on social media. Those patients that did use social media appreciated this option, because it made the information even more readily available and accessible. However, they also considered that the campaign was not active enough on social media. Furthermore, some patients indicated that they preferred social media over a website, because it is more interactive, allows for easier contact and information sharing with professionals and other patients. One patient stated: *"Facebook is more effective than a website. All the information is just there when you open it. ... You can read it or take action." (Patient 12).* Some patients were less interested to use social media, because they doubted confidentiality and reliability of the information provided and shared, but mostly because they did not use social media at all. Overall, 'open' social media (e.g., Facebook) was preferred over 'closed' social media (e.g., forum on protected login website).

Perceived benefits of intervention

Patients stated that they experienced various benefits of the website. For example, they noted that the information provided was reassuring, increasing their knowledge, providing insight and awareness, and improving their mental attitude about their LBP (e.g. by hearing about others' experiences with LBP). The website was seen as a second opinion for the information patients had already received from their healthcare provider, and in that way the information was either complementary to their treatment, or a reminder for the information they had already received. Patients also felt that the website alerted them to the importance of exercise in LBP recovery, and it motivated them to start exercising. Equally important to the patients was the fact that the website was always available if they wanted to look up exercises or other sorts of information, and they felt that their LBP was taken seriously. One participant stated: *"Imagine that the physio has no time for you, then you can do the exercise at home. In the evening or at any time, and that's great. So that is definitely the added value." (Patient 23).*

In order to perceive the benefits of the website, patients indicated that it was important that they trusted the information on the website. Patients also stated that the opinion of their healthcare provider about this website was important to them: if he/she refers a patient to the website, the website is perceived as trustworthy and helpful, leading to an increased number of visits to the website. Involvement of the healthcare provider led to increased perceived trustworthiness and use of the website.

Usage of intervention

The majority of patients stated that they visited the website only once, and the visits usually lasted 10 to 30 min. The main reason for patients not to return to the website was that they did not experience LBP anymore, and patients with chronic or recurring LBP were already familiar with the information provided on the website. Some patients also noted that the information on the website was not applicable to their personal situation: *"There were a lot of things for me that I already knew or tried, that don't apply to me, or I knew that they would not help me." (Patient 24)*. Other barriers for usage of the website were not remembering to visit the website, a lack of time, difficulty with the language, and dissatisfaction with the medium used.

Patients that indicated visiting the website repeatedly mentioned experiencing several triggers for returning. Most often, receiving the monthly newsletter reminded them of the website and stimulated a return visit. Another important trigger was the need to refresh their memory about the exercises or other information, such as tips and tricks to reduce pain, or to see if any new information was available.

Satisfaction with medium used

Many patients indicated that their dissatisfaction with the medium used was a barrier for repeated or regular use of the website. Several components of the medium attributed to this, of which the layout of the website was one. Patients indicated that the website was perceived to be functional, but it was not attractive and did not draw attention, because of its design and structure. Another hindering component was the usability of the website. The website was not entirely responsive on some mobile devices, leading to discontinued visits in these cases. Many patients also indicated the necessity of protected login to be a barrier for visiting the website. They often forgot or lost their login credentials, and noted that logging in limited them in visiting the website, and sharing information from the website with others who did not participate in this study. This also led to discontinued visits and the preference of other, non-protected websites for information, illustrated by one participant by stating: *"It [login] obstructed me. I wanted to visit the website, so I looked it [login credentials] up, but actually I wanted to drop out because of it." (Patient 28)*.

While most patients indicated that they were content with the information provided via the website, some patients would prefer additional facilities. These included personalised information, more frequent and instant triggers and reminders (e.g. push notifications), and the possibility to directly connect with a healthcare professional. Most non-native respondents appreciated the translated parts of the website, and indicated that translations were important to involve a broader target group of patients, e.g. ethnic minorities who do not understand the Dutch language. These translations made these patients feel welcomed and valued, which increased their willingness to participate in the study, to visit the website, and to make use of the information provided. For the translations to be even more helpful, patients indicated that they should be translated professionally, into more languages/dialects, and, most importantly, that all components of the intervention should be fully translated.

Comparison between groups

The satisfaction and experiences with the content of the intervention did not vary much between the various ethnic groups. Non-western patients (i.e. from Moroccan, Turkish/Iraqi or Surinamese/Indonesian origin) were more often not satisfied with the medium used, and indicated that they would have preferred a more modern, quick and on-the-go approach to information transfer than a website, for example using a mobile app that they could consult easier and more often. Non-western patient also viewed the exercises more often, and attached more importance to the translation of strategy materials than native Dutch patients.

Discussion

This process evaluation showed that the protocolled strategy components were performed as planned to a dose delivered degree of 78%. Login registration data showed that 170 unique patients (55% of intervention group) logged on to the website, while a total of 302 logins was registered (1.8 visits per patient on average). Self-reported usage of the website (dose received) by patients showed that most patient only logged in once ($n = 91$, 42.9%). Although the majority of the patients who logged in did not view a large part of the website (i.e. video-messages, links, exercises), 70% ($n = 99$) of those patients perceived the website of added value and would recommend it to others ($n = 100$). Patients' overall rating of the website was reasonable (6.7 out of 10). However many barriers for use, including information saturation and lack of translations, were identified in this evaluation. The reach of patients for this study was low, with only 14.1% ($n = 753$) participating patients.

Interpretation of findings and comparison to other studies

The low reach found in the present study is in line with other implementation studies, for example that performed by Tonnon et al. [17], where the implementation of a lifestyle intervention in a workplace setting reached only 2.4% of the target population. The reach of the current study was not as high as for example the study performed by Buist et al., where the reach was 22.4% in an integrated healthcare system [18]. It must be noted that assessing the actual reach of a target population in implementation research is hard to measure, as is also discussed by Van Vilsteren et al. in their process evaluation of a workplace intervention for workers with rheumatoid arthritis [19]. For example, the amount of patients that were invited to participate could have been an overestimation, since the HCPs inviting the patients could have excluded patients without reporting exclusions to the research team. The reach of this implementation study can be compared to awareness levels of back pain mass media campaigns that have been conducted in other countries. For example, an effective Australian campaign reported that up to 86% of survey respondents reported having seen the mass media campaign [20]. While this is a high percentage, similar studies from Norway, Canada, and Scotland have reported awareness levels of 40, 50, and 60% respectively [21–23].

The results of this study suggest several possible reasons for the low use of the intervention. One explanation could be the quick recovery from LBP by some patients, after one visit to the website, or even before the visit. Another barrier might be the fact that the HCPs rarely discussed the website with their patients, and slightly more patients, although only 5%, were actually referred to the website by their HCP. This is supported by the qualitative results, in which patients indicated that referral to the website by their HCP leads them to trust the website more. This implicates that eHealth interventions should be blended in usual care, so called blended eHealth intervention. Thereby, involvement of HCPs may increase use of the campaign. These findings are in line with other studies in comparable primary care settings, for example a study performed by De Jong et al. [24], who offered a web-based counselling program for employees on sick leave due to non-specific low back pain or neck pain, and their occupational physicians (OPs). Although their participants appreciated the program, actual program utilization by the employees as well as by the OPs was low in the study by De Jong [24]. However, the low use in the current study was not in line with the aims and expectations of the intervention providers. Since the HCPs also received a multifaceted implementation strategy, and played an important role in including patients for the study, it was expected that they would play a bigger role in activating patients to use the eHealth campaign [13]. A literature review on public engagement with eHealth has suggested that health professionals play an important role in endorsement and promotion of eHealth services to patients [25]. The same review also suggested that trust might influence patients' perception of eHealth services, for example concerns about scientific sources of the information provided [25]. An observational study on self-management of chronic neck and LBP showed that adherence to non-

pharmacologic self-management strategies increased when patients received information about their illness and the effectiveness of the self-management strategy during the clinical course from their HCP [26]. From the current study it seems that involvement of the HCP and the perceived trustworthiness of the eHealth service may be related and their combination could be a factor in the use of the eHealth campaign. Unfortunately, both barriers seem to have influenced the use of this campaign in the current study.

Another barrier for usage of the eHealth campaign might be the dissatisfaction with the content and layout of the website. Many patients indicated that the information provided on the website was already known to them, and that the layout and design of the website did not trigger return visits. This is in line with the importance of both content and design of eHealth intervention that has been shown in previous studies [27, 28]. It seems not only important that patients receive the intervention (i.e. the information) in a timely manner (at the start of their first episode of LBP), but that the information also be communicated in a state-of-the-art manner. Designing eHealth intervention with high levels of interactivity in an interpersonal, dynamic, and engaging digital environment seems to be an important aspect in increasing the usage and effectiveness of eHealth interventions [24, 28, 29]. In the current study, mainly non-western immigrant patients were dissatisfied with the medium used. This may be explained by the difference in mean age and gender of the patients. Non-western immigrant patients were on average 18 years younger (mean age 38.8 years) than native or western-immigrant patients, and were mostly female ($n = 18$). The Centres for Disease Control and Prevention have shown that women are more likely than men to use the Internet for health information [30]. National statistics from the United States and the United Kingdom have shown that Internet use among 15–44 year olds is highest, and that usage decreases with the increase of age [31, 32], although there is no evidence that this is true for health information seeking specifically. Research has also shown that health care utilisation is higher among the immigrant population than among the native Dutch population [33–35], and that ethnicity is a predictor for health care utilisation regardless of health status [35, 36]. It also seems that immigrant patients with LBP have a worse prognosis than their native Dutch counterparts [37]. A possible explanation for these differences between ethnic groups might be that health care interventions insufficiently take the various needs and perspectives of immigrant patients into account. Therefore, to better cater to the needs of this population group, it is important to account for these ethnic differences. This could be done by targeting health care interventions specifically to this population and their beliefs.

For non-western immigrant patients, the lack of full translation of all intervention components also seemed to be an important barrier for intervention use. By translating the most important items of the intervention (i.e. the video-messages and home page information), the current study aimed to actively involve these patients. Although it might seem common sense to ensure that interventions are linguistically understandable to a broad group of patients, research has shown that it is not the only important aspect playing a role in involvement of culturally diverse patients [38, 39]. In all phases of the research process, from recruitment through staff that reflects cultural diversity to the use of linguistically and culturally appropriate materials, it is important to dwell upon the needs of various patient groups in order to involve them in health research and intervention. Assessing the needs of these patients prior to the development of healthcare interventions might increase the usefulness and effectiveness of these interventions.

Strengths and Limitations
When interpreting the results of this study, some limitations have to be taken into account. Although effort was put into the recruitment of LBP patients with non-western ethnic backgrounds (especially Turkish, Moroccan, and Surinamese patients) in the trial, most participating patients were native Dutch or western immigrants. This led to ad-hoc recruitment of these ethnic patients for the sole purpose of the current process evaluation. The patients in the qualitative evaluation only received access to parts of the intervention (i.e. the website and social media), and thus did not have the full-experience of the entire intervention. This might have influenced their satisfaction and experiences with the website. Furthermore, it is plausible that illiterate and thus low or non-educated respondents were underrepresented in this study. Another notable finding in this study was that the majority of patients had a high educational level. Although this is in line with other research [40], it is important to put effort into the recruitment and participation of lower educated patients. The fact that the majority of patients that participated in the quantitative process evaluation had a high educational background might have influenced the results, as these patients may have different needs and opinions than lower educated patients. Also, the dose delivered component should be interpreted with caution, as it is an arbitrary quantification of parts of the full strategy, and has its own limitations. For example, due to planning issues, only 11 out of 12 video-messages, and 17 out of 24 newsletters were delivered on the planned date.

This is also true for the dose received, which was defined as the proportion of patients who logged into the website at least once. Whether these measures reflect effective doses is debatable, but it makes a first step in increasing the quality of the current study. Ideally, if technical opportunities allow for this, intervention providers should collect data on actual use, for example by tracking time spent on the website or website components used. To further increase the quality of this process evaluation, a mixed methods approach to data collection and analysis was applied. Triangulation of these methods (i.e. descriptive quantitative analysis, regression modelling, and qualitative data analysis) improved the quality of this evaluation. Furthermore, to ensure correct analysis and interpretation of qualitative data, a large random sample of all interviews were coded and discussed by two independent researchers.

Implication of findings
The results of this study showed that many patients did not use the intervention at all or only once, and this is an important finding in the light of the future effect evaluation of this implementation study. As this patient based eHealth campaign was part of a larger implementation study, it was designed to support the HCP based implementation of a guideline that advocates reduced referral rates for diagnostic imaging and consultations with medical specialists [13]. The current process evaluation showed that HCPs rarely discussed the eHealth campaign with their patients, indicating that the patient based and the HCP based campaigns were too independent of each other. This may be reflected in the final results of the implementation study (i.e. reduced referral rates for LBP). HCPs should discuss with and stimulate the use of eHealth interventions by their patients, and implementation strategies that are targeted at changing patient outcomes should ideally also pay more attention in their strategy to the improvement of HCP behaviour and attitude towards these interventions.

Conclusion
This process evaluation showed that the multifaceted implementation strategy was used by only a small proportion of the patients with non-specific LBP. It seemed that the campaign was offered to the patients too late, that the lay-out of the campaign did not meet the needs of the patients, and that healthcare providers rarely discussed this campaign with the patients, while involvement of those providers seemed to improve trustworthiness of the campaign and increase its usage. As the current study showed that the satisfaction of the intervention increased with more visits to the website, it probably pays off to invest in motivating HCPs to

activate patients to use eHealth interventions at the right timing (i.e. at patients' initial consultation with the HCP). Needs assessment research might contribute to the development of (more) serviceable eHealth interventions. Future researchers and practitioners may benefit from including patient perspectives and expectations, and adapting interventions to the targeted population in terms of language, content, and delivery method, while health care providers could aid in promotion of eHealth interventions and self-management.

Abbreviations
CME: Continuing medical education; HCP: Healthcare provider; LBP: Low back pain; OP: Occupational physician; RCT: Randomized controlled trial

Acknowledgements
The authors would like to thank dr. Cécile R.L. Boot for her valuable comments on this manuscript, and Margo Altena and Rosan Kreuzen for their help in data collection and analysis. We also thank dr. Marjan Westerman for the valuable discussions regarding the qualitative data analysis.

Funding
This paper is part of a project funded by The Netherlands Organisation for Health Research and Development (ZonMw; grant number 837003005). The funding party did not have any role in design of the study, in collection, analysis, and interpretation of data, or in writing the manuscript.

Author's contributions
AS, FGS, MWvT, and JRA were involved in the design of the study. AS and BJ were involved in the acquisition of data. AS, FGS, JB, MWvT, and JRA were involved in the interpretation of data. AS drafted the manuscript, and FGS, JB, MWvT, and JRA revised the manuscript. AS, FGS, JB, MWvT, and JRA agreed to be accountable for all aspects of the work, and have read and approved the final manuscript.

Competing interests
The authors declare that they have no competing interests.

Consent for publication
The patients' quotes, and participant information, used to illustrate the themes that emerged from the current study are anonymised in a way that prevents the identification of individual patients. Therefore, consent for publication was not required.

Author details
[1]Amsterdam Public Health research institute, Department of Public and Occupational Health, VU University Medical Centre, PO Box 70571007 MB Amsterdam, The Netherlands. [2]Department of Public and Occupational Health, Research Centre for Insurance Medicine, Collaboration between AMC-UMCG-UWV-VUmc, VU University medical centre, PO Box 70671007 MB Amsterdam, The Netherlands. [3]Faculty of Earth & Life Sciences, Department of Health Sciences, Student Health Sciences at the VU University Amsterdam, De Boelelaan 1085, 1081 HV Amsterdam, The Netherlands. [4]Amsterdam Public Health research institute, Faculty of Earth & Life Sciences, Department of Health Sciences, VU University Amsterdam, De Boelelaan 1085, 1081 HV Amsterdam, The Netherlands.

References
1. Global Burden of Disease Study 2013 Collaborators. Global, regional, and national incidence, prevalence, and years lived with disability for 301 acute and chronic diseases and injuries in 188 countries, 1990–2013: a systematic analysis for the Global Burden of Disease Study 2013. Lancet. 2015;386:743–800.
2. Williams JS, Ng N, Peltzer K, Yawson A, Biritwum R, Maximova T, et al. Risk Factors and Disability Associated with Low Back Pain in Older Adults in Low- and Middle-Income Countries. Results from the WHO Study on Global AGEing and Adult Health (SAGE). PLoS One. 2015;10(6):e0127880.
3. Dagenais S, Caro J, Haldeman S. A systematic review of low back pain cost of illness studies in the United Stated and internationally. Spine J. 2008;1:20.
4. Duthey B. Update on 2004 Background Paper, BP 6.24 Low back pain. Geneva: World Health Organization; 2013.
5. Hoy D, Brooks P, Buchbinder R. The Epidemiology of low back pain. Best Pract Res Clin Rheumatol. 2010;4(6):69–781.
6. Kemper SJ, Apeldoorn AT, Chiarotto A, Smeets RJEM, Ostelo RWJG, Guzman J, van Tulder MW. Multidisciplinary biopsychosocial rehabilitation for chronic low back pain: Cochrane systematic review and meta-analysis. BMJ. 2015;350:h444.
7. Van Tulder MW, Custers JWH, de Bie RA, Hammelburg R, Hulshof CTJ, Kolnaar, et al. Ketenzorgrichtlijn aspecifieke lage rugklachten. The Netherlands: KKCZ; 2010.
8. Francke AL, Smit MC, de Veer AJE, Mistiaen P. Factors influencing the implementation of clinical guidelines for health care professionals: A systematic meta-review. BMC Med Inform Decis Mak. 2008;8:38.
9. Moore GF, Audrey S, Barker M, Bond L, Bonell C, Hardeman W, Moore L, O'Cathain A, Tinati T, Wight D, Baird J. Process evaluation of complex interventions: Medical Research Council guidance. BMJ. 2015;19(350):h1258.
10. Grol R, Wensing M. Implementatie: effective verbetering van de patiëntenzorg. (Improving Patient Care. The Implementation of Change in Health Care). Amsterdam: Reed Business Education; 2013.
11. Linnan L, Steckler A. Process evaluation for public health interventions and research. San Francisco: Jossey-Bass; 2002.
12. Suman A, Schaafsma FG, Buchbinder R, Van Tulder MW, Anema JR. Implementation of a multidisciplinary guideline for low back pain: process-evaluation among health care professionals. J Occup Rehabil. 2016. doi:10. 1007/s10926-016-9673-y.
13. Suman A, Schaafsma FG, Elders PJM, van Tulder MW, Anema JR. Cost-effectiveness of a multifaceted implementation strategy for the Dutch multidisciplinary guideline for nonspecific low back pain: design of a stepped-wedge cluster randomised controlled trial. BMC Public Health. 2015;15:522.
14. Centraal Bureau voor de Statistiek Nederland (Statistics Netherlands). www.cbs.nl. Accessed 23 Sept 2013.
15. Trotter RT. Qualitative research sample design and sample size: Resolving and unresolved issues and inferential imperatives. Prev Med. 2012;55(5):398–400.
16. Boeije H. Analyseren in kwalitatief onderzoek. Denken en doen. (Analysis in Qualitative Research.). The Hague: Boom Lemma; 2008.
17. Tonnon SC, Proper KI, van der Ploeg HP, Anema JR, van der Beek AJ. Process Evaluation of the Nationwide Implementation of a Lifestyle Intervention in the Construction Industry. J Occup Environ Med. 2016;58(1):e6–14.
18. Buist DS, Knight Ross N, Reid RJ, Grossman DC. Electronic health risk assessment adoption in an integrated healthcare system. Am J Manag Care. 2014;0(1):62–9.
19. Van Vilsteren M, Boot CRL, Voskuyl AE, Steenbeek R, Van Schaardenburg D, Anema JR. Process Evaluation of a Workplace Integrated Care Intervention for Workers with Rheumatoid Arthritis. J Occup Rehabil. 2016;26(3):382–91.
20. Buchbinder R, Jolley D. Effects of a mass media campaign on back beliefs is sustained 3 years after its cessation. Spine. 2005;30(11):1323–30.
21. Werner EL, Ihlebaek C, Laerum E, Wormgoor ME, Indahl A. Low back pain media campaign: no effect on sickness behaviour. Patient Educ Couns. 2008;71(2):198–203.
22. Gross DP, Russell AS, Ferrari R, Battié M, Schopflocher D, Hu R, et al. Evaluation of a Canadian back pain mass media campaign. Spine. 2010;35(8):906–13.
23. Waddell G, O'Connor M, Boorman S, Torsney B. Working Backs Scotland: a public and professional health education campaign for back pain. Spine. 2007;32(19):2139–43.
24. De Jong T, Heinrich J, Blatter BM, Anema JR, Van der Beek AJ. The feasibility of a web-based counselling program for occupational physicians and employees on sick leave due to back or neck pain. BMC Med Inform Decis Mak. 2009;9:46.
25. Hardiker NR, Grant MJ. Factors that influence public engagement with eHealth: A literature review. Int J Med Inform. 2011;80(1):1–12.

26. Escolar-Reina P, Medina-Mirapeix F, Gascón-Cánovas JJ, Montilla-Herrador J, Valera-Garrido JF, Collins SM. Self-management of chronic neck and low back pain and relevance of information provided during clinical encounters: an observational study. Arch Phys Med Rehabil. 2009;90(1):1734–9.

27. Cline RJ, Haynes KM. Consumer health information seeking on the internet: the state of the art. Health Educ Res. 2001;16(6):671–92.

28. Carey M, Noble N, Mansfield E, Waller A, Henskens F, Sanson-Fisher R. The role of eHealth in optimizing preventive care in the primary care setting. J Med Internet Res. 2015;17(5):e126.

29. Kreps GL, Neuhauser L. New directions in eHealth communication: opportunities and challenges. Patient Educ Couns. 2010;78(3):329–36.

30. Cohen RA, Adams PF. Use of the Internet for Health Information: United States, 2009, NCHS data brief, no 66. Hyattsville: National Center for Health Statistics; 2011.

31. Office for National Statistics. Internet users in the UK Statistical bulletins. Office for National Statistics, UK. 2015. http://www.ons.gov.uk/businessindustryandtrade/itandinternetindustry/bulletins/internetusers/2015. Accessed 4 Aug 2016.

32. File T, Ryan C. Computer and Internet use in the United States: 2013, American Community Survey Reports, ACS-28. Washington DC: U.S. Census Bureau; 2014.

33. Stronks K, Ravelli ACJ, Reijneveld SA. Immigrants in the Netherlands: Equal acces for equal needs? J Epidemiol Community Health. 2001;55:701–7.

34. Uiters E, Devillé WL, Foets M, Groenewegen PP. Use of health care services by ethnic minorities in The Netherlands: do patterns differ? Eur J Public Health. 2006;16(4):388–93.

35. Stronks K. Etnische herkomst van patiënten blijft belangrijk (Ethnicity of patients remains important). Ned Tijdschr Geneeskd. 2013;157:A6182.

36. Menezes CostaLda C, Maher CG, McAuley JH, Hancock MJ, Herbert RD, Refshauge KM, Henschke N. Prognosis for patients with chronic low back pain: inception cohort study. BMJ. 2009;339:b3829.

37. Sloots M, Dekker JHM, Bartels EAC, Geertzen JHB, Dekker J. Reasons for drop-out in rehabilitation treatment of native patients and non-native patients with chronic low back pain in the Netherlands: a medical file study. Eur J Phys Rehabil Med. 2010;46:505–10.

38. Anderson LM, Scrimshaw SC, Fullilove MT, Fielding JE, Normand J. and the Task Force on Community Preventive Services. Culturally competent healthcare systems: a systematic review. Am J Prev Med. 2003;24(3S):68–79.

39. Somnath S, Beach MC, Cooper LA. Patient centeredness, cultural competence and healthcare quality. J Natl Med Assoc. 2008;100(11):1275–85.

40. Higgins O, Sixsmith J, Barry MM, Domegan C. A literature review on health information-seeking behaviour on the web: a health consumer and health professional perspective. Stockholm: ECDC; 2011.

41. Roland M, Fairbank J. The Roland-Morris Disability Questionnaire and the Oswestry Disability Questionnaire. Spine. 2000;5(24):3115–24.

Implementing the Keele stratified care model for patients with low back pain: an observational impact study

Adrian Bamford[1], Andy Nation[1], Susie Durrell[1], Lazaros Andronis[2], Ellen Rule[3] and Hugh McLeod[2*]

Abstract

Background: The Keele stratified care model for management of low back pain comprises use of the prognostic STarT Back Screening Tool to allocate patients into one of three risk-defined categories leading to associated risk-specific treatment pathways, such that high-risk patients receive enhanced treatment and more sessions than medium- and low-risk patients. The Keele model is associated with economic benefits and is being widely implemented. The objective was to assess the use of the stratified model following its introduction in an acute hospital physiotherapy department setting in Gloucestershire, England.

Methods: Physiotherapists recorded data on 201 patients treated using the Keele model in two audits in 2013 and 2014. To assess whether implementation of the stratified model was associated with the anticipated range of treatment sessions, regression analysis of the audit data was used to determine whether high- or medium-risk patients received significantly more treatment sessions than low-risk patients. The analysis controlled for patient characteristics, year, physiotherapists' seniority and physiotherapist. To assess the physiotherapists' views on the usefulness of the stratified model, audit data on this were analysed using framework methods. To assess the potential economic consequences of introducing the stratified care model in Gloucestershire, published economic evaluation findings on back-related National Health Service (NHS) costs, quality-adjusted life years (QALYs) and societal productivity losses were applied to audit data on the proportion of patients by risk classification and estimates of local incidence.

Results: When the Keele model was implemented, patients received significantly more treatment sessions as the risk-rating increased, in line with the anticipated impact of targeted treatment pathways. Physiotherapists were largely positive about using the model. The potential annual impact of rolling out the model across Gloucestershire is a gain in approximately 30 QALYs, a reduction in productivity losses valued at £1.4 million and almost no change to NHS costs.

Conclusions: The Keele model was implemented and risk-specific treatment pathways successfully used for patients presenting with low back pain. Applying published economic evidence to the Gloucestershire locality suggests that substantial health and productivity outcomes would be associated with rollout of the Keele model while being cost-neutral for the NHS.

Keywords: Low back pain, Stratified care model, STarT Back Screening Tool, IMPaCT Back, Implementation study, Physiotherapy, Economic evaluation

* Correspondence: h.s.t.mcleod@bham.ac.uk
[2]University of Birmingham, Birmingham, UK
Full list of author information is available at the end of the article

Background

Low back pain (LBP) has reached epidemic proportions, affecting a large number of people each year and with a lifetime prevalence of up to 80% [1, 2]. Each year in England, about 2.3 million people, 4.2% of the population, consult a general practitioner (GP) at least once for LBP [3], and these individuals represent about 20% of those with LBP [4]. Back pain causes considerable discomfort and is a leading cause of work absence and economic loss [1, 5]. UK costs associated with back pain were conservatively estimated in 1998 prices as follows: NHS treatment £1.1 billion, private treatment £0.6 billion, informal care £1.6 billion, employment-related productivity loss costs £3.4 billion [1]. These figures underline the impact of LBP on society.

A wide range of therapies have been used for treatment of LBP [6], although clinicians' views on appropriate therapies have varied [7] along with reported uncertainty about the value of treatment options [8] and calls for research on cost-effectiveness [9]. The type of treatment for which there is most economic evidence is combined physical and psychological interventions. These include those that are physiotherapist-led (spanning the use of the Keele stratified care model [10–13], group exercise and education sessions [14], two pain-management programmes [15, 16] and spinal stabilisation physiotherapy [16]), multidisciplinary (with input from different combinations of physiotherapists, nurses, psychologists or professional counsellors) [17–20], and a psychologist-led intervention [21]. With one exception [15], the interventions have been compared to usual care and found to be cost-effective. However, the main evaluation perspectives taken in these studies vary from healthcare system (such as the NHS) to healthcare (system and private) to societal (healthcare and productivity losses), and this makes it difficult for clinicians and local commissioners to compare treatment options.

The Keele stratified care model

The Keele stratified care model for management of LBP comprises use of the prognostic STarT Back Screening Tool to allocate patients into one of three risk-defined categories [22] followed by delivery of associated risk-specific treatment pathways [10]. All patients receive a 30-min session with a physiotherapist comprising reassurance, education, and treatment specific to the patient's screening tool score [23]. Low-risk patients receive no further intervention. Medium-risk patients present with predominantly physical prognostic indicators and are referred for further physiotherapy. The high-risk patients are also referred for further physiotherapy which is designed to address the high psychosocial indicators, such as anxiety and fear, with which they present. A training package is required for the physiotherapists to enable them to deliver the treatment pathways [23]. The intention of the stratified care model was to change the pattern of treatment such that it would better target appropriate interventions and improve patient outcomes. The initial randomised controlled trial (the STarT Back trial) comparing the stratified care model to usual care was designed so that all eligible LBP patients identified from routine general practice records were seen in a physiotherapy clinic [10]. This does not reflect usual practice, where GPs are the first-contact clinician and only a minority of LBP patients are referred to physiotherapy [10]. The subsequent IMPaCT Back study was a sequential comparison study designed to explore the impact of the Keele stratified care model when implemented by GPs [12, 13]. Both the STarT Back and IMPaCT Back studies found that the stratified care model's treatment pathways change the pattern of usual treatment resulting in an increase in the number of treatment sessions provided as the risk-classification increases. The IMPaCT Back study found that over a 6-month post-implementation period (phase 3) the stratified care model was associated with a gain in mean quality-adjusted life years (QALYs) of 0.003 per patient compared to a 6-month pre-implementation period (phase 1) [12]. An increase in mean back-related NHS costs over 6 months of £1.75 per patient was associated with stratified care compared to a reduction in mean costs of £33.54 when private treatment costs were included [12, 13]. Stratified care was also associated with a mean saving in indirect productivity loss costs associated with LBP-related work absence of £400 per employed patient over the 6-month period [12].

Aims

The Keele stratified care model has attracted considerable NHS [24] and international [25] interest since the initial randomised controlled trial findings were published in 2011 [10], but there is little published information on its performance and usefulness in everyday practice [24, 25]. With this in mind, we set out to assess the impact of the model following its implementation as a pilot by physiotherapists at Gloucestershire Hospitals NHS Foundation Trust (GHT), an acute hospital physiotherapy department setting in Gloucestershire, England, in 2013. Use of the stratified care model is assessed in terms of three criteria: evidence of i) whether it was associated with the anticipated treatment pathways as represented by the number of risk-specific treatment sessions provided, ii) the physiotherapists' views on the usefulness of the stratified care model because the model is more likely to inform clinical behaviour if it is viewed as useful by the physiotherapists, and iii) the potential consequences for NHS and private treatment costs, QALYs, and societal productivity losses associated with the rollout of the stratified care model in Gloucestershire.

Methods

Design and setting

Treatment for LBP in Gloucestershire is provided by physiotherapists in the outpatient departments of both the local acute hospital and community care provider Trusts. Referrals to both services are received either from a GP or patient self-referral. The acute hospital physiotherapy service introduced the Keele stratified care model in Spring 2013, when patients presenting with LBP at one of the two acute hospital sites started to complete the prognostic STarT Back Screening Tool to determine their risk-rating at the first physiotherapy appointment. In order to audit this service innovation, an audit was undertaken during 15 weeks from March 2013 and repeated during 8 weeks from June 2014, by AN as part of the Trust's empowered leadership programme. The audit data were essential for the study because diagnostic codes are not routinely recorded on electronic systems for outpatient attendances at the Trust and so in their absence it would have been necessary to examine paper patient physiotherapy records to identify patients.

The GHT audit data allow an observation cohort design for the study, which also draws on the findings of the IMPaCT Back sequential comparison study to assess two of the study's aims: whether the introduction of the stratified care model was associated with the anticipated treatment pathways, and what the potential consequences of rolling out the model in Gloucestershire would be for NHS and private treatment costs, QALYs, and societal productivity losses.

Data

In each audit, physiotherapists were requested to complete an audit form on 100 consecutive patients for whom the patients' risk-rating had been determined. The sample size was determined on pragmatic grounds to be logistically feasible. The data recorded included: patient hospital number, Keele STarT Back Screening Tool score (1 to 9), risk-defined category (low, medium, high), clinical impression/differential diagnosis, number of treatment sessions, type of treatment, outcome, 'yes' or 'no' response to the question 'In your opinion did the risk category accurately reflect the patient?', free text response to 'Reflection - usefulness of the tool/did it guide patient management etc'. The audit forms were logged on a summary sheet that included a physiotherapist identifier code and the date on which the patient was first seen by a physiotherapist. A classification code for the physiotherapists' seniority was added to the dataset on the basis of the recorded physiotherapist identifier code by the head of service (SD), to distinguish physiotherapists up to grade 5 from those in higher grades. Where possible, the patient hospital number and the initial attendance date were used to determine the patient gender and age in years from the electronic patient administration system. The 2013 audit data for a small number of patients were recorded before the patient was discharged and so, where possible, the patient hospital number and the initial attendance date were used to determine the number of physiotherapy sessions undertaken from the patient administration system.

Analysis

Statistical analyses was used to assess whether implementation of the stratified care model was associated with the anticipated treatment pathways as represented by the number of risk-specific treatment sessions provided. This involved i) generating descriptive statistics for the number of treatment sessions provided and comparing them to those for the STarT Back and IMPaCT Back studies, ii) carrying out regression analysis using a multilevel linear mixed-effects model to examine the relationship between the patient-level number of treatment sessions and the risk-defined category, controlling for patient age, gender, year of audit, physiotherapists' seniority and physiotherapist. The risk-defined category was included as a fixed-effect categorical variable, and the patient age in years was included as a fixed-effect continuous variable. Gender (1 = female, 2 = male), year of audit (1 = 2013, 2 = 2014), and physiotherapists' seniority (1 = up to grade 5, 2 = higher grades) were included as fixed-effect dichotomous variables. Physiotherapist was included as a random-effect categorical variable in order to account for a possible physiotherapist-level cluster effect. Log transformation of the treatment session data was undertaken in order to reduce the right-skewness of the distribution due to the small number of patients receiving a comparatively large number of treatment sessions. The Kernel density estimate of the treatment session square root transformation was closer to normality compared to the Kernel of either the square root transformation or the natural units. The exponential of each fixed-effect coefficient is reported, as it represents the expected percent change in the number of treatment sessions associated with a one unit change in the independent variable [26]. Statistical significance was set at the 5% level. STATA version 12 software was used for the analysis. In order to provide an alternative measure of physiotherapist-level effects, a linear fixed-effects regression model was also run. However, the results were not sensitive to choice of model and so the results of the linear fixed-effects regression model are not reported here. Sensitivity analysis included omitting physiotherapist as an independent variable. A small-scale data validation exercise was undertaken for six patients to check the extent to which the physiotherapist's record of the number of physiotherapy sessions matched the medical records and number of sessions recorded in the electronic patient administration system. No evidence of discrepancies was found.

Audit data on whether the physiotherapist thought the risk category accurately reflected the patient were analysed to assess the percentage of patients and mean number of treatments by risk group to see if there was a link between valuing the tool and adopting a treatment strategy that reflected the risk category it produced. To further explore the physiotherapists' views on the usefulness of the stratified care model, the free text data on this question were analysed using framework methods [27]. Framework uses a thematic structure to summarise and classify case-based data that are organised in a series of matrices. Text is coded to represent key topics/themes and recorded in columns, with rows representing individual informants. This facilitates exploration of themes and patterns across the range of informants. In this study, the physiotherapists' views were first classified by whether the physiotherapist viewed the risk-rating tool as accurately reflecting the patient. The physiotherapists' comments were then coded as 'useful' or 'not useful' before associated attributes were identified.

The potential consequences for NHS and private back-related treatment costs, QALYs, and societal productivity losses associated with the rollout of the stratified care model in Gloucestershire were modelled by applying the local audit data on the proportion of patients by risk classification and estimates of local incidence to the published 6-month parameter estimates from the IMPaCT Back study [13]. Costs included consultations with GPs and practice nurses, consultations with other healthcare professionals, hospital-based procedures, prescribed medication, and out-of-pocket expenditures on treatments and/or aids [13]. The impact on treatment costs is reported from the perspectives of the NHS, private, and healthcare (NHS and private). Productivity losses are reported from a societal perspective. The impact of the stratified care model can be expressed in terms of net monetary benefit (NMB). The incremental benefit is rescaled into monetary value using the cost-effectiveness threshold to value each unit of benefit, and the incremental cost is subtracted from this value to give the NMB [28]. The cost-effective threshold used by the National Institute of Health and Care Excellence (NICE) is £30,000 per QALY, and this value is used in our analysis [28]. As a sensitivity analysis we also apply a cost-effective threshold of £15,500 per QALY which was empirically estimated for musculoskeletal treatment by Claxton et al. [29] and reported by Drummond et al. [28] table 4.3.

The proportions of patients by risk classification were estimated from the GHT audit data. The annual number of LBP patients referred from general practice for physiotherapy treatment was estimated as 20% [12, 30] of the consulting prevalence for LBP from an observational study of primary care consultations [3], applied to Gloucestershire gender and age-specific population rates

from Office for National Statistics mid-year estimates for 2013 [31]. The estimate of 20% of the consulting prevalence was increased to 25% in a sensitivity analysis. The 2008/9 back-related costs from the IMPaCT Back study [13] were translated into 2013/14 values using the hospital and community health services (HCHS) index to account for pay and price inflation [32]. A sensitivity analysis of the percentage of patients in each risk-category was undertaken assuming the percentages from the IMPaCT Back study in place of the GHT audit findings.

Results

The GHT audits included 201 patients presenting with LBP, of whom 59% (118/201) were female. Patient age was recorded for 92% (184/201) of the patients and the mean age was 51 years (range 16 to 90 years). The 201 patients were seen by 29 physiotherapists; 23 participated in the 2013 audit, 18 in 2014, and 12 in both audits. Patients were randomly allocated to a physiotherapist and on average each participating physiotherapist saw 6.9 patients (range 1 to 36 patients).

Treatment pathways

After the introduction of the Keele model, 2.7 physiotherapy sessions were provided to the LBP patients, on average, and the trend was for more sessions to be provided on average as the risk-rating increased (Table 1). Similarly, the trend was that more sessions were provided on average in 2014 compared to 2013.

The experience of the GHT audit patients was similar to that of patients in the IMPaCT Back study, such that the trend was for more sessions to be provided on average as the risk-rating increased (Table 2). This comparison is based on the 57% (314/554) of patients in the IMPaCT Back phase 3 for whom data on resource use was available (Table 2) [13]. Table 2 also illustrates the impact of the introduction of the stratified care model in the IMPaCT Back study, in terms of the increase in the mean number of treatment sessions, particularly for patients in the medium- and high-risk categories.

Overall, 33% (66/201) of the patients in the GHT audits were classified as high-risk, compared to 38% medium-risk and 29% low-risk (Table 1). The GHT experience was for a larger proportion of patients to be classified as high-risk compared to the 20% (108/554) experienced in the post-implementation phase of the IMPaCT Back study (Table 2). The chi-squared test indicates that the proportions in each risk category in the GHT audits compared to the post-implementation phase of the IMPaCT Back study were significantly different ($p < 0.01$) (Tables 1 and 2).

The multilevel linear mixed-effects model was used to examine the relationship between the number of treatment sessions and the risk-defined category, while controlling for patient and physiotherapist-level variables

Table 1 GHT audits: the number of LBP patients and NHS physiotherapy treatment sessions by risk category and year

stratified care model risk category	2013		2014		total	
	number (%) of patients	mean number (sd) of treatment sessions	number (%) of patients	mean number (sd) of treatment sessions	number (%) of patients	mean number (sd) of treatment sessions
Low	30 (30)	1.63 (1.2)	29 (29)	2.31 (1.9)	59 (29)	1.97 (1.6)
Medium	36 (36)	2.31 (1.4)	40 (40)	3.18 (3.2)	76 (38)	2.76 (2.5)
High	35 (35)	3.09 (3.0)	31 (31)	3.42 (2.5)	66 (33)	3.24 (2.8)
Total	101 (100)	2.38 (2.1)	100 (100)	3.00 (2.7)	201 (100)	2.69 (2.4)

sd standard deviation

Table 2 IMPaCT Back study: the number of LBP patients and NHS physiotherapy treatment sessions by risk category

stratified care model risk category	pre-implementation: phase 1			post-implementation: phase 3			% change in mean number of treatment sessions between phases 1 and 3
	all patients[a]	patients providing data at 6 months[b]		all patients[a]	patients providing data at 6 months[b]		
	number (%)	number (%)	mean number (sd) of treatment sessions	number (%)	number (%)	mean number (sd) of treatment sessions	
Low	136 (37)	81 (35)	1.05 (2.3)	214 (39)	110 (35)	1.14 (3.3)	9
Medium	151 (41)	104 (45)	1.45 (0.8)	232 (42)	143 (46)	2.08 (3.0)	43
High	81 (22)	48 (21)	1.87 (2.8)	108 (20)	61 (19)	2.67 (3.9)	43
Total	368 (100)	233 (100)	1.40	554 (100)	314 (100)	1.87	33

sd standard deviation
[a]Source: risk-category level data from Hill et al., [10, Table 1]
[b]Source: risk-category level data from Whitehurst et al., [13, web appendix table 3b]

(Table 3). The audit year, patient gender and physiotherapists' seniority were not significant explanatory variables (Table 3). However, compared to patients in the low-risk category, patients in the medium- and high-risk categories received on average 29.3% and 54.6% more treatment sessions, respectively, and these differences were statistically significant (Table 3). This finding confirms that GHT experienced treatment patterns, in terms of the number of physiotherapy sessions provided, in line with the expectations of the stratified care model.

Running the model with patient age for the 184 patients for whom the data were available did not change the results. In order to provide an alternative measure of physiotherapist-level effects, a linear fixed-effects regression model was also run. The risk-category results were not sensitive to choice of model (patients in the medium- and high-risk categories received on average 31.0% or 61.9% more treatment sessions, respectively, compared to patients in the low-risk category, and these differences were significant at the 5% level), although the audit year variable was also significant and indicated that patients in the 2014 audit received 24.7% more treatment sessions than those in the 2013 audit. Omitting physiotherapist as an independent variable altogether in a fixed-effects model found patients in the high-risk category receiving on average 55.3% more treatment sessions, compared to patients in the low-risk category, and the difference was significant ($p = 0.01$), but the 25.8% increase for medium-risk patients was not significant ($p = 0.06$).

Physiotherapists' views on the usefulness of the stratified care model

The audits requested the physiotherapist to record their view on whether or not the risk category accurately reflected the patient, in other words whether they thought that the prognostic risk-rating had aided them in managing the condition, and any comment on the usefulness of the screening tool. These data for the high-risk patients in the 2013 audit were not available for the study and so the analysis of these data is limited to the 2014 audit. In 67% (67/100) of cases the physiotherapist indicated that the screening tool had accurately reflected the patient, compared to 15% taking the opposite view, and 18% not responding to the question (Table 4). When the physiotherapist noted that the screening tool had accurately reflected the patient, the pattern of mean treatment sessions was in line with the expectations of the stratified care model: more sessions were provided to higher-risk patients (Table 4). However, this was not the case when physiotherapist noted that the screening tool had not accurately reflected the patient, or had not responded to the question (Table 4).

In the 2014 audit, comments were recorded by 13 of the 18 physiotherapists on their views of the usefulness of the screening tool for 43 of the 100 patients, and other comments were reported for a further 12 cases. Our analysis of the comments focuses first on those cases where the screening tool was viewed as having accurately reflected the patient, before considering those cases where the screening tool was not viewed as having accurately reflected the patient. In the two-thirds of cases when the physiotherapist had indicated that the screening tool had accurately reflected the patient, the comments on usefulness were positive in 93% (28/30) cases. The positive comments applied across risk categories, patient ages, physiotherapist seniority, diagnoses and treatments, and they suggest benefits for both the patient, for example *"prompted discussion about concerns – enabling reassurance"*, and physiotherapist, for example *"v useful, guided me to give advice & d/c [discharge]"*. For low-risk patients the feedback suggests that use of the tool guided management and discharge, while for medium- and high-risk patients it facilitated communication between physiotherapists and patients which led to anxiety being identified and then addressed.

Table 3 GHT audits multilevel linear regression model coefficients for log of the number of treatment sessions

fixed effects	coefficient	exponential of coefficient	p value	95% CIs
audit year	0.146	1.157	0.160	−0.058 to 0.350
patient gender	0.061	1.063	0.529	−0.130 to 0.253
physio seniority	−0.132	0.876	0.351	−0.410 to 0.145
Risk (low)				
medium	0.257	1.293	0.032	0.022 to 0.492
high	0.435	1.546	<0.001	0.192 to 0.679
intercept	0.389	1.475	0.184	−0.184 to 0.961
Random effects	estimate		95% CIs	
physiotherapist				
sd cons	0.191		0.077 to 0.470	
sd residual	0.667		0.601 to 0.741	

Table 4 GHT 2014 audit: physiotherapists' view on whether the risk category accurately reflected the patient by risk category and number of patients and NHS treatment sessions

stratified care model risk category	'yes'		'no'		'no response'	
	number (%) of patients	mean number (sd) of treatment sessions	number (%) of patients	mean number (sd) of treatment sessions	number (%) of patients	mean number (sd) of treatment sessions
Low	19 (28)	1.6 (1.1)	4 (27)	4.5 (2.4)	6 (33)	3.2 (2.2)
Medium	26 (39)	2.4 (2.3)	6 (40)	2.0 (1.5)	8 (44)	6.6 (4.4)
High	22 (33)	3.5 (2.7)	5 (33)	3.0 (2.4)	4 (22)	3.3 (2.2)
Total	67 (100)	2.5 (2.3)	15 (100)	3.0 (2.2)	18 (100)	4.7 (3.6)

sd standard deviation

Two comments were not positive; one was for a low-risk patient presenting with posterior/lateral derangement who received five treatment sessions before being discharged and the physiotherapist's comment was *"Due to symptoms & progressions of HEP [home exercise programme] needed low category did not reflect no. of treatments needed. Also had hip issue which needed clarification"*. The other case was a medium-risk patient presenting with mechanical LBP who received one treatment session before being discharged and the physiotherapist's comment was *"No it didn't guide management"*.

Comments on usefulness were made for 13 of the 15 cases where the physiotherapist had indicated that the screening tool had not accurately reflected the patient. In the four low-risk cases, the physiotherapist viewed the patient as being more anxious or requiring more clinical support than that indicated by the low-risk classification, and in each case the patient received more than one treatment session. Of the six medium-risk cases, comments on two indicated that the risk-rating may not be optimal; being either too high *"More easily reassured than tool score suggested"* or too low *"I feel high risk category may have been more appropriate"*. In two cases, the comments indicated that the use of any care model was not relevant; *"Did not guide treatment as pt v specific about what she wanted"* and *"Not useful as pt seeking advice about falls protection"*. In the other two cases, the comments do not provide insight into why the screening tool was *"not helpful"* or *"not relevant for this pt"*. Of the high-risk patients, two cases suggest that initial patient anxiety was addressed such that the high-risk classification may not have been warranted: *"Anxious due to acute onset but able to reassure"* was the comment for one of patients, who did not attend a second treatment session. The third high-risk case appeared to illustrate inappropriate completion of the screening tool: *"Main problem OA hip & pt misinterpreted tool by answering re hip pain"*. Overall, where the physiotherapist had indicated that the screening tool had not accurately reflected the patient, their comments suggest the risk-rating was viewed as too low in five cases and too high in three cases.

Potential economic consequences associated with the rollout in Gloucestershire

The IMPaCT Back study estimated the incremental change in NHS costs and healthcare costs (NHS and private) associated with the introduction of the stratified care model using data imputation methods for its full patient sample ($n = 922$) (Table 5) [12]. The changes in these costs by risk category up-rated to 2014/15 values are summarised in Table 5, which shows that applying the percentage of patients in each risk-category

experienced in the GHT audits (Table 1), generates an estimated aggregate incremental back-related NHS cost saving of £0.65 per patient associated with the stratified care model. Similarly, applying the IMPaCT Back study's estimated incremental change in QALYs to the percentages of patients in each risk-category experienced in the GHT audits gives an estimated aggregate incremental QALY gain of 0.006 per patient associated with the stratified care model (Table 5). The estimated annual number of patients referred for LBP physiotherapy treatment in Gloucestershire is 5217 patients (Table 5), which suggests a NHS cost saving of approximately £3400 per annum and an associated gain of approximately 30.2 QALYs and a net monetary benefit of approximately £909,000. The NMB is based on the cost-effectiveness threshold associated with NICE of £30,000 per QALY, and an alternative empirically estimated threshold of £15,500 per QALY for musculoskeletal treatments implies associated NMB of £471,000.

The estimate of the annual number of patients referred for LBP physiotherapy treatment may be conservative; it assumes that 20% of the estimated annual consulting prevalence for LBP in primary care is referred. In practice, for example, some LBP patients may be referred for physiotherapy more than once in a year. If 25% of the estimated annual consulting prevalence for LBP in primary care is referred, the annual NHS cost saving would be approximately £4200 with an associated gain of 37.7 QALYs and NMB of £1,136,000 (or £589,000 based on the alternative empirically estimated cost-effectiveness threshold).

These findings are sensitive to the percentage of patients in each risk-category; applying those for all patients in the post-implementation phase of IMPaCT Back study (Table 2) result in an overall increase in mean back-related NHS costs of £1.13 per patient (£1.03 up-rated to 2014/15 values). This indicates an increase in NHS costs of approximately £5900 and an increase in 14.1 QALYs and NMB of £418,000 (or £213,000 based on the empirically estimated threshold) in Gloucestershire.

The IMPaCT Back study reported productivity losses associated with LBP-related work absence following the introduction of the stratified care model [13], which suggests a mean saving of £545 per employed patient (in 2014 values) (Table 6). Applying the IMPaCT study's estimates of the percentage of LBP patients in work, and the mean change in the number of days of LBP-related work absence during the 6 months following the introduction of the stratified care model, to the estimated annual number of patients referred for LBP physiotherapy treatment in Gloucestershire, suggests a saving of approximately 10,500 days of work absence valued at £1.4 million (Table 6).

Table 5 Estimated change to back-related NHS costs and QALYs associated with introducing stratified care in Gloucestershire

stratified care model risk category	% patients in risk category[a]	mean incremental costs and QALYs per patient over 6 months associated with the stratified care model[b]				annual referrals for LBP physio. in Glos.[c]	annual incremental impact for Gloucestershire:		
		Costs (£)			QALYs		NHS cost (£ 1000)	QALY gain	NMB[d] (£ 1000)
		NHS	private	total					
Low	29	−6.58	9.85	3.27	0.003	1531	−10.1	4.6	147.9
Medium	38	14.96	−23.52	−8.56	−0.007	1973	29.5	−13.8	−443.8
High	33	−13.33	−122.61	−135.93	0.023	1713	−22.8	39.4	1204.8
Total	100	−0.65	−46.26	−46.91	0.006	5217	−3.4	30.2	909.0

physio physiotherapy, *Glos* Gloucestershire, *NMB* net monetary benefit
[a]Source: GHT audits (Table 1)
[b]Source: IMPaCT Back study [13, Table 3]. Costs up-rated to 2014/15 values using the HCHS index [31]: private costs extrapolated from NHS and total (healthcare) costs
[c]Source: 20% [10, 30] of 26,085, the estimated annual consulting prevalence for LBP in primary care [3] applied to Gloucestershire gender and age-specific population rates for 2013 [31]
[d]assuming a cost-effectiveness threshold of £30,000 per QALY

Table 6 Estimated change to productivity costs associated with introducing stratified care in Gloucestershire

Risk category	IMPaCT Back study estimates[a]			Gloucestershire estimates		
	% of LBP patients in work	change in mean no days off work for employed patients	Change in mean cost of LBP-related work absence[b] (£)	Number of LBP patients in work[c]	mean change in no of days of LBP-related work absence	Change in cost of LBP-related work absence (£ million)
Low	57	0.3	94	873	288	0.1
Medium	48	−6.1	−909	947	−5785	−0.9
High	48	−6.1	−805	822	−4975	−0.7
Total	51	−4.0	−545	2642	−10,472	−1.4

[a]Source: [13, Table 4]

[b]Costs over 6 months up-rated to 2014 prices using the retail price index [32]

[c]Applying the IMPaCT Back study's estimate of the percentage of LBP patients in work and the annual estimated annual referrals for LBP physiotherapy in Gloucestershire (Table 5)

As above, assuming a higher estimate of incidence of 25% of the annual consulting prevalence indicates a productivity loss saving of approximately 13,100 days of work absence valued at £1.8 million. Alternatively applying the percentage of patients in each risk-category from the IMPaCT Back study post-implementation phase (Table 2) result in a mean saving of £461 per employed patient (in 2014 values), and an aggregate productivity loss saving of approximately 9000 days of work absence valued at £1.2 million.

Discussion

In 2013, the physiotherapy department at GHT started to use the stratified care model for LBP patients, with the expectation that prognostic screening and matched treatment pathways would improve the pattern of activity, such that at the extremes low-risk patients would be appropriately discharged after a single treatment session, and high-risk patients would receive a psychologically-informed treatment package to address psychosocial obstacles to recovery as well as physical symptoms and function [10]. The analysis of the GHT audit data indicates that the use of the stratified care model was broadly associated with the anticipated pattern of treatment sessions. On the whole, patients received more treatment sessions as the patients' risk-rating increased, having controlled for patient and physiotherapist characteristics, which suggests that the stratified care model was supporting the intended treatment practice.

The physiotherapists' audit feedback on the model confirmed that the risk-rating was viewed as accurately reflecting the patient in 82% (67/82) of the cases where data were reported. Comments on the cases where the patient was not viewed as being accurately reflected by the risk-rating indicated a few cases where the physiotherapist felt that a different rating would have been appropriate. One of the factors cited relates to patient anxiety, and to the extent that its impact can be addressed, the findings suggest that it is important for physiotherapists to have appropriate specialist training. When the physiotherapists viewed the prognostic risk-rating as having aided them in managing the LBP, the mean number of treatment sessions was 1.6, which indicates that many of these low-risk patients were discharged after one session in line with expectations of the Keele model. The audit data also show that there were a few instances where the model was not viewed as relevant because, for one reason or another, the patient was not primarily seeking treatment for LBP. This issue may have influenced the omission of recording a response to the audit question on whether or not the tool accurately reflected the patient. If we assume that all non-responses to this question indicated that the risk-rating was not viewed as accurately reflecting the patient, then in 67%

(67/100) of the cases the audit feedback on the model confirmed that the risk-rating was viewed as accurately reflecting the patient. When the physiotherapists' gave feedback on the prognostic screening tool it was dominated by positive views, which represent an important component of this impact assessment.

The potential economic consequences associated with the introduction of the stratified model in Gloucestershire were estimated by applying published economic evaluation findings on back-related NHS costs, QALYs and societal productivity losses to the local experience of the proportion of patients in each risk category, and estimates of local incidence. This approach suggests that the introduction of the model could achieve an annual incremental gain of about 30 QALYs generating a net monetary benefit of £471,000, on the basis of an empirically-estimated cost-effectiveness threshold of half the level indicated by NICE. Looking beyond benefits associated with health-related quality of life, the economic evaluation evidence suggests that a societal benefit from fewer work days lost because of LBP corresponds to a productivity loss saving of £1.4 million which could be achieved by rolling out the model in Gloucestershire. The economic evaluation evidence suggests that these benefits are associated with almost no impact on NHS costs.

The strengths of the study lie in its analysis combining local audit data and published economic evaluation results to assess the potential of the stratified care model in a physiotherapy department setting. The analysis of the physiotherapists' views of the risk-rating is a strength of the study, albeit limited by the necessity to focus on the 2014 audit data. The analysis demonstrates a pragmatic approach to applying trial findings to a real world scenario. The analysis is limited by its reliance on the audits to collect data on use of the stratified care model, and literature-based estimates of the number of LBP patients receiving physiotherapy. While our findings may not be generalisable to other settings, our analytical approach could be widely employed to assess the potential impact of the stratified care model.

The extent to which the IMPaCT Back study can inform the potential impact of introducing the stratified care model in a setting such as Gloucestershire depends on the extent to which the study's experience is likely to be relevant. The general context is similar in terms of both settings being in the NHS in England, and the IMPaCT Back study being based on largely urban general practices in Staffordshire, while the Gloucestershire audits were based on patients mostly from the Gloucester locality. However, the IMPaCT Back study involved GPs administering the screening tool and hence their decisions to refer patients for physiotherapy, whereas in Gloucestershire the tool was administered by physiotherapists following GP referral, or in some cases, patient self-referral.

This means that the denominator in each setting is different; the GHT patients represent a subset of comparatively higher-risk referred patients, compared to those in the IMPaCT Back study. This difference in context may account for the 39% low-risk patients in the phase 3 IMPaCT Back study compared to 29% in the GHT audits. The consequences are appreciable; the GHT risk-specific percentages are associated with an additional net monetary benefit of £201,000 compared to the phase 3 IMPaCT Back study, based on the conservative empirically-estimated cost-effectiveness threshold. To the extent that the stratified care model may for logistical reasons be more likely to be implemented by physiotherapists for referred patients, rather than by GPs in primary care, the GHT experience provides new insight into the scale of the stratified care model's potential benefits. Having noted the similarities and differences in context between the IMPaCT Back study and the use of the tool in Gloucestershire, we view that the risk-level treatment effects found in the IMPaCT Back study provide a reasonable, and certainly the best available, basis for estimating the potential consequences for rolling out the stratified care model in Gloucestershire. The IMPaCT Back study found that pre-implementation of the Keele model, the mean number of treatment sessions increased with the risk rating, and that after the introduction of the Keele model, patients with higher risk-ratings received comparatively more treatment sessions. We assume that GHT will experience similar risk-level treatment effects. Better estimates of impact would require a local cost-utility analysis, entailing collection of data on resource use, costs and health-related quality of life, both before and after the introduction of the Keele model and for a suitable control group.

Being a sequential comparison study, rather than a randomised trial, the IMPaCT Back study must be considered with caution. Nevertheless, its findings about the risk-specific incremental impact on NHS costs and outcomes offer a guide for likely experience in Gloucestershire. From a commissioner's decision-making perspective, the IMPaCT Back study's main analysis would have been even more informative if it had been undertaken from an NHS perspective, in line with NICE guidance [33], rather than a healthcare perspective. The reported healthcare cost savings are due to a reduction in mean private treatment costs largely experienced by high-risk patients (Table 5). The inclusion of private costs in the main Keele economic evaluations mean that the analysis of uncertainty, using cost-utility planes and cost-effectiveness acceptability curves, may be of comparatively limited value for commissioners. Furthermore, while the IMPaCT Back study's reporting at risk-defined subgroup level emphasises the dominance of the intervention for high-risk patients, and the opposite for medium-risk patients, our analysis indicates that the stratified care model is dominant for the whole

patient group represented by the GHT audits (i.e. reduced NHS costs, albeit very slightly, and gains in health-related quality of life). Economic theory indicates that the uncertainty relating to this outcome, where differences in cost and QALYs are not statistically significant [13] should not impede implementation, but should prompt consideration of commissioning a value of information study to assess whether further research should be undertaken [34]. In this instance, a pragmatic response would be to focus future local quality improvement effort on ensuring that the treatment package for medium-risk patients has an optimal impact on health-related quality of life. This would be facilitated by routine coding of outpatient attendances by clinical diagnosis and, when used, the risk-stratification scores.

The estimated net monetary benefit associated with the adoption of the stratified care model is substantial, despite the estimated mean incremental QALY gain being modest over 6 months (0.006), because of the large number of patients and small cost consequences (Table 5). This raises the question of whether other LBP interventions are associated with larger impact on health-related quality of life. The NHS advice, assessment and group cognitive behavioural therapy (CBT) intervention reported by Lamb et al. [19, 35, 36] stands out for achieving a comparatively large incremental QALY gain of 0.099 over 12 months. However, comparison with the stratified care model is not straightforward. First, a follow-up study of 56% (395/701) of the original trial participants, who were older and had less disability and pain at baseline compared to the full patient cohort, found no incremental gain in EQ5D scores at 3, 6, 12 or the average follow-up period of 34 months [36]. This suggests that as for the stratified care model, QALY gains may be mostly attributable to those patients with a poorer prognosis. Second, the CBT study reported a secondary analysis of costs, aiming to reflect the likely costs for NHS rather than those associated with the delivery of the trial, which estimated a £96 incremental NHS cost over 12 months largely due to the £126 intervention cost per patient [35]. These costs represent a considerable additional resource requirement in comparison to the stratified care model of about £497,000 in Gloucestershire. Commissioners may favour the stratified care model in this case because of the NHS resource consequences. However, the CBT intervention's estimated costs may not be readily comparable with those of other non-group-based interventions. This is because it allocated session costs to the number of patients that attended, so the cost of resource allocated to the patients who did not attend sessions were included. In contrast, the cost of resource allocated to the patients who did not attend booked physiotherapy sessions in the stratified care model studies were not included. Furthermore, it may be that the CBT intervention could be targeted and delivered in fewer sessions, as only 62% of participants attended at least 3 of the 6 group sessions held [35]. Overall, it would be interesting to see whether the stratified care model's impact on health-related quality of life could be enhanced by combining the risk-stratification tool with targeted use of group CBT. The draft guideline on the management of non-specific LBP published by the National Clinical Guideline Centre in February 2016 endorsed consideration of the STarT Back risk assessment tool for risk stratification along with a range of potential treatment options including psychological therapies for managing LBP as part of multi-modal treatment packages or combined physical and psychological programme for people with persistent LBP [37].

Conclusion

The Keele stratified care model was implemented and risk-specific treatment pathways successfully used for patients presenting with LBP for physiotherapy in Gloucestershire. The physiotherapists' feedback on using the prognostic screening tool was very positive. Applying published economic evidence to the Gloucestershire locality suggests that substantial health and productivity outcomes would be associated with rollout of the Keele model while being largely cost-neutral for the NHS.

Abbreviations
CBT: Cognitive behavioural therapy; GHT: Gloucestershire Hospitals NHS Foundation Trust; GP: General practitioner; HCHS: Hospital and community health services; HEP: Home exercise programme; LBP: Low back pain; NICE: National Institute of Health and Care Excellence; NMB: Net monetary benefit; QALYs: Quality-adjusted life years

Acknowledgements
We thank Dr Karla Hemming of the University of Birmingham for statistical advice and Zara Strinati of GHT for support with extracting information from the patient administration system.

Funding
No specific funding was provided for this study.

Authors' contributions
HM, LA and SD designed the study. AN undertook the GHT audits. AB collated the data and undertook the analysis with supervision by LA and HM. HM and AB led the writing of the manuscript to which LA, SD, AN and ER contributed. All authors read and approved the final manuscript.

Authors' information
Part of this study was undertaken as a MSc in Health Economics and Health Policy dissertation at the University of Birmingham by AB supervised by HM and LA. HM was seconded to Gloucestershire Clinical Commissioning Group between May and October 2015.

Competing interests
The authors declare that they have no competing interests.

Consent for publication
Not applicable.

Author details
[1]Gloucestershire Hospitals NHS Foundation Trust, Gloucester, UK. [2]University of Birmingham, Birmingham, UK. [3]Gloucestershire Clinical Commissioning Group, Gloucester, UK.

References
1. Maniadakis N, Gray A. The economic burden of low back pain in the United Kingdom. Pain. 2000;84(1):95–103.
2. Newton JN, Briggs AD, Murray CJ, Dicker D, Foreman K, Wang H, et al. Changes in health in England, with analysis by English regions and areas of deprivation, 1990–2013: a systematic analysis for the Global Burden of Disease Study 2013. Lancet. 2015;386:2257–74.
3. Jordan K, Kadam U, Hayward R, Porcheret M, Young C, Croft P. Consultant prevalence of regional musculoskeletal problems in primary care: an observational study. BMC Musculoskelet Di. 2010;11:144–51.
4. Savigny P, Kuntze S, Watson P, Underwood M, Ritchie G, Cotterell M, et al. Low Back Pain: early management of persistent non-specific low back pain. London: National Collaborating Centre for Primary Care and Royal College of General Practitioners; 2009.
5. Chartered Institute of Personnel and Development. Absence Management 2015 Annual Survey Report. London: Chartered Institute of Personnel and Development; 2015.
6. Chou R, Huffman LH. Nonpharmacologic therapies for acute and chronic low back pain: a review of the evidence for an American Pain Society/ American College of Physicians clinical practice guideline. Ann Intern Med. 2007;147(7):492–504.
7. Bishop A, Foster NE, Thomas E, Hay EM. How does the self-reported clinical management of patients with low back pain relate to the attitudes and beliefs of health care practitioners? A survey of UK general practitioners and physiotherapists. Pain. 2008;135(1–2):187–95.
8. Royal College of General Practitioners. In: Guidance NIfHaCE, editor. Low Back Pain: Early Management of Persistent Non-specific Low Back Pain. London: Royal College of General Practitioners (UK); 2009.
9. Costa LCM, Koes BW, Pransky G, Borkan J, Maher CG, Smeets RJEM. Primary care research priorities in low back pain: an update. Spine. 2013;38(2):148–56.
10. Hill JC, Whitehurst DG, Lewis M, Bryan S, Dunn KM, Foster NE, et al. Comparison of stratified primary care management for low back pain with current best practice (STarT Back): a randomised controlled trial. Lancet. 2011;378(9802):1560–71.
11. Whitehurst DGT, Bryan S, Lewis M, Hill J, Hay E. Exploring the cost-utility of stratified primary care management of low back pain compared with current best practice within risk-defined subgroups. Ann Rheum Dis. 2012;10:1136.
12. Foster N, Mullis R, Hill J, Lewis M, Whitehurst D, Doyle C, et al. Effect of stratified care for low back pain in family practice (impact back): a prospective population-based sequential comparison. Ann Fam Med. 2014;12(2):102–11.
13. Whitehurst DGT, Bryan S, Lewis M, Hay E, Mullis R, Foster N. Implementing stratified primary care management for low back pain: cost-utility analysis alongside a prospective population-based. sequential comparison study. Spine. 2015;40(6):405–14.
14. Johnson RE, Jones GT, Wiles NJ, Chaddock C, Potter RG, Roberts C, et al. Active exercise, education, and cognitive behavioral therapy for persistent disabling low back pain: a randomized controlled trial. Spine. 2007;32(15):1578–85.
15. Whitehurst DG, Lewis M, Yao GL, Bryan S, Raftery JP, Mullis R, et al. A brief pain management program compared with physical therapy for low back pain: results from an economic analysis alongside a randomized clinical trial. Arthritis Rheum. 2007;57(3):466–73.
16. Critchley DJ, Ratcliffe J, Noonan S, Jones RH, Hurley MV. Effectiveness and cost-effectiveness of three types of physiotherapy used to reduce chronic low back pain disability: a pragmatic randomized trial with economic evaluation. Spine. 2007;32(14):1474–81.
17. Rogerson MD, Gatchel RJ, Bierner SM. A cost utility analysis of interdisciplinary early intervention versus treatment as usual for high-risk acute low back pain patients. Pain Pract. 2010;10(5):382–95.
18. Skouen JS, Grasdal AL, Haldorsen EM, Ursin H. Relative cost-effectiveness of extensive and light multidisciplinary treatment programs versus treatment as usual for patients with chronic low back pain on long-term sick leave: randomized controlled study. Spine. 2002;27(9):901–9.
19. Lamb SE, Hansen Z, Lall R, Castelnuovo E, Withers EJ, Nichols V, et al. Group cognitive behavioural treatment for low-back pain in primary care: a randomised controlled trial and cost-effectiveness analysis. Lancet. 2010;375(9718):916–23.

Implementing the Keele stratified care model for patients with low back pain: an observational impact...

85

20. Norton G, McDonough CM, Cabral H, Shwartz M, Burgess JF. Cost-utility of cognitive behavioral therapy for low back pain from the commercial payer perspective. Spine. 2015;40(10):725–33.

21. Schweikert B, Jacobi E, Seitz R, Cziske R, Ehlert A, Knab J, et al. Effectiveness and cost-effectiveness of adding a cognitive behavioral treatment to the rehabilitation of chronic low back pain. J Rheumatol. 2006;33(12):2519–26.

22. Hill JC, Dunn KM, Lewis M, Mullis R, Main C, Foster N, Hay E. A primary care back pain screening tool: identifying patient subgroups for initial treatment. Arthritis Rheum. 2008;59:632–41.

23. Hay EM, Dunn KM, Hill JC, Lewis M, Mason E, Konstantinou K, et al. A randomised clinical trial of subgrouping and targeted treatment for low back pain compared with best current care. The STarT Back Trial Study Protocol. BMC Musculoskelet Dis. 2008;9:58. doi:10.1186/1471-2474-9-58.

24. West Midlands Academic Health Science Network. Person-centred care STarT Back. http://www.wmahsn.org/programmes/view/start-back. Accessed 5 Apr 2016.

25. Keele University. STarT Back Commissioners Impact. https://www.keele.ac.uk/sbst/commissioners/impact/. Accessed 5 Apr 2016.

26. Wooldridge J. Introductory Econometrics. A modern approach. 4th ed. Mason: South Western College; 2009.

27. Ritchie J, Spencer L, O'Connor W. Carrying out qualitative analysis. In: Ritchie J, Lewis J, editors. Qualitative research practice: A guide for social science students and researchers. London: Sage; 2003.

28. Drummond M, Sculpher M, Claxton K, Stoddart G, Torrance G. Methods for the economic evaluation of health care programmes. 4th ed. Oxford: Oxford University Press; 2015.

29. Claxton K, Martin S, Soares M, Rice N, Spackman E, Hinde S, et al. Methods for the estimation of the NICE cost effectiveness threshold. York: CHE Research Paper 81; 2013.

30. Dunn K. Epidemiology of low back pain in primary care: a cohort study of consulters PhD thesis. Staffordshire: Keele University; 2004.

31. Office for National Statistics. Annual mid year population estimates: 2013. http://www.ons.gov.uk/peoplepopulationandcommunity/populationandmigration/populationestimates/bulletins/annualmidyearpopulationestimates/2014-06-26. Accessed 5 Apr 2016.

32. Curtis L, Burns A. Unit Costs of Health and Social Care 2014. Canterbury: Personal Social Services Research Unit; 2015.

33. National Institute for Health and Care Excellence. Guide to the methods of technology appraisal 2013. https://www.nice.org.uk/process/pmg9/chapter/foreword. Accessed 5 Apr 2016.

34. Claxton K. The irrelevance of inference: a decision-making approach to the stochastic evaluation of health care technologies. J Health Econ. 1999;18:341–64.

35. Lamb S, Lall R, Hansen Z, Castelnuovo E, Withers EJ, Nichols V, et al. A multicentred randomised controlled trial of a primary care-based cognitive behavioural programme for low back pain. The back skills training (BeST) trial. Health Technol Asses. 2010;14(41):iii–253.

36. Lamb S, Mistry D, Lall R, Hansen Z, Evans D, Withers E, et al. Group cognitive behavioural interventions for low back pain in primary care: extended follow-up of the Back Skills Training Trial (ISRCTN54717854). Pain. 2012;153(2):494–501.

37. National Clinical Guideline Centre. Low back pain and sciatica: management of non-specific low back pain and sciatica. Draft for consultation. London: National Clinical Guideline Centre; 2016.

7

Are paraspinous intramuscular injections of botulinum toxin a (BoNT-A) efficient in the treatment of chronic low-back pain?

Mélanie Cogné[1,2,3]*, Hervé Petit[2], Alexandre Creuzé[2], Dominique Liguoro[4] and Mathieu de Seze[2,3]

Abstract

Background: Treatment for patients with chronic low-back pain (LBP) is a public health issue. Intramuscular injections of botulinum toxin A (BoNT-A) have shown an analgesic effect on LBP in two previous randomized controlled studies. The objective of the study was to verify the efficacy of paravertebral injections of BoNT-A in patients with LBP.

Methods: Patients were included in this phase 3 randomized double-blinded trial comparing the efficacy of BoNT-A versus placebo in a crossover study on LBP. Both groups received 200 units of BoNT-A in paravertebral muscles or a placebo, and vice versa at Day 120. The main judgment criterion was LBP intensity 1 month after the injections, evaluated by using a visual pain scale (VAS). Secondary assessment criteria included: LBP intensity 90 and 120 days after injection day; number of days when an allowed antalgic oral treatment was needed in between each evaluation; functional disability measured by the Quebec Back Pain Disability Scale; quality of life; inability to work; patient satisfaction in relation to the treatment's effect; spinal mobility; and strength of spinal muscles, measured by isokinetic technique.

Results: Nineteen patients completed the study. There was no significant difference between the groups' average LBP during the last 8 days at Day30 ($p = 0.97$). There was no significant difference between the two groups regarding the secondary assessment criteria ($p > 0.05$).

Conclusions: Injections of BoNT-A in the paravertebral muscles were not found to be effective to relieve chronic LBP. The limits of the study are that the dose of BoNT-A used was lower than in other studies, and that the limited number of patients included may explain the negative results.

Keywords: Low-back pain, Botulinum toxin, Disability, Function, Quality of life, Work

Background

Chronic low-back pain (LBP) is a public health problem that concerns 5 to 7% of the general occidental population [1] and has a significant impact on the quality of life of its sufferers [2].

Since the significance of lumbar stiffness in relation to contraction of the erector spinae muscles has been linked to the level of intensity of LBP [3], the lumbar erector spinae muscles have become a therapeutic target. Many recent arguments purport that paravertebral muscles have a predominant pathogenic role in perpetuating chronic back pain. During spinal movements, paravertebral muscles' activity, recorded by electromyography, show abnormalities in subjects with low-back pain compared to subjects without LBP. A decrease in the power ratio between the erector spinae and flexor spinal muscles, measured by isokinetic techniques, is associated with chronic low-back pain. Finally, the significance of lumbar stiffness in relation to the erector spinae muscles contracting is linked to the level of intensity of low-back pain [3].

* Correspondence: melaniecogne@hotmail.fr
[1]Service de Médecine Physique et de Réadaptation, hôpital Raymond Poincaré, 92380 Garches, France
[2]Service de Médecine Physique et de Réadaptation, CHU de Bordeaux, 33076 Bordeaux, France
Full list of author information is available at the end of the article

Local muscular treatments have already been tried such as physiotherapy, massage, infrared therapy and botulinum toxin A (BoNT-A) [4–6].

In addition to its muscle-relaxing effect, local intramuscular injections of BoNT-A have also shown an analgesic effect on pain related to dystonia, tension headaches, myofascial pain syndrome and chronic neck pain [7–11]. This effect is usually reversible after 3 months. Foster et al. [4] used BoNT-A A for its peripheral muscle relaxant action as a local intramuscular treatment of chronic LBP. This double-blinded, placebo, controlled trial in 31 patients showed that paravertebral administration of BoNT-A in patients with chronic LBP relieved pain and improved function at 3 and 8 weeks after treatment. Machado et al. [6] showed also in a randomized controlled trial that BoNT-A injections relieved pain and improved quality of life of 19 patients at 4 weeks. Further open studies have been performed to value the efficacy of BoNT-A in patients with chronic LBP [12–15] but all of them aimed to establish predictive factors of pain relief, and the efficacy was limited to 3 months. A Cochrane meta-analysis [16] concluded that "there was low quality evidence in the short term, and very low quality in the intermediate term, that BoNT-A injections reduced pain intensity more effectively than saline injections in participants with LBP" and that "there was very low quality evidence that BoNT-A injections compared to corticosteroid injections could reduce chronic LBP intensity in the short term".

Studying the therapeutic effect of paravertebral injections of BoNT-A requires further studies to confirm the reported short-term therapeutic effect and to determine potential predictive factors of efficacy.

Objectives of this trial

Main objective: To evaluate the analgesic effect 1 month after a single injection of 200 IU of BoNT-A in 10 bilateral paravertebral intramuscular points for treating chronic LBP.

Secondary objectives

- To evaluate the analgesic effect of paravertebral injections of BoNT-A 3 months after its administration in chronic LBP sufferers.
- To measure the impact of paravertebral injections of 200 IU of BoNT-A in a single administration on lumbar stiffness and on spinal extensor muscle strength in patients with chronic LBP.
- To search for predictive factors of the analgesic effect of BoNT-A injections.

Materials and methods

This study was a randomized, double-blinded, placebo-controlled phase 3 trial comparing BoNT-A Type A injections (Botox) to a placebo in patients with chronic LBP (Level 2, OCEBM Levels of Evidence Working Group*, "The Oxford 2011 Levels of Evidence"). This superiority trial obtained support from the French Hospital Clinical Research Project (PHRC).

The number of participants included in the study was similar as those included in the previous study (see [4]), that showed a strong positive effect of BoNT-A injections on LBP. Furthermore, the design of our study (i.e. a crossover) increased the power of the statistical analysis. In this context, 60 inclusions were planned (30 in each group). Nevertheless, regular intermediary analyses were planned by an independent scientific committee, to ensure that the trial did not present any secondary effect, or that we could conclude in an intermediary step that BoNT-A was inefficient in pain relief. After obtaining a similar number of injections than Foster, the study was stopped by the scientific committee, because there was no trend in pain relief.

Ethics, consent and permissions

This trial obtained the approval of a French ethics Committee (2003/02) and all participants received an information note and gave their written informed consent. The clinical trial registration number was: Identifiers: NCT03181802, Unique Protocol ID: CHUBX2003.

Population

The patients included were consulted by Physical and Rehabilitation Medicine spinal pathology specialists at the University Hospital of Bordeaux, met the eligibility criteria, and volunteered to participate in the study.

Inclusion criteria were: LBP defined as a pain located between the thoracic lumbar hinge and the gluteal sulcus, where pain had evolved over a period of 6 months despite well conducted medical treatment, self-assessed lumbar pain intensity over 50 mm long on a visual analogue scale of 100 mm (0 = no pain; 100 = maximal pain), having been on sick leave for 60 or more days in the year preceding the inclusion (in order to include patients with high consequences of chronic low-back pain on their work), the same long-term chronic pain treatment for at least 6 weeks, and a paravertebral painful point pressure.

Exclusion criteria were: age under 18 or over 55 years (to avoid secondary causes of low back pain, like spinal tumor), ongoing pregnancy or breast-feeding, a neuromuscular pathology (myasthenia gravis, amyotrophic lateral sclerosis, myopathy, polymyositis), aminoglycoside treatment at the time of inclusion, skin infection at injection points, diabetes and alcoholism (in order to avoid other etiologies of chronic pain), a history of injecting BoNT-A A, anticoagulation treatment, sciatica, suspected spinal inflammatory disorder (spondylitis, inflammatory rheumatism, tumoral pathology), a failed back surgery syndrome (when surgery failed to relieve low-back pain), incapacity to stand, cardiorespiratory deficiency which does not allow the isokinetic exploration of the spinal muscles, cognitive disorders limiting patient participation, conflicts of interest owing to existing pain (unconsolidated work accident, ongoing damage compensation). Spine infection, tumour or trauma had been specifically excluded by an MRI done by all patients before the inclusion in the present study. Some of risk factors associated with going from acute low-back pain to chronic low-back pain are linked to the socio-professional context, notably with the job dissatisfaction [17, 18]. Furthermore, 2 studies [17, 19] showed that there was a significant positive association between a damage compensation and chronic incapacity. In general, patients with unconsolidated work accident or ongoing damage compensation have a higher probability to be at risk of chronic disease; they also have a lower probability to positive response to treatment in general. That is why we excluded them from the study. We measured it by asking to each participant: "are you currently in an unconsolidated work accident?" and "are you currently ongoing a damage compensation?". As a High Authority of Health in France (l'Agence Nationale d'Accréditation et d'Evaluation en Santé, Diagnostic, Prise en charge et suivi des malades atteints de lombalgie chronique, Décembre 2000) classified the beginning of a LBP after the age of 55 as an « alert sign », we excluded them from the study.

No patient was allowed to take opiates during the time of the study, and facet joint injections were also not permitted during the study period. Physiotherapy programs offered during the study period were isometric exercises and core muscle strengthening exercises one or twice per week (usual physiotherapy in chronic low-back pain, that patients made before the study, and which was not modified during the study).

Experimental procedure
Task
The design of this study was a crossover. The subjects were randomized into two groups and successively received the two treatments of the study: patients in group 1 received intramuscular paravertebral injections of BoNT-A during the first sequence of treatment, then a placebo during the second sequence of treatment 120 days later; patients in group 2 received a placebo during the first sequence of treatment, then intramuscular paravertebral injections of BoNT-A during of the second sequence of treatment 120 days later. The crossover was performed 120 days after the inclusion in the study, because most patients with initial improvement induced by BoNT-A injections reported in previous studies [12] that the beneficial effect waned at four months.

A paper table of randomization was used by the pharmacist at the University Hospital of Bordeaux (block randomization with block size of 6). The pharmacist who performed the randomization was blinded to the patient's characteristics.

Therapeutic procedure: For each group, the injected solution was prepared by the hospital pharmacist in order that both the patients and the injectors were blinded to the nature of the injected solution. The treatments compared were: 200 IU of BoNT-A diluted in 4 ml of physiological saline injected intramuscularly in the paravertebral lumbar muscles, versus 4 ml of physiological saline injected intramuscularly in the paravertebral lumbar muscles (placebo). The injector administered the solution in 10 intramuscular puncture points (0.4 mL/point) equally distributed from L1 to L5, bilaterally. The site of injection was detected by electromyography using the injection needle. No complementary pain treatment was prescribed after the injections.

Follow-up: patients were examined at inclusion Days 0, 30, 90, 120 (Day of the crossover), 150, 210 and 240, i.e., D0, D30, D90 and D120 after both sessions of injection. The follow-up was done in person. Patients were blinded throughout the entire study.

Measures
The main judgment criterion was the level of LBP intensity at D30 (when the maximal effect of BoNT-A injections is anticipated). Pain intensity was measured on a horizontal visual analogue scale 100 mm long, with « no pain » written on one end and « maximum pain » on the other (0 = no pain; 100 = maximal pain). The question asked was: "How was the intensity of your LBP over the last 8 days?" To consider the pain decrease as clinically significant, we used the guidelines of Pham et al. [20], who suggested that a change of 40 mm could be clinically significant.

Secondary judgment criteria

– Initial pain was detailed as follows: Immediate average LBP was recorded on VAS at the first injection (D0). Average pain intensity over the last week and the last month were also recorded at D0, with the same horizontal visual analogue scale.
– Lumbar pain intensity at D90 and D120 was measured on a horizontal visual analogue scale 100 mm long, with « no pain » written on one end and "maximum pain" on the other. The question asked was: "How was the intensity of your LBP over the last 8 days?" (0 = no pain; 100 = maximal pain).
– The number of days when oral pain treatment (antalgic or non-steroid anti-inflammatory, opiates were not permitted) between evaluation times was

taken. Days when treatment was taken were noted as they occurred by the patient in a calendar, which was distributed at D0. We thought that a change of 25% would be significant.

- Functional disability related to LBP was measured by the Quebec Back Pain Disability Scale at each evaluation time. The higher the score (/100), the higher the disability. We considered as determined by Ostelo et al. [21] 20 points of change of the Quebec score as clinically significant.
- Quality of life was measured at each evaluation time on a horizontal visual analogue scale 100 mm long. The question asked was: "In your opinion, how was your quality of life over the last month?" (0 = no impact to 100 = major deterioration). We considered as clinically significant a change of 0.2 standard deviation (small change), 0.5 standard deviation (moderate change) and 0.8 standard deviation (large change) [22, 23].
- Inability to work was measured by a compendium of data indicating the number of sick leave days due to LBP in the 8 months preceding inclusion and during follow-up. A change of 25% was considered as clinically significant.
- Patient satisfaction regarding the effect of the treatment was measured on a horizontal visual analogue scale 100 mm long at each evaluation time. The question asked at each evaluation was: "In your opinion, how is the overall efficacy of the treatment that you have received?"(0 = no efficacy; 100 = high efficacy). A change superior than 50% was considered as clinically significant.
- Spinal mobility was measured at each evaluation time by using Schober & Macrae's test (Miller 1984). Two lines were drawn 10 cm above the postero superior iliac spine and 5 cm below the postero superior iliac spine. The distances in a standing position and in anteflexion were measured. A difference less than 4 cm was considered as a spine stiffness.
- Spinal muscle strength was measured by flexion and extension isokinetic technique at a speed of 60° per second before the injections, at D30, D120, D150 and D240. A variation of strength up to 20% or a reversal of the flexor/extensor ratio was considered as clinically significant.
- MODIC classification of discopathy and Hadar classification of the rector spinae muscles were based on MRI performed in the previous year. The MODIC measures are divided in 3 classes: [24]: there were type 1 (inflammatory phase), type 2 (fatty phase) and type 3 (marked sclerosis adjacent to the endplates). We collected the data in order to look for predictive factors for efficacy of BoNT-A.

- Tolerance to BoNT-A injections was studied by actively asking at each visit for possible side effects (pain at injection points, sensation of general weakness, falling, nausea, diplopia, dry mouth).

Statistical analysis

Comparisons were made by a paired Student t-test after verifying the conditions of validity of the test (normal distribution, homogeneous variances). The Chi square test was used in order to compare the gender distribution of the two groups. Paired t-tests and Chi square tests were performed on cumulative data from 19 patients following placebo (19 patients) and BoNT-A injections (19 patients) after a crossover. Linear regression analysis was also planned. Risk of type 1 error was $\alpha = 5\%$ at each statistical analysis. To run the statistical analyses, we used the Excel software, version 15.32. The statistician who decided the kind of statistics used was blinded. The author who made the statistical analyses was not blinded, but he/she did not compile the data into the statistical software.

Results

The group who began the injections with BoNT-A was named group 1; the group who began the injections with a placebo was named group 2. As planned, in order to increase the power of the statistical analysis of the crossover, we pooled post-BoNT-A follow-up and post-placebo follow-up. The group with BoNT-A injections was named group A and the group with placebo injections was named group B. The follow-up of groups A and B was performed at D30, D90 and D120 following each injection time.

Flow diagram (Figure 1)

In this study, 19 patients were approached and eligible to the study. No patient declined participation in the study. The inclusion period was about 23 months. All patients included were randomized in one of the two groups. Nine of them received BoNT-A at D0, 10 of them received placebo at D0. In the BoNT-A group (group 1), all patients were followed at D30, D90, all of them received placebo at D120, were followed at D150, D210 and D240 and completed the trial. In the placebo group (group 2), one patient was lost during the follow-up at D90 and one patient was lost during the follow-up at D210; 8 patients received BoNT-A at D120, all of them were followed at D150, D210 and D240 and completed the trial. We excluded the 2 lost patients from the statistical analysis, because they did not benefit from the 2 injections (BoNT-A and placebo). Patients' distribution is presented in Fig. 1.

Description of the population at baseline (standard deviations are noted in parentheses) (Table 1)

The group who initially received BoNT-A was named group 1; the group who initially received the placebo

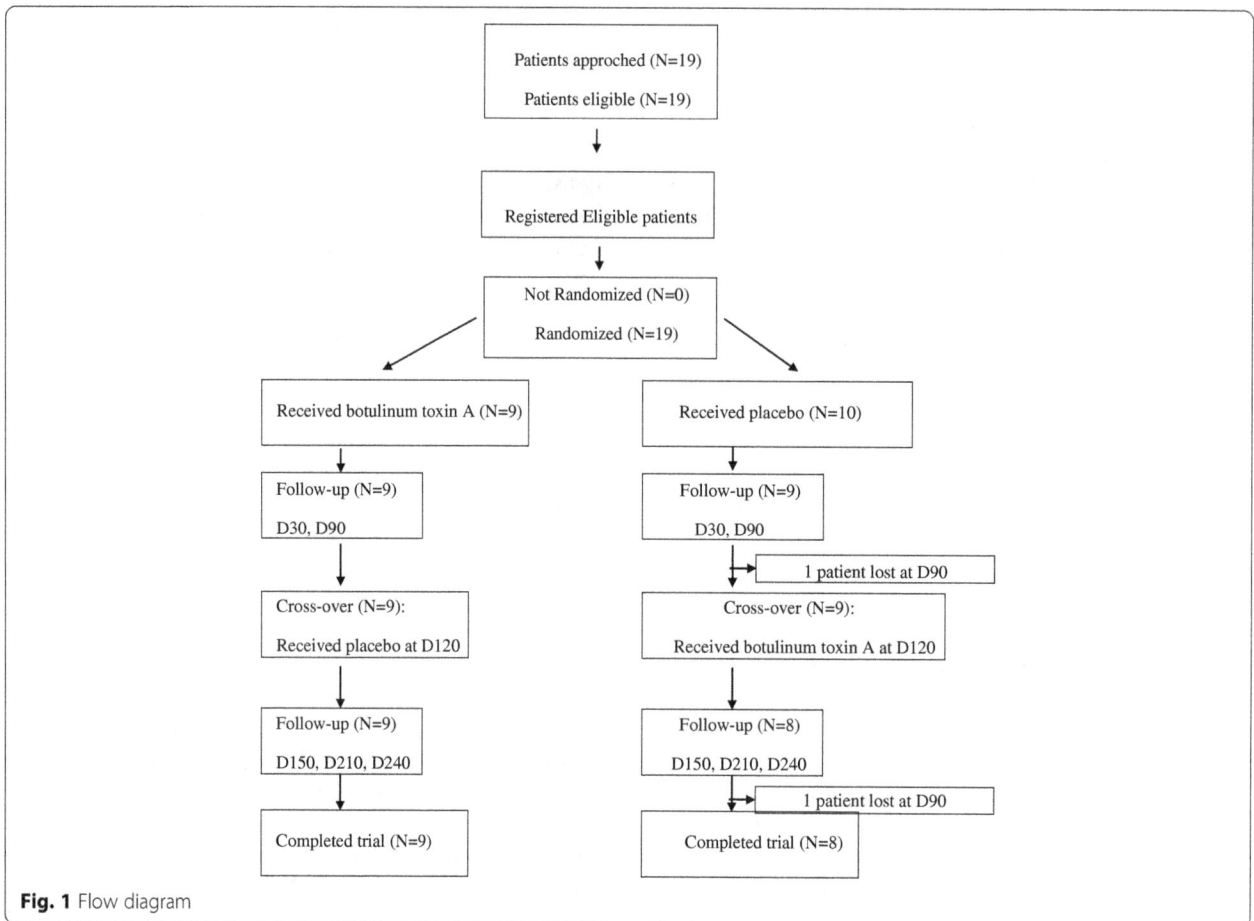

Fig. 1 Flow diagram

was named group 2. The group 1 contained 6 women and 3 men, and the group 2 contained 10 women (Chi square = 3.96, $p = 0.047$). There was no significant difference concerning the mean age of group 1 (38.1($\pm$5.94)) and group 2 (38.2($\pm$10.27)) ($p = 0.98$). The mean usual spinal pain intensity of group 1 was 59.33 mm ($\pm$15.71) and the one of group 2 was 58.70 ($\pm$15.89) ($p = 0.93$). The usual root pain intensity did not differ between groups either ($p = 0.26$) (mean pain intensity in group 1: 42.89 mm ($\pm$26.98); mean pain intensity in group 2: 28.40 mm ($\pm$27.16)). The mean pain intensity during the last month was 63.11 mm ($\pm$25.70) in group 1 and 66.70 mm ($\pm$24.50) in group 2 ($p = 0.76$); the mean pain intensity during the last 8 days was 67.67 mm ($\pm$22.37) in group 1 and 57.50 mm ($\pm$25.63) in group 2 ($p = 0.37$). There was no significant difference concerning the mean Quebec initial score between group 1 (52.56 mm ($\pm$11.64)) and group 2 (51.70 mm ($\pm$16.55)) ($p = 0.90$). There was no significant difference concerning the mean disability during the last month between group 1 (7.44 mm ($\pm$12.99)) and group 2 (13.4 mm ($\pm$14.55)) ($p = 0.36$); but the disability during the last 8 months was higher in the group 2 (151.6 mm ($\pm$96.56)) than in the group 1 (58.22 mm ($\pm$82.29)) ($p = 0.03$). The quality of life

at inclusion was estimated at 76.56 mm ($\pm$16.41) for group 1 and at 65.00 mm ($\pm$17.80) for group 2 ($p = 0.16$). There was no significant difference concerning the number of days with painkillers or anti-inflammatories between group 1 (19.67 days ($\pm$13.44)) and group 2 (14.1 days ($\pm$12.57)) ($p = 0.36$). In group 1, 4 patients had a right-, 3 had a left- and 2 had a bilateral paravertebral painful point pressure; in group 2, 4 patients had a right- and 6 patients had a bilateral paravertebral painful point pressure. In group 1, 8 patients and 6 patients of group 2 had a stiffness ($p = 0.17$). The Schober's test was measured at 4.22 cm ($\pm$1.30) for group 1 and 3.95 cm ($\pm$1.77) for group 2 ($p = 0.71$). The hand-ground distance was about 28.60 cm ($\pm$13.60) in group 1 and 20.60 ($\pm$15.60) for group 2 ($p = 0.25$). The mean number of localization of spinal pain was 3.13 ($\pm$1.46) in group 1 and 3.60 ($\pm$1.84) in group 2 ($p = 0.55$), and the mean number of localization of paravertebral pain was 5.00 ($\pm$1.51) in group 1 and 4.60 ($\pm$2.32) in group 2 ($p = 0.67$). No patients presented a Lasegue sign at the inclusion; 2 patients presented a pseudo-Lasegue sign in group 1 and 5 presented a pseudo-Lasegue sign in group 2 ($p = 0.30$). Only one patient in group 2 presented a disco-radicular conflict ($p = 0.34$). The isokinetic evaluation revealed a maximum

Table 1 Demographic data of 19 randomized patients (mean or number are noted, standard deviations are in parentheses) at Day 0 (D0)

Patients	Botulinum toxin	Placebo	t-test (p)
Sample size	$N = 9$	$N = 10$	
Men/Women	3/6	0/10	0.047
Age: mean (SD) in years	38.1 (5.94)	38.2 (10.27)	0.49
Spinal pain intensity: mean (SD) /100 mm	59.33 (15.71)	58.70 (15.89)	0.47
Radicular pain intensity: mean (SD) /100 mm	42.89 (26.98)	28.40 (27.16)	0.13
Pain intensity during last month: mean (SD) /100 mm	63.11 (25.70)	66.70 (24.50)	0.38
Pain intensity during last week: mean (SD) /100 mm	67.67 (22.37)	57.50 (25.63)	0.18
Quebec initial score mean (SD) /100 mm	52.56 (11.64)	51.70 (16.55)	0.45
Disability during last 8 months: mean (SD) /100 mm	58.22 (82.29)	151.6 (96.56)	0.018
Disability during last month: mean (SD) /100 mm	7.44 (12.99)	13.4 (14.55)	0.18
Quality of life at inclusion: mean (SD) /100 mm	76.56 (16.41)	65.00 (17.80)	0.08
Number of days with painkillers or anti-inflammatories: number (SD)	19.67 (13.44)	14.1 (12.57)	0.18
Paravertebral painful point pressure Right/Left/Bilateral	4/3/2	4/0/6	
Stiffness: number	8	6	0.08
Tendency to cough: number	5	7	0.27
Instability: number	9	8	0.08
Schober's test: centimeter (SD)	4.22 (1.30)	3.95 (1.77)	0.35
Hand-ground distance: centimeter (SD)	28.60 (13.60)	20.60 (15.60)	0.13
Spinal pain: mean (SD)	3.13 (1.46)	3.60 (1.84)	0.27
Paravertebral pain: number	2	5	0.33
Lasegue sign: number	0	0	
Pseudo-Lasegue sign: mean (SD)	0.25 (0.46)	0.5 (0.53)	0.15
Disco-radicular conflict: number	0	1	0.17
MODIC L1-L2 0/1/2/3	9/0/0/0	9/0/1/0	0.17
MODIC L2-L3 0/1/2/3	9/0/0/0	9/0/1/0	0.17
MODIC L3-L4 0/1/2/3	9/0/0/0	9/0/1/0	0.17
MODIC L4-L5 0/1/2/3	9/0/0/0	9/0/0/1	0.17
MODIC L5-S1 0/1/2/3	5/3/1/0	4/3/2/1	0.15
HADAR L1-L2 0/1/2/3	8/1/0/0	8/2/0/0	0.31
HADAR L2-L3 0/1/2/3	6/3/0/0	7/3/0/0	0.44
HADAR L3-L4 0/1/2/3	4/5/0/0	7/1/2/0	0.33
HADAR L4-L5 0/1/2/3	1/6/2/0	3/4/3/0	0.37
HADAR L5-S1 0/1/2/3	1/4/4/0	0/4/6/0	0.18
Isokinetic maximum strength: n/m (SD)	115.33 (58.63)	114.44 (37.63)	0.49
Isokinetic endurance: n/m (SD)	89.11 (62.50)	77.33 (53.86)	0.34
Flexors/extensors ratio at 60°: % (SD)	123.63 (37.56)	119.36 (49.51)	0.42

strength at 115.33n/m (±58.63) in group 1 and at 114.44n/m (±37.63) in group 2 ($p = 0.97$); the endurance was calculated at 89.11n/m (±62.50) in group 1 and 77.33n/m (±53.86) in group 2 ($p = 0.67$); the flexors/extensors ratio at 60° was calculated at 123.63% (±37.56) in group 1 and 119.36 (±49.51) in group 2 ($p = 0.84$). Population at baseline is described in Table 1.

Between-group comparisons (Table 2)
Level of LBP intensity
Between-group comparisons are presented in Table 2.

- LBP intensity during the last 8 days (Fig. 2):

There was no significant difference concerning the mean of the LBP intensity during the last 8 days between

Table 2 Presentation of averages, standard deviations and p-values of judgment criteria for group A and group B

		Number of patients (n) A/B	Mean group A	Standard deviation group A	Mean group B	Standard deviation group B	p-value
Average lumbar pain over last 8 days by visual analogue scale (/100 mm)	D0	18/19	67.70	24.64	60.35	28.07	p = 0.43
	D30	18/19	63.12	18.92	63.12	18.92	p = 0.75
	D90	15/16	62.60	27.39	58.43	24.66	p = 0.80
	D120	15/16	60.87	26.83	55.87	32.50	p = 0.70
Average root pain over last month by visual analogue scale (/100 mm)	D30	18/19	60.29	22.99	53.47	33.88	p = 0.45
	D90	15/16	42.07	37.40	27.57	33.05	p = 0.52
	D120	15/16	56.73	25.33	46.20	30.42	p = 0.70
Number of days with significant or very significant pain	D30	18/19	13.29	9.88	15.18	12.82	p = 0.55
	D90	15/16	11.43	10.45	11.71	16.94	p = 0.44
Functional disability related to low-back pain by Quebec Back Pain Disability Scale (/100)	D0	18/19	51.53	16.19	52.35	20.16	p = 0.89
	D30	18/19	53.76	13.18	52.29	20.74	p = 0.77
	D90	15/16	53.07	17.75	45.93	22.82	p = 0.47
	D120	16/16	52.87	21.69	42.93	23.70	p = 0.48
Inability to work during last 30 days (/30)	D0	18/19	11.00	14.56	11.06	14.55	p = 0.99
	D30	18/18	12.41	15.17	9.56	14.25	p = 0.35
	D90	15/16	12.41	14.59	9.69	17.93	p = 0.46
	D120	15/16	8.00	13.73	12.00	15.21	p = 0.34
Estimated impact of low-back pain on quality of life (/100)	D0	18/19	71.41	21.70	64.47	24.61	p = 0.37
	D30	18/19	68.71	18.85	64.06	23.33	p = 0.44
	D90	15/16	63.47	23.72	58.57	23.33	p = 0.38
	D120	15/16	61.00	30.01	60.67	29.63	p = 0.96
Number of days when pain medication or anti-inflammatories were necessary in last 30 days (/30)	D0	18/19	17.06	13.65	15.35	14.69	p = 0.71
	D30	18/19	16.06	13.21	13.41	13.44	p = 0.51
	D90	15/16	15.73	13.85	11.50	13.82	p = 0.79
	D120	15/16	14.80	14.87	13.53	14.54	p = 0.86
Patients' assessment of efficacy of treatment (/100)	D30	18/19	0.76	1.15	0.94	1.14	p = 0.62
	D90	15/16	1.33	1.80	1.43	1.60	p = 1.00
	D120	15/16	1.47	1.77	1.73	1.62	p = 1.00
Spinal flexibility measured by Schoeber Macrae's test (cm)	D0	18/19	5.00	2.34	4.21	1.86	p = 0.22
	D30	18/19	4.76	1.88	4.32	1.67	p = 0.48
	D90	15/16	4.00	1.18	4.54	1.31	p = 0.23
	D120	15/16	4.23	1.55	5.53	2.28	p = 0.18
Hand-ground distance (cm)	D0	18/19	26.17	13.32	25.64	14.03	p = 0.93
	D30	18/19	26.35	14.02	26.85	12.89	p = 0.92
	D90	15/16	24.87	14.51	16.79	10.17	p = 0.35
	D120	15/16	27.53	12.18	21.93	13.08	p = 0.25
Isokinetic maximum strength (n/m)	D0	16/17	116.00	45.53	126.40	63.41	p = 0.78
	D30	15/18	120.93	53.30	134.40	63.67	p = 0.70
	D120	13/14	126.69	67.20	135.07	50.35	p = 0.70
Isokinetic endurance (n/m)	D0	16/17	100.27	51.63	102.33	63.24	p = 0.81
	D30	15/17	96.07	53.38	108.73	69.00	p = 0.76
	D120	15/14	103.17	63.74	111.79	57.67	p = 0.65

Table 2 Presentation of averages, standard deviations and *p*-values of judgment criteria for group A and group B *(Continued)*

		Number of patients (n) A/B	Mean group A	Standard deviation group A	Mean group B	Standard deviation group B	*p*-value
Isokinetic maximum force ratio flexors/extensors (%)	*D0*	16/17	115.85	31.13	119.72	38.95	*p* = 0.36
	D30	15/17	122.93	33.83	107.86	24.41	*p* = 0.16
	D120	13/14	111.54	24.29	102.88	23.53	*p* = 0.72

Group A: all 17 patients assessed during 120 days after BoNT-A injections, group B: all 17 patients assessed during 120 days after placebo injections

group 1 and group 2 at D30 (*p* = 0.59), at D90 (*p* = 0.94), at D120 (*p* = 0.73), at D150 (*p* = 0.92), at D210 (*p* = 0.80) and at D240 (*p* = 0.36).

There was no significant difference concerning the mean of the LBP intensity during the last 8 days between group A and group B at D30 (*p* = 0.75), at D90 (*p* = 0.80) and at D120 (*p* = 0.70).

- Root pain intensity over the last month:

There was no significant difference concerning the mean root pain over last month between group 1 and group 2 at D30 (*p* = 0.31), at D90 (*p* = 0.23), at D120 (*p* = 0.54), at D150 (*p* = 0.92), at D210 (*p* = 0.77) and at D240 (*p* = 0.46).

There was no significant difference concerning the mean root pain over last month between group A and group B at D30 (*p* = 0.45), at D90 (*p* = 0.51) and at D120 (*p* = 0.70).

- Number of days with significant or very significant pain:

There was no significant difference concerning the number of days with significant or very significant pain between group 1 and group 2 at D30 (*p* = 0.63), at D90 (*p* = 0.94), at D120 (*p* = 0.94), at D150 (*p* = 0.27), at D210 (*p* = 0.68) and at D240 (*p* = 0.64).

There was no significant difference concerning the number of days with significant or very significant pain between group A and group B at D30 (*p* = 0.55), at D90 (*p* = 0.44) and at D120 (*p* = 0.35).

Functional disability related to LBP evaluated by Quebec back pain disability scale (figure 3)

There was no significant difference concerning the score of the Quebec scale between group 1 and group 2 at D30 (*p* = 0.86), at D90 (*p* = 0.89), at D120 (*p* = 0.94), at D150 (*p* = 0.65), at D210 (*p* = 0.35) and at D240 (*p* = 0.13).

There was no significant difference concerning the score of the Quebec scale between group A and group B at D30 (*p* = 0.77), at D90 (*p* = 0.47) and at D120 (*p* = 0.48).

Inability to work during the last 30 days

There was no significant difference concerning the number of days with inability to work during the last 30 days between group 1 and group 2 at D30 (*p* = 0.35), at D90 (*p* = 0.46), at D120 (*p* = 0.27), at D150 (*p* = 0.10), at D210 (*p* = 0.47) and at D240 (*p* = 0.86).

There was no significant difference concerning the number of days with inability to work during the last 30 days between group A and group B at D30 (*p* = 0.35), at D90 (*p* = 0.46) and at D120 (*p* = 0.34).

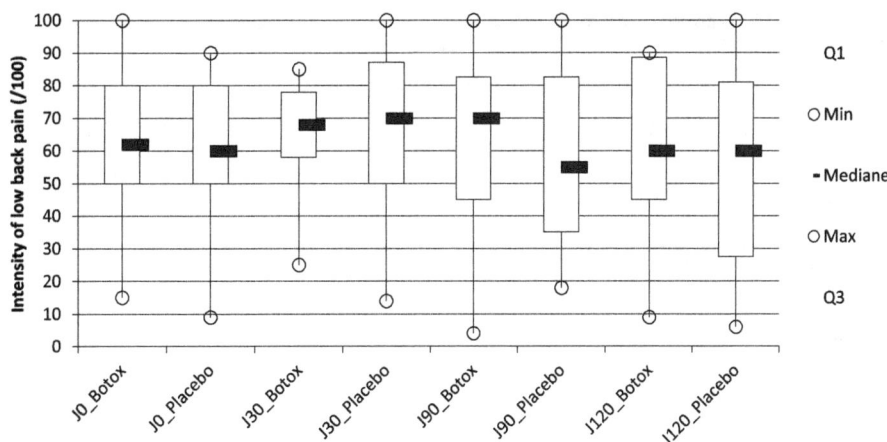

Fig. 2 Pain intensity at D0,30, 90 and 120 for patients treated by Botulinum toxin A (BoNT-A) (group A) or by placebo (group B). Pain intensity was measured on a horizontal visual analogue scale 100 mm long, with « no pain » written on one end and « maximum pain » on the other. The question asked was: "How was the intensity of your low-back pain over the last 8 days?"

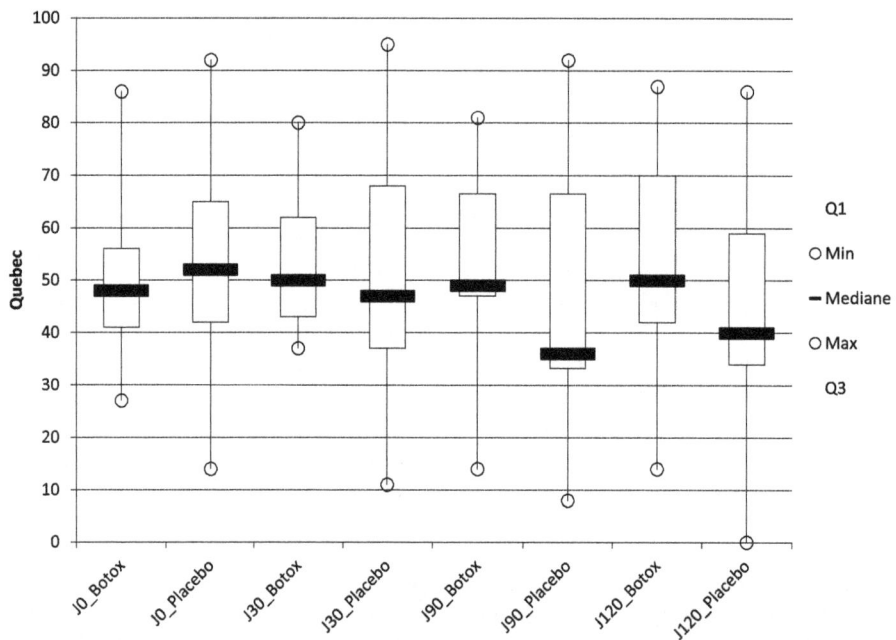

Fig. 3 Quebec Back Pain Disability Scale at D0, 30, 90 and 120 for patients treated by Botulinum toxin A (group A) or by placebo (group B)

Estimated impact of LBP on quality of life (figure 4)

There was no significant difference concerning the estimating impact of LBP on quality of life during the last month between group 1 and group 2 at D30 ($p = 0.38$), at D90 ($p = 0.56$), at D120 ($p = 0.90$), at D150 ($p = 0.98$), at D210 ($p = 0.98$) and at D240 ($p = 0.93$).

There was no significant difference concerning the estimating impact of LBP on quality of life during the last month between group A and group B at D30 ($p = 0.44$), at D90 ($p = 0.38$) and at D120 ($p = 0.95$).

Number of days when pain medication or anti-inflammatories were necessary in last 30 days

There was no significant difference concerning the number of days when pain medication or anti-inflammatories were necessary in the last 30 days between group 1 and

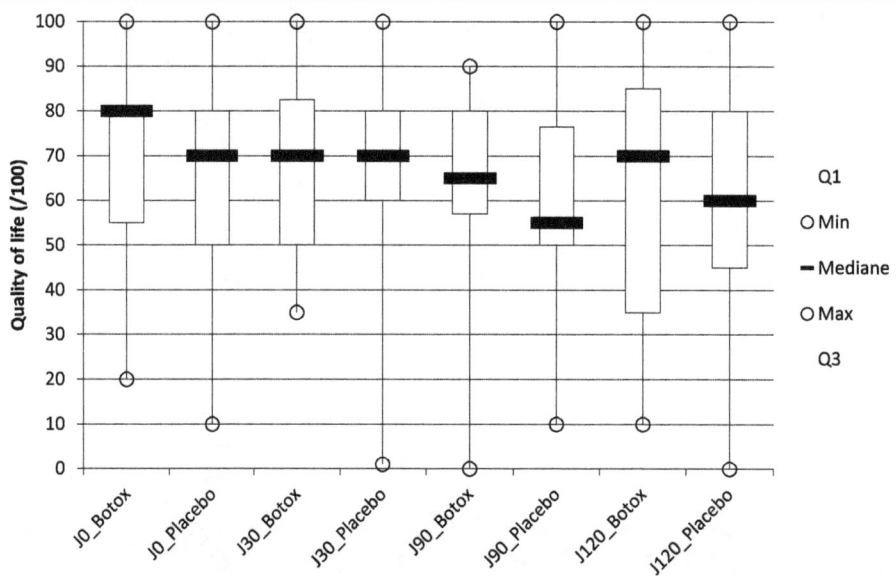

Fig. 4 Estimated impact of low-back pain on quality of life at D0, D30, D90 and D120 for patients treated by Botulinum toxin A (group A) or by placebo (group B). It was measured on a horizontal visual analogue scale 100 mm long. The question asked was: "in your opinion, how was your quality of life over the last month?" (0 = no impact to 100 = major deterioration)

group 2 at D30 ($p = 0.82$), at D90 ($p = 0.51$), at D120 ($p = 0.73$), at D150 ($p = 0.57$), at D210 ($p = 0.58$) and at D240 ($p = 0.92$).

There was no significant difference concerning the number of days when pain medication or anti-inflammatories were necessary in the last 30 days between group A and group B at D30 ($p = 0.51$), at D90 ($p = 0.79$) and at D120 ($p = 0.86$).

Patients' assessment of efficacy of treatment
There was no significant difference concerning the patients' assessment of efficacy of treatment between group 1 and group 2 at D30 ($p = 0.73$), at D90 ($p = 0.69$), at D120 ($p = 0.89$), at D150 ($p = 0.91$), at D210 ($p = 0.64$) and at D240 ($p = 0.51$).

There was no significant difference concerning the patients' assessment of efficacy of treatment between group A and group B at D30 ($p = 0.62$), at D90 ($p = 1.00$) and at D120 ($p = 1.00$).

Spinal flexibility measured by Schoeber Macrae's test
There was no significant difference concerning the spinal flexibility measured by Schoeber Macrae's test between group 1 and group 2 at D30 ($p = 0.49$), at D90 ($p = 0.06$), at D120 ($p = 0.30$), at D150 ($p = 0.64$), at D210 ($p = 0.47$). There was a significant difference between group 1 and group 2 concerning the spinal flexibility at D240 ($p = 0.04$).

There was no significant difference concerning the spinal flexibility measured by Schoeber Macrae's test between group A and group B at D30 ($p = 0.48$), at D90 ($p = 0.23$) and at D120 ($p = 0.18$).

Hand-ground distance
There was no significant difference concerning the hand-ground distance between group 1 and group 2 at D30 ($p = 0.64$), at D90 ($p = 0.10$), at D120 ($p = 0.33$), at D150 ($p = 0.41$) and at D210 ($p = 0.81$). There was a significant difference concerning the hand-ground distance between group 1 and group 2 at D240 ($p = 0.58$).

There was no significant difference concerning the hand-ground distance between group A and group B at D30 ($p = 0.92$), at D90 ($p = 35$) and at D120 ($p = 0.25$).

Isokinetic maximum strength
There was no significant difference concerning the isokinetic maximum strength between group 1 and group 2 at D30 ($p = 0.34$), at D120 ($p = 0.30$) and at D150 ($p = 0.11$). There was a significant difference concerning the isokinetic maximum strength between group 1 and group 2 at D240 ($p = 0.04$).

There was no significant difference concerning the isokinetic maximum strength between group A and group B at D30 ($p = 0.70$) and at D120 ($p = 0.70$).

Isokinetic endurance
There was no significant difference concerning the isokinetic endurance between group 1 and group 2 at D30 ($p = 0.26$), at D120 ($p = 0.21$) and at D150 (0.08). There was a significant difference between group 1 and group 2 concerning the isokinetic endurance between group 1 and group 2 at D240 ($p = 0.03$).

There was no significant difference concerning the isokinetic endurance between group A and group B at D30 ($p = 0.76$) and at D120 ($p = 0.65$).

Isokinetic maximum force ratio flexors/extensors
There was no significant difference concerning the isokinetic maximum force measured by the radio flexors/extensors at 60° between group 1 and group 2 at D30 ($p = 0.90$), at D120 (0.89), at D150 (0.08), at D240 (0.19).

There was no significant difference concerning the isokinetic maximum force measured by the radio flexors/extensors at 60° between group A and group B at D30 ($p = 0.16$) and at D120 ($p = 0.72$).

Within-group comparisons
There was no significant difference in group A and in group B concerning the pain intensity between D0 and D120 ($p = 0.58$ for group A and $p = 0.70$ for group B).

Symmetric carryover effect
There was a symmetric carryover effect between group 1 and group 2 concerning the main judgement criterion, i.e. pain intensity at D30.

Adverse effects
The adverse effects were actively asked at each visit. No patients declared an adverse effect during the present study. No complications were experienced in this study.

Discussion
This randomized controlled trial did not find any advantage for injections of BoNT-A versus placebo in the paravertebral muscles of patients with LBP at 30, 90 et 120 days with regard to pain relief, functional disability, sick leave, quality of life, consumption of oral antalgics, spinal flexibility and isokinetic strength or endurance. Indeed, there was no significant difference between the two groups regarding the main criterion, i.e., average lumbar pain over the last 8 days at D30 ($p = 0.97$), nor was there any significant difference between the two groups regarding secondary judgment criteria ($p > 0.05$, see Table 2).

Our results differ largely from those of two previous studies [4, 6]. Since LBP is a complex phenomenon involving heavy lifting, twisting and trauma which is sometimes work-related [25] psychological factors [26], smoking, alcoholism, biomechanical and psychosocial professional factors, the difference in results could be due to differences in the populations of the two studies. Indeed, in a previous study [4], 3 patients had a discectomy compared to none in our study. In addition, no patient had any MRI evidence of acute disc pathology in the two previous studies [4, 6], whereas 6 patients in our study had a MODIC 1. Furthermore, in our study, only 3 male patients were included. Nevertheless, there was no difference between groups concerning the gender. Furthermore, the present literature is not uniform about the role of the gender on the chronicity of low-back pain [27, 28].

In our study, we used 200 units of Botox for bilateral injections. But we assume that the negative results of our study could also be secondary to the lower dose of botulinum toxin A used on each injection point compared to Foster et al.'s study. Indeed, we decided to inject bilaterally the paravertebral muscles, because there is usually a bilateral injury in both paravertebral muscles after an acute low back-pain, which leads to chronic low-back pain [29]. More precisely, we think that LBP could be secondary to an over-activity of muscles compensating multifidus' atrophy. The dose used in Machado et al.'s study (1000UI of Dysport in case of bilateral injections) was also superior to ours, which could explain the difference between the results.

Reporting a negative study is still an interesting point, because the efficiency of BoNT-A on chronic low-back pain is still not proved at this time, and because it could make reconsider on one part in researchers' further studies about BoNT-A and LBP, and one the other part in clinicians using BoNT-A injections for chronic LBP.

The strength of this trial is its randomized, controlled crossover design. A limitation is the small sample. Nevertheless, the number of patients treated was similar to that in previous studies [4, 6, 14], which showed a strong positive effect of BoNT-A on LBP. While some differences between the groups became apparent before the crossover (hand-ground distance, Schober's test, isokinetic measures), they disappeared when the data were aggregated after the crossover (group A and group B), perhaps owing to variations due to the size of groups 1 and 2. Indeed, group 1 demonstrated more spine stiffness and less strength than group 2, a finding that was unexpected.

The main result of the study is the absence of any significant difference or trend to feel pain relief with injections of BoNT-A A compared to placebo injections. A larger sample of patients now needs to be studied in order to identify those who would benefit most from BoNT-A injections for LBP.

Conclusions

Botulinum toxin injections did not show any efficacy in relieving pain in patients with chronic low-back pain in this randomised controlled trial using a cross-over. Result is in contradiction with the existing literature. With 200UI of Botox injected bilaterally, we did not find any pain relief. But this negative result could also be explained by the lower dose used compared to other studies, and by the low number of patients included. Nevertheless, this negative result could be useful being included in a meta-analysis.

Abbreviations

BoNT-A: Botulinum Toxin A; LBP: Low-back pain

Acknowledgements

The authors thank Briane Marie Sheperd, Ray Cooke and Anna Moraitis for helping with the English syntax. The authors thank also Dr. Jean-François Knebel for his help with the statistical analyses.
This work was supported by the French Hospital Clinical Research Project (PHRC).

Funding

The authors thank the Allergan company for co-funding this study (co-financing with 13,700 euros) within the French Hospital Clinical Research Project (PHRC Project) framework (42,000 euros). The Allergan company did not interfere with the collection, the analysis and the interpretation of data, nor with the writing of the manuscript.

Authors' contributions

MC made the statistical analysis and wrote the paper. HP and AC included some patients, helped for the interpretation of the statistical analyses and were involved in drafting the manuscript. MDS helped for promoting the study, included the patients and helped for the statistical analysis. DL helped for designing and promoting the study. She was also involved in drafting the manuscript. All authors discussed the results and commented on the manuscript. All authors read and approved the final manuscript.

Consent for publication

Not applicable

Competing interests

The authors declare that they have no competing interests.

Author details

[1]Service de Médecine Physique et de Réadaptation, hôpital Raymond Poincaré, 92380 Garches, France. [2]Service de Médecine Physique et de Réadaptation, CHU de Bordeaux, 33076 Bordeaux, France. [3]EA4136 Handicap, Activité, Cognition, Santé, Bordeaux University, Bordeaux, France. [4]Neurosurgical Unit, University Hospital, Bordeaux, France.

References

1.   Andersson GB. Epidemiological features of chronic low-back pain. Lancet. 1999;354:581–5.
2.   Rossignol M, Abenhaim L, Séguin P, Neveu A, Collet JP, Ducruet T, Shapiro S. Coordination of primary health care for back pain. Spine. 2000;25:251–9.

3. Mellin G. Decreased joint and spinal mobility associated with low back pain in young adults. J Spinal Disord. 1990;3:228–43.
4. Foster L, Clapp L, Erickson M, Jabbari B. BoNT-a A and chronic low back pain: a randomized, double blind study. Neurology. 2001;56:1290–993.
5. Jazayeri SM, Ashraf A, Fini HM, Karimian H, Nasab MV. Efficacy of botulinum toxin type a for treating chronic low back pain. Anesh Pain Med. 2011;1:77–80.
6. Machado D, Kumar A, Jabbari B. Abobotulinum toxin a in the treatment of chronic low back pain. Toxins. 2016;8:374.
7. Cheshire WP, Abashian SW, Mann JD. BoNT-A in the treatment of myofascial pain syndrome. Pain. 1994;59:65–9.
8. Dutton JJ. BoNT-A in treatment of crabiocervical muscle spasms short and long term, local and sistemic effects. Surv Ophthalmol. 1996;41:51–65.
9. Grazko MA, Polo KB, Jabbari B. BoNT-a A for spaticity muscle spasms, and rigidity. Neurology. 1995;45:712–7.
10. Greene P, Kang U, Fahn S, Brin M, Moskowitz C, Flaster E. Double blind, placebo controlled trial of botulinum injection for the treatment of spasmodic torticollis. Neurology. 1990;40:1213–8.
11. Wheeler A, Goelkusian PA, Gretz SS. Randomised double blind, prospective pilot study of boutilinum toxin injection for refractory unilateral, cervicothoracic, paraspinal, myofacial pain syndrome. Spine. 1998;23:1662–7.
12. Herskowitz A. BOTOX (BoNT-a type A) treatment of patients with sub-acute low back pain: a randomized, double blind, placebo-controlled study. *The journal of Pain* Supplement 1 2004; 5(1), S62.
13. Jabbari B, Ney J, Sichani A, Monacci W, Foster L, Difazio M. Treatment of refractory, chronic low back pain with botulinum neurotoxin a: an open-label, pilot study. Pain Med. 2006;7:260–4.
14. Ney JP, Difazio M, Sichani A, Monacci W, Foster L, Jabbari B. Treatment of chronic low back pain with successive injections of BoNT-a a over 6 months: a prospective trial of 60 patients. Clin J Pain. 2006;22:363–9.
15. Subin B, Saleemi S, Morgan GA, Zaviska F, Cork RC. Treatment of chronic low back pain by local injection of BoNT-a A. Internet Journal of Anesthesiology. 2003;6:8.
16. Waseem Z, Boulias C, Gordon A, Ismail F, Sheean G, Furlan AD. BoNT-A injections for low-back pain and sciatica. *Cochrane database syst Rev* 2011 19; Issue 1. Art no.CD008257.
17. Coste J, Delecoeuillerie G, De Lara AC, LeParc JM, Paolaggi JB. (1994). Clinical course and prognostic factors in acute low back pain: an inception cohort study in primary care practice. BMJ 1994; 308,577-580.
18. Williams RA, Pruitt SD, Doctor JN, Epping-Jordan JE, Wahlgren DR, Grant I, ... & Atkinson JH. (1998). The contribution of job satisfaction to the transition from acute to chronic low back pain. Arch Phys Med Rehabil *1998*; 79, 366-374.
19. Gatchel RJ. (2004). Comorbidity of chronic pain and mental health disorders: the biopsychosocial perspective. Am Psychol 2004; 59, 795.
20. Pham T, Tubach F. Etat sympomatique acceptable ou Patient Acceptable Symptomatic State (PASS). Rev Rhum. 2009;76:602–4.
21. Ostelo RW, Deyo RA, Stratford P, Waddell G, Croft P, Von Korff M, Bouter LM, de Vet HC. Interpreting change scores for pain and functional status in low back pain: towards international consensus regarding minimal important change. Spine. 2008;33:90–4.
22. Cohen J. Statistical Power Analysis for the Behavioral Sciences. 1988. 2nd ed. Hillsdale, NJ: Lawrence Erlbaum Associates.
23. Guyatt GH, Osoba D, Wu AW, Wyrwich KW, Norman GR. Clinical Significance Consensus Meeting Group. Methods to explain the clinical significance of health status measures. Mayo Clin Proc. 2002;77:371–83.
24. Modic MT, Steinberg PM, Ross JS, Masaryk TJ, Carter JR. Degenerative disk disease: assessment of changes in vertebral body marrow with MR imaging. Radiology. 1988;166:193–9.
25. Biering-Sørensen F. A prospective study of low back pain in a general population. III. Medical service–work consequence. Scand J Rehabil Med. 1983;15:89–96.
26. Joukamaa M. Psychological factors in low back pain. Ann Clin Res. 1987;19:129–34.
27. Valat JP, Goupille P, Védere V. Low back pain: risk factors for chronicity. Rev Rhum Engl Ed. 1997;64:189–94.
28. Wáng YXJ, Wáng JQ, Káplár Z. Increased low back pain prevalence in females than in males after menopause age: evidences based on synthetic literature review. Quantitative imaging in medicine and surgery. 2016;6:199.
29. Danneels LA, Vanderstraeten GG, Cambier DC, Witvrouw EE, De Cuyper HJ. CT imaging of trunk muscles in chronic low back pain patients and healthy control subjects. Eur Spine J. 2000;9:266–72.

8

Leg pain location and neurological signs relate to outcomes in primary care patients with low back pain

Lisbeth Hartvigsen[1]* , Lise Hestbaek[1,2], Charlotte Lebouef-Yde[3,4], Werner Vach[5] and Alice Kongsted[1,2]

Abstract

Background: Low back pain (LBP) patients with related leg pain and signs of nerve root involvement are considered to have a worse prognosis than patients with LBP alone. However, it is unclear whether leg pain location above or below the knee and the presence of neurological signs are important in primary care patients. The objectives of this study were to explore whether the four Quebec Task Force categories (QTFC) based on the location of pain and on neurological signs have different characteristics at the time of care seeking, whether these QTFC are associated with outcome, and if so whether there is an obvious ranking of the four QTFC on the severity of outcomes.

Method: Adult patients seeking care for LBP in chiropractic or general practice were classified into the four QTFC based on self-reported information and clinical findings. Analyses were performed to test the associations between the QTFC and baseline characteristics as well as the outcomes global perceived effect and activity limitation after 2 weeks, 3 months, and 1 year and also 1-year trajectories of LBP intensity.

Results: The study comprised 1271 patients; 947 from chiropractic practice and 324 from general practice. The QTFC at presentation were statistically significantly associated with most of the baseline characteristics, with activity limitation at all follow-up time points, with global perceived effect at 2 weeks but not 3 months and 1 year, and with trajectories of LBP. Severity of outcomes in the QTFC increased from LBP alone, across LBP with leg pain above the knee and below the knee to LBP with nerve root involvement. However, the variation within the categories was considerable.

Conclusion: The QTFC identify different LBP subgroups at baseline and there is a consistent ranking of the four categories with respect to outcomes. The differences between outcomes appear to be large enough for the QTFC to be useful for clinicians in the communication with patients. However, due to variation of outcomes within each category individuals' outcome cannot be precisely predicted from the QTFC alone. It warrants further investigation to find out if the QTFC can improve existing prediction tools and guide treatment decisions.

Keywords: Classification, Quebec Task Force classification, Cohort studies, Low back pain, Primary care, Radiculopathy, Referred leg pain, Sciatica

Background

Low back pain (LBP) is the leading cause of disability worldwide contributing more than 10 of total years lived with disability [1] and the cost for society is huge. In the United States alone the estimated direct medical cost for all back-related conditions was $253 billion in 2009 to 2011 and back pain resulted in more than 290 million lost workdays [2]. Most of the money is spent on the small minority of patients with persistent work disability [3], and the need for prognostic assessment is highlighted in evidence-based guidelines for nonspecific low back pain in primary care [4]. Feasible assessment tools to identify prognostic indicators are needed that can facilitate clinical decision-making with the ultimate goal of preventing persistent problems and reducing costs.

Many attempts have been made to develop such back pain classification systems and screening tools [5–7]. One tool is the Quebec Task Force (QTF) classification

* Correspondence: lhartvigsen@health.sdu.dk
[1]Department of Sports Science and Clinical Biomechanics, University of Southern Denmark, Odense, Denmark
Full list of author information is available at the end of the article

of spinal disorders, proposed in 1987 [7]. The classification in its original form includes 11 categories. Categories 1 to 3 are based on the location of pain ('LBP alone', 'LPB + leg pain above the knee', 'LBP + leg pain below the knee'), whereas category 4 requires the presence of signs of nerve root involvement (NRI) in the clinical examination ('LBP + NRI'). QTF categories 5 to 7 are based on the results of imaging, categories 8 to 10 on the response to treatment, and category 11 is based on paraclinical tests.

Although the QTF classification was originally developed as a guideline to the management of patients with spinal disorders, the QTF categories 1 to 4, which are based on pain distribution and signs of NRI, have been evaluated in different settings for their discriminative and predictive ability [8–13]. These categories have been shown to differ on baseline patient profiles, generally with increasing severity from category 1 to 4 [11, 12] and also on outcomes [10, 11, 13, 14]. In workers on sick leave, leg pain below the knee and signs of NRI were shown to be strong predictors of prolonged disability and greater back-related costs [9]. Signs of NRI has been associated with greater improvement, but at the same time poorer absolute outcomes than LBP +/– leg pain above or below the knee in patients in a secondary care setting [13]. Two primary care studies found that radiating leg pain was associated with more severe pain and disability than 'LBP alone' both at presentation and after 6 months, and it was worse for patients with pain radiating below the knee compared to patients with pain above the knee [14, 15]. None of these studies investigated neurological signs as prognostic factors.

A systematic review of the literature on LBP-related leg pain reported consistent evidence for worse health outcomes and increased utilization of health care with radiation of leg pain below the knee and with neurological findings [16]. However, in a systematic review concerning non-surgically treated sciatica, findings on neurological deficit as a significant prognostic factor of poor outcome were inconsistent [17].

Although several studies have shown LBP-related leg pain to be a poor prognostic factor, studies often either fail to define leg pain/sciatica/radiculopathy or use LBP with leg pain below the knee as a proxy for nerve root pain [14]. No primary care studies have investigated whether LBP with leg pain below the knee has as different prognosis than LBP with nerve root involvement. Clinical guidelines for LBP recommend that, as part of the initial clinical history, pain distribution should be addressed and that the initial examination should include a neurological screening [4, 18]. However, the impact of both pain distribution in itself and neurological findings as well as the clinical relevance of differentiating between each of the four QTF categories remain to be investigated in primary care.

The objectives of this study are to explore 1) if the four QTF categories ('LBP alone', 'LBP + leg pain above the knee', 'LBP + leg pain below the knee', and 'LBP + NRI') have different characteristics at the time of care seeking; 2) whether the QTF categories are associated with the outcomes global perceived effect (GPE) and activity limitation after 2 weeks, 3 months, and 1 year and also 1-year trajectories of LBP intensity; if so, 3) whether this association is independent of socio-demographic factors; and lastly, 4) if there is an obvious ranking of the four QTF categories on the severity of outcomes. In studying the degree of association, we focus on the differences in expected outcomes i.e. the separative capacity of the QTF categories [19] and whether they reach a clinically relevant degree. In our opinion this requires that the group differences are large enough to add meaningful and useful information to patients or clinicians about the average future course of patients in the different QTF categories.

Methods

Design and setting

Patients with LBP were recruited by chiropractors and general practitioners to participate in a prospective observational study.

Thirty-six chiropractors (17 clinics), in a research network of the Nordic Institute of Chiropractic and Clinical Biomechanics that were geographically spread across Denmark, agreed to include consecutive patients with LBP from September 2010 till January 2012. Participating chiropractors attended a 1-day course introducing study procedures and a research assistant visited all clinics prior to study start to ensure that the clinical examination procedures related to the study were adequately standardized.

All 800 general practitioners in the Region of Southern Denmark were invited to participate in a quality development initiative by the Audit Project Odense [19]. Of the general practitioners, 88 agreed to participate and include patients over 10 weeks in 2011. No attempt was made to standardize the clinical examination procedures in general practice. Patient recruitment has been described in more detail elsewhere [19, 20].

As the study was observational, treatment was not affected by participation. Patients received 'usual care' from their chiropractor/general practitioner.

Participants

Patients were invited to participate if they sought care for LBP with or without leg pain, were 18 to 65 years of age, could read and understand Danish, had access to a mobile phone and were able to use text messaging (as one of the outcome measures was based on responses to text messages). Patients were not included if pathology or inflammatory pain was suspected or if their condition required acute referral for surgery.

Chiropractic patients were also excluded if they were pregnant or if they had had more than one health care consultation for their LBP within the previous 3 months.

Data collection

Chiropractic patients completed a baseline questionnaire in the reception area before the first consultation and returned it in a sealed envelope to the clinic secretary who sent it to the research unit. Patients consulting a general practitioner were given an envelope with information on the project and a baseline questionnaire following the first consultation. If they consented to participate, they were asked to complete the questionnaire at home and send it to the research unit in a prepaid envelope. In both settings, the included patients were given the 2-week follow-up questionnaire and a prepaid envelope at the initial consultation.

The clinical examination by the chiropractor followed a standardized examination protocol thoroughly described elsewhere [21] including questions on pain localization ('LPB alone', 'LBP + leg pain above the knee', 'LBP + leg pain below the knee') and a lumbar neurological examination (straight leg raise, femoral nerve stretch test, muscle strength, deep tendon reflexes, and sensitivity to touch or pinprick). On the basis of these variables, the chiropractors classified patients according to the QTF categories 1 to 4.

Data collection in general practice consisted of a practitioner-completed questionnaire including questions on pain localization ('LPB alone', 'LPB + leg pain above the knee', 'LBP + leg pain below the knee') and a yes/no question on the presence of abnormal neurological findings. On the basis of these variables, we classified patients according to the QTF categories 1 to 4.

Follow-up questionnaires were posted to the participants 3 months and 1 year after the initial consultation and non-responders were contacted by phone. Each Sunday for 52 weeks, patients received an SMS question asking about LBP intensity during the preceding week. Patients replied to the SMS question by sending a return text message that went directly into a data file accessible to the researchers.

Baseline characteristics

The Quebec Task Force classification

The QTF categories 1–4 ('LPB alone', 'LBP + leg pain above the knee', 'LBP + leg pain below the knee', or 'LBP + NRI') [7].

To investigate whether the four QTF categories had different characteristics at the time of care seeking the following variables were considered:

Socio-demographics

Information on age, sex, physical work load (mainly sitting, sitting and walking, light physical work, or hard physical work), sick leave (the proportion reporting any days off work due to LBP within the previous month), educational level (no qualification, vocational training, higher education of < 3 years, higher education of 3–4 years, or higher education of >4 years), and activity limitation (Roland Morris Disability Questionnaire (RMDQ) proportional score (0–100) [22]).

LBP characteristics

Duration of pain (<2 weeks, 2–4weeks, 1–3months, or >3 months), previous LBP episodes (0, 1–3, or > 3), LBP last year (≤30 days or > 30 days), LBP intensity (typical intensity of back pain during the last week measured on a Numeric Rating Scale (NRS) 0–10 (0: no pain, 10: worst imaginable pain) [23]), leg pain intensity (typical intensity of leg pain during the last week measured on NRS 0–10 (0: no pain, 10: worst imaginable pain) [23]).

Psychological factors

Recovery expectations 0–10 ("How likely do you think it is that you will be fully recovered in 3 months?" 0: no chance, 10: high chance) [24]), depressive symptoms (Major Depression Inventory 0–50, sum score) [25], *Fear-Avoidance Beliefs Questionnaire* (FABQ) physical activity scale (0–24, sum score), *FABQ* work scale (0–42, sum score) [26].

General health

Self-perceived general health measured by the EuroQol-5D Visual Analogue Scale 0–100 (0: worst imaginable health state, 100: best imaginable health state) [27].

STarT Back Tool

The STarT Back Tool (SBT) (three prognostic profiles: low, medium, and high-risk groups for persisting LBP disability) [28].

Outcome measures

To investigate whether the QTF categories were associated with outcome and, if so, whether there was a obvious ranking of the four QTF categories on the severity of outcomes the following outcome measures were used:

Global perceived effect (GPE)

Measured on a 7-point Likert scale ("much better" to "much worse") [29] at 2 weeks, 3 months and 12 months follow-up. Dichotomized to improved/not improved (improved = much better or better).

Activity limitation

Measured by the 23-item RMDQ at 2 weeks, 3 months and 12 months follow-up and converted to a proportional score (0%: no activity limitation, 100%: maximum activity limitation [22]).

LBP intensity trajectories

Five LBP trajectories have previously been identified in this cohort by latent class analysis (labelled 'recovery', 'recovery with mild relapses', 'slow improvement', 'moderate on-going or relapsing', and 'severe on-going') [20]. These were based on weekly measures of LBP intensity (0: no pain, 10: severe pain) collected by SMS for 12 months [30, 31]. To make sure that patients' individual course matched these trajectories well, only patients with at least 95% posterior probability of belonging to their assigned trajectory were included in the analyses involving this outcome variable. The posterior probabilities were obtained directly from the latent class analysis.

Data analyses

Preliminary analyses indicated that the QTF categories were differently distributed and differently associated with the baseline characteristics in chiropractic and general practice patients. Consequently, we decided to stratify all analyses according to practice types. Baseline characteristics were reported in each QTF category and significance of differences between the categories was assessed. Continuous variables were summarized using median and 10th and 90th percentiles. For binary, categorical, and ordinal variables proportions were reported with 95% confidence intervals (95% CI). Statistical significance of differences between groups was assessed by the Chi-Square-test for binary and categorical variables and by the Kruskal-Wallis-test for ordinal and continuous variables.

Associations between QTF categories and outcomes

The statistical analyses were performed in four steps. 1) Mixed models with clinics as random effects were applied to test for potential clustering within clinics. Because the random effect of clinics did not improve the model fits significantly we ignored such clustering in our further analyses. 2) Crude associations between the QTF categories and the three outcomes were evaluated using linear and logistic regression analyses and statistical significance of differences was assessed at each follow-up time point. The association between the QTF categories and RMDQ scores was illustrated in box plots and distributions within categories described as medians with 95% CI. The association with GPE was described as the proportion (with 95% CI) of patients improved at each time point. The association with the LBP trajectories was described as the proportion (with 95% CI) of patients in each LBP trajectory within each QTF category. To facilitate the interpretation of this analysis, we additionally merged the five LBP trajectories into three

trajectory groups of good outcome ('recovery' trajectory), intermediate outcome ('recovery with mild relapses' + 'slow improvement' trajectories) and poor outcome ('moderate on-going or relapsing' + 'severe on-going' trajectories), which were illustrated in stacked bar charts. We reported the observed difference between the QTF categories in relation to the outcomes and performed a subjective assessment of the relevance of the magnitude. We did not specify limits for when to regard an observed degree of separation as clinically relevant, as we are not aware of any previous work considering a minimal clinically important difference (MCID) to be used when informing patients or clinicians on expected outcomes. Established MCIDs for the RMDQ and pain scales [32, 33] relate to individuals' change over time and cannot be directly applied for the interpretation of group differences.

Nevertheless they may be kept in mind when judging clinical relevance in our study. The GPE is used in many studies as an anchor to determine MCDIs, so here it is even more obvious that the question of clinical relevant differences in expected outcomes (i.e. probability of experiencing GPE) has to be judged in a different manner. We hence tried to interpret the observed difference in expected outcomes in the sense of obtaining a separation among patients [34], which is large enough to be taken into account in communication with patients and in decision making. 3) Adjusting the linear and logistic regression analyses for socio-demographic factors (age, sex, educational level) we investigated whether observed associations could be explained by the confounding effects of these factors. We did not adjust for factors that may be part of the causal pathway (mediators) between the QTF categories and the outcomes considered. 4) We investigated whether there is an obvious ranking of the four QTF categories on the severity of outcomes by comparing neighbouring categories across all outcomes and follow-up time points:

- 'LBP alone' was thus compared to 'LBP + leg pain above the knee',
- 'LBP + leg pain above the knee' was compared to 'LBP + leg pain below the knee'
- 'LBP + leg pain below the knee' was compared to 'LBP + NRI'.

A simple count was performed on how many times observed differences between neighbouring categories went in the same direction. For example: did patients with 'LBP + NRI' consistently have poorer outcome than patients with 'LBP + leg pain below the knee'. We excluded the 3 intermediate LBP trajectories ('recovery with mild relapses', 'slow improvement' and 'moderate on-going or relapsing') from this analysis as the order of severity across those trajectories could not be unequivocally determined.

We did two analyses to describe dropout: one comparing those who could be classified using the four QTF categories to those who could not, and one comparing responders at follow-up to non-responders.

For all analyses the significance level was $p < 0.05$. Analyses were performed using STATA 14.

Results

Study cohorts

A total of 1271 patients were included, 947 chiropractic patients and 324 patients from general practice (Fig. 1). Each of the chiropractic clinics recruited from 14 to189 patients, 45% of whom were women and the median age was 43 years. General practitioners each included from 1 to 27 patients; 55% were women and the median age was 46 years.

Of the included patients, 97% of chiropractic patients and 62% of patients from general practice could be classified according to the QTF categories. Patients who were not classified according to the QTF categories did not differ significantly on any baseline characteristics from patients who were classified, except for the median age being 1.6 years lower in the non-classified general practice patients ($p < 0.05$) (Table 1a and b).

At the 1-year follow-up, 73 and 76% responded to questionnaires in chiropractic and general practice respectively. The dropout rates did not differ between the four QTF categories. In chiropractic practice, non-responders were on average 6 years younger and were more often male (45% vs. 39%), had slightly lower recovery expectations, slightly more depressive symptoms and marginally higher fear avoidance beliefs than responders ($p < 0.05$). General practice non-responders were more often male (60% vs. 38%) and more of them had heavy physical work (38% vs. 23%) as compared to responders ($p < 0.05$). On all other baseline characteristics, non-responders did not differ significantly from responders.

In total, 27% of the chiropractic patients and 38% from general practice could not be allocated to a LBP intensity trajectory with at least 95% probability. General practice patients with no assigned LBP intensity trajectory were marginally less depressive ($p < 0.05$) and were less frequently in the SBT high-risk group ($p < 0.01$). There were no other statistically significant differences between patients with and without an assigned trajectory in the two cohorts.

Baseline characteristics of the four QTF categories (objective 1)

The majority of chiropractic patients presented with 'LBP alone' (67%) and only 2% presented with 'LBP + NRI'

whereas 48% of patients in general practice presented with 'LBP alone' and 11% with 'LBP + NRI'. In both settings, the majority of the 17 baseline characteristics differed significantly between the four QTF categories with effects in the same direction and of similar magnitude (Table 1a and b). Generally, those with 'LBP alone' had the least severe profile and patients with 'LBP + NRI' were most severely affected on the largest number of parameters.

Crude associations between QTF categories and outcomes (objective 2)

Activity limitation

Statistically significant associations between the QTF categories and activity limitation were present at all follow-up time points in both cohorts (Fig. 2a and b). Generally, 'LBP alone' had the least activity limitation at all time points and 'LBP + NRI' had the most activity limitation. Differences were substantial with for example an expected median score of 35/100 after 3 months for patients with 'LBP + NRI' compared to an expected score of 13/100 in patients with 'LBP + leg pain below the knee' and 4/100 for patients with 'LBP alone' in chiropractic practice (tables in the lower part of Fig. 2a and b). However, activity limitation scores varied within each QTF category, implying that some individuals would experience outcomes that differed substantially from the mean score of their QTF category.

Global perceived effect

In both settings, there was a statistically significant association between the QTF categories and GPE at 2 weeks follow-up with the largest proportion of improved patients in the 'LBP alone' and the 'LBP + leg pain above the knee' categories (Table 2). A larger proportion of patients with 'LBP + leg pain above the knee' compared to patients with 'LBP + leg pain below the knee' improved in both cohorts and in chiropractic practice the probability of being improved further decreased considerably for patients with 'LBP + NRI'. There were no statistically significant associations at the later follow-up time points.

LBP intensity trajectories

The QTF categories were statistically significantly or borderline significantly associated with the 'recovery', 'moderate on-going' and 'severe on-going trajectories' in both settings. The table in the lower part of Fig. 3 shows the distribution of the five trajectories within each QTF category. In the chiropractic cohort, the majority of patients were in the 'recovery' trajectory (38%) and only 6% had 'severe on-going pain', whereas only 15% of general practice patients were in the 'recovery' trajectory and 29% had 'severe on-going pain'. The upper part of Fig. 3

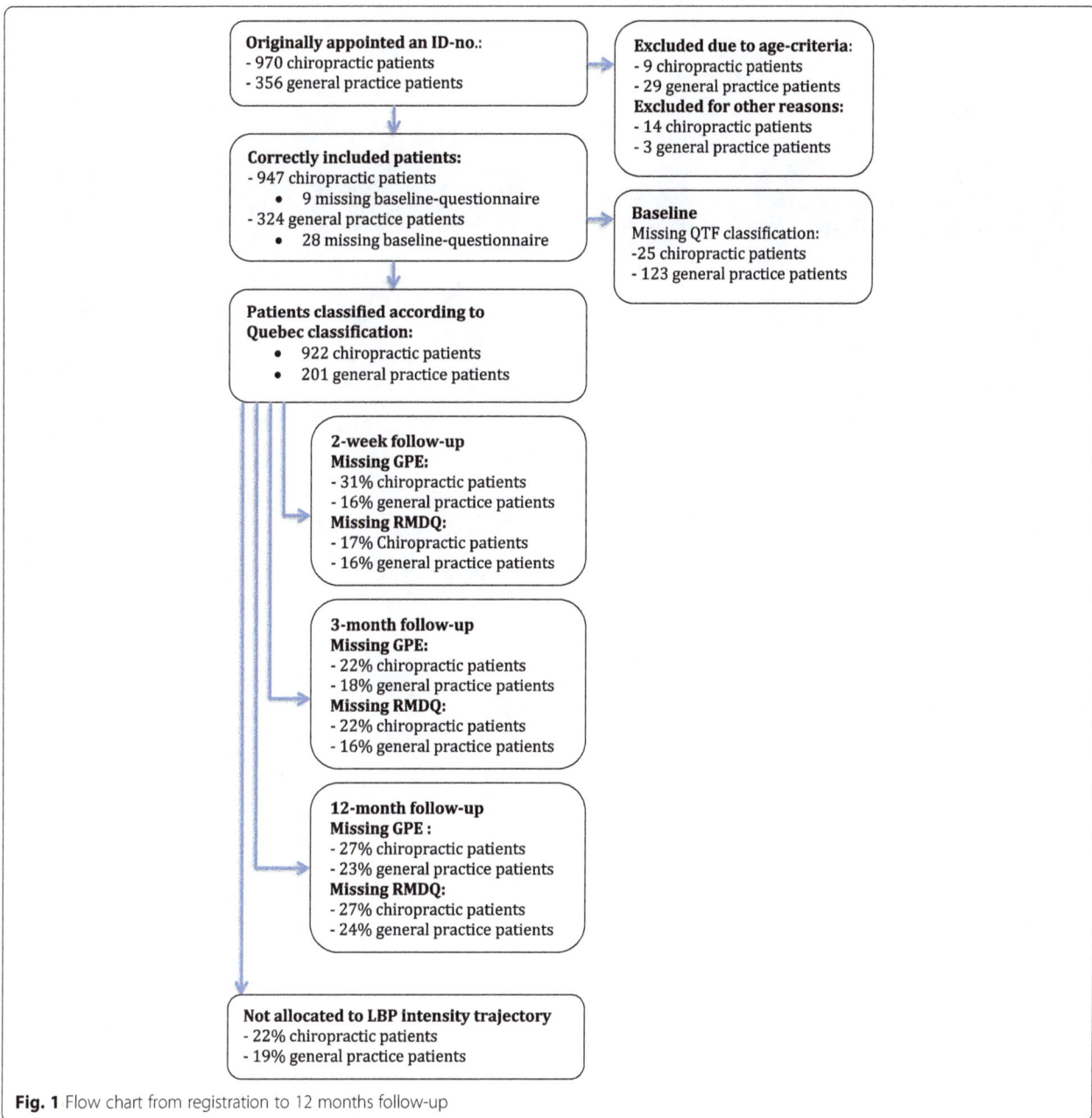

Fig. 1 Flow chart from registration to 12 months follow-up

shows the mean LBP intensity in each week within the five trajectories.

The distribution across the five trajectories was similar for patients with 'LBP alone' and patients with 'LBP + leg pain above the knee' in both cohorts, whereas for patients with 'LBP + leg pain below the knee' and in particular for patients with 'LBP + NRI' we observed a larger proportion of patient in the trajectories with on-going pain. The ranking across the QTF categories became even more visible when merging the five LBP trajectories into three trajectory groups of good, intermediate, and poor outcome

(Fig. 4). In chiropractic practice there was a decreasing proportion of patients in the good outcome trajectory and an increasing proportion of patients in the poor outcome trajectory going from 'LBP alone', across 'LBP + leg pain above the knee' and 'LBP + leg pain below the knee', to 'LBP + NRI'. In general practice patients with 'LBP alone' and patients with 'LBP + leg pain above the knee' had similar distributions across the three trajectory groups, whereas the proportion of patients in the poor outcome trajectory was substantially larger in patients with 'LBP + leg pain below the knee' and even more so for patients with 'LBP + NRI'.

Table 1 Patient-reported baseline characteristics of chiropractic patients (a) and general practice patients (b)

	All chiropractic patients (a)	'LBP alone'	'LBP + pain above knee'	'LBP + pain below knee'	'LBP + signs of nerve root involvement'	Quebec missing	p-values[§]
	n = 947	n = 614 (67%)	n = 219 (24%)	n = 69 (7%)	n = 20 (2%)	n = 25 (3%)	
Age in years[a]	43 (28, 59)	42 (27, 58)	45 (30, 60)	47 (32, 63)	48 (33, 66)	37 (23, 62)	<.01
Females[b]	45 (42–48)	42 (38–45)	52 (45–58)	52 (40–64)	55 (32–76)	40 (22–61)	0.03
Physical work load[b]							0.82
- Sitting	23 (21–26)	23 (20–27)	25 (19–31)	22 (13–34)	18 (5–46)	22 (9–45)	
- Sitting/walking	34 (31–37)	34 (30–38)	34 (28–41)	38 (27–52)	41 (19–67)	22 (9–45)	
- Light physical work	21 (19–24)	22 (19–25)	20 (15–26)	17 (9–29)	6 (1–37)	35 (17–57)	
- Heavy physical work	21 (19–24)	21 (18–24)	21 (16–27)	23 (14–36)	35 (15–62)	22 (9–45)	
Sick leave[b]	22 (19–25)	20 (17–24)	26 (20–32)	28 (18–41)	24 (8–52)	14 (4–37)	0.23
Educational level[b]							0.04
- No qualification	9 (7–11)	9 (7–12)	10 (6–15)	6 (2–16)	11 (2–39)	-	
- Vocational training,	26 (23–29)	26 (23–30)	24 (18–30)	32 (22–45)	33 (14–60)	25 (11–47)	
- Higher education < 3 y	16 (13–18)	14 (12–17)	21 (16–27)	8 (3–18)	28 (11–55)	13 (4–34)	
- Higher education 3–4 y	34 (31–38)	33 (30–37)	36 (31–43)	37 (26–50)	28 (11–55)	42 (23–63)	
- Higher education >4 y	15 (13–18)	17 (14–21)	9 (6–14)	17 (9–28)	-	21 (8–43)	
Duration of pain[b]							0.02
- 0–2 weeks	62 (59–66)	66 (62–70)	58 (52–65)	55 (42–66)	39 (18–65)	50 (30–70)	
- 2–4 weeks	14 (12–16)	14 (11–17)	13 (9–18)	11 (5–21)	22 (8–49)	17 (6–39)	
- 1–3 months	10 (9–13)	9 (7–11)	14 (10–20)	12 (6–23)	17 (5–44)	8 (2–30)	
- >3 months	13 (11–16)	11 (9–14)	14 (10–20)	23 (14–35)	22 (8–49)	25 (11–47)	
Previous LBP episodes[b]							0.03
- 0 episodes	16 (14–19)	17 (14–20)	17 (12–22)	6 (2–15)	18 (51–46)	21 (8–43)	
- 1–3 episodes	35 (32–38)	37 (33–41)	33 (27–40)	27 (18–40)	24 (8–52)	29 (14–52)	
- >3 episodes	49 (45–52)	46 (42–50)	50 (44–57)	67 (54–77)	59 (33–81)	50 (30–70)	
LBP last year[b]							<0.001
- ≤30 days	74 (72–77)	79 (76–82)	68 (61–74)	58 (46–70)	53 (27–78)	75 (53–89)	
- >30 days	26 (23–28)	21 (18–24)	32 (26–39)	42 (30–54)	47 (22–73)	25 (11–47)	
LBP intensity[a]	7 (3, 9)	7 (3, 9)	7 (4, 9)	8 (3, 9)	7 (3, 9)	8 (2, 10)	0.07
Leg pain intensity[a]	2 (0, 7)	0 (0, 5)	4 (1, 7)	6 (2, 9)	8 (4, 9)	0 (0, 6)	<0.001
Recovery expectations[a]	9 (4, 10)	10 (4, 10)	9 (4, 10)	8 (2, 10)	9 (1, 10)	10 (4, 10)	<0.001
Depressive symptoms[a]	6 (1, 18)	5 (1, 17)	7.5 (2, 21)	9.5 (2, 21)	6 (2, 34)	7 (2, 19)	<0.001
Fear avoidance beliefs physical activity[a]	13 (6, 20)	13 (6, 20)	12 (5, 19)	14 (2, 20)	12 (5, 20)	14 (6, 22)	0.08

Table 1 Patient-reported baseline characteristics of chiropractic patients (a) and general practice patients (b) (Continued)

	All general practice patients (b) n=324	'LBP alone' n=97 (48%)	'LBP + pain above knee' n=42 (21%)	'LBP + pain below knee' n=39 (19%)	'LBP + signs of nerve root involvement' n=23 (11%)	Quebec missing n=123 (38%)	p-values§
Fear avoidance beliefs work[a]	11 (3, 26)	10 (3, 26)	13 (2, 24)	12 (2, 31)	17.5 (5,31)	11 (4, 33)	0.10
Start Back Tool[b]							<0.001
- Low risk	54 (51–57)	60 (56–64)	41 (34–48)	44 (32–57)	35 (15–62)	46 (26–67)	
- Medium risk	38 (35–41)	34 (30–38)	47 (40–54)	48 (35–60)	41 (19–67)	42 (23–63)	
- High risk	8 (6–10)	6 (4–8)	13 (8–18)	8 (3–18)	24 (8–52)	13 (4–34)	
Activity limitation[a]	52 (17, 83)	52 (13, 83)	56 (26, 83)	57 (17, 83)	74 (17, 90)	59 (15, 85)	0.01
General health[a]	70 (35, 90)	75 (37, 90)	70 (30, 90)	67 (34, 90)	70 (28, 97)	72 (40, 92)	<.01
Age in years[a]	46 (27–59)	46 (23–61)	47 (31–60)	49 (34–61)	45 (34–60)	44 (26–58)	0.48
Females[b]	55 (49–60)	54 (43–63)	64 (48–78)	46 (31–62)	39 (21–61)	58 (49–67)	0.20
Physical work load[b]							0.45
- Sitting	14 (11–19)	19 (11–29)	6 (1–21)	11 (3–30)	37 (17–62)	18 (11–26)	
- Sitting/walking	32 (27–38)	33 (24–44)	34 (20–52)	36 (20–56)	-	30 (22–39)	
- Light physical work	28 (23–33)	23 (15–34)	23 (11–40)	32 (17–52)	32 (14–57)	31 (22–40)	
- Heavy physical work	25 (21–31)	25 (16–35)	37 (22–55)	21 (9–42)	32 (14–57)	22 (15–31)	
Sick leave[b]	40 (34–46))	34 (25–45)	54 (37–70))	39 (23–58)	56 (31–78)	37 (29–47)	0.12
Educational level[b]							0.47
- No qualification	20 (16–25)	16 (10–26)	26 (14–42)	26 (13–43)	20 (7–45)	19 (13–28)	
- Vocational training,	18 (14–23)	16 (10–26)	23 (12–40)	17 (8–34)	20 (7–45)	18 (12–26)	
- Higher education < 3 y	22 (18–27)	19 (12–29)	26 (14–42)	17 (8–34)	30 (13–55)	23 (16–31)	
- Higher education 3–4 y	29 (24–34)	31 (22–41)	18 (9–34)	34 (20–52)	25 (10–50)	31 (23–40)	
- Higher education >4 y	6 (4–9)	14 (8–23)	3 (0–17)	3 (0–19)	-	3 (1–8)	
Duration of pain[b]							0.03
- 0–2 weeks	39 (33–44)	42 (32–53)	51 (35–67)	20 (9–37)	20 (7–45)	41 (32–50)	
- 2–4 weeks	14 (10–18)	15 (9–25)	5 (1–20)	17 (8–34)	15 (4–40)	14 (8–21)	
- 1–3 months	16 (12–21)	20 (13–30)	8 (2–23)	14 (6–31)	20 (7–45)	15 (10–23)	
- >3 months	32 (27–37)	22 (15–33)	35 (21–52)	49 (32–65)	45 (24–68)	31 (23–40)	
Previous LBP episodes[b]							0.03
- 0 episodes	14 (11–19)	23 (15–34)	8 (2–23)	6 (1–21)	5 (1–32)	14 (9–22)	
- 1–3 episodes	24 (19–29)	16 (10–26)	37 (23–54)	23 (11–40)	25 (10–50)	25 (18–34)	
- >3 episodes	62 (56–67)	60 (50–70)	55 (39–71)	71 (54–84)	70 (45–87)	60 (51–69)	

Table 1 Patient-reported baseline characteristics of chiropractic patients (a) and general practice patients (b) (Continued)

							p-value
LBP last year[b]							0.29
- ≤30 days	51 (45–56)	56 (45–66)	53 (36–68)	37 (22–55)	45 (24–68)	51 (42–60)	
- >30 days	49 (44–55)	44 (34–55)	47 (32–64)	63 (45–78)	55 (32–76)	49 (40–58)	
LBP intensity[a]	7 (4, 9)	7 (4, 9)	8 (5, 10)	7 (4, 9)	7 (3, 10)	7 (4, 9)	0.35
Leg pain intensity[a]	3 (0, 9)	0 (0, 6)	5 (0, 9)	7 (3, 9)	6 (4, 10)	3 (0, 9)	<0.001
Recovery expectations[a]	6 (0, 10)	7 (2, 10)	8 (0, 10)	3 (0, 9)	5 (0, 7)	7 (1, 10)	<0.001
Depressive symptoms[a]	9 (2, 26)	8 (2, 22)	7 (1, 27)	15 (2.6, 39)	10 (4, 28)	9 (2, 25)	0.09
Fear avoidance beliefs physical activity[a]	14 (6, 21)	13 (3, 21)	15 (8, 20)	14.5 (5, 22)	17 (9, 24)	13.5 (6, 21)	0.01
Fear avoidance beliefs work[a]	14 (3, 28)	11 (3, 27)	18 (6, 27)	16 (4, 30)	23 (12, 38)	14 (3, 29)	0.001
Start Back Tool[b]							<0.001
- Low risk	41 (36–47)	51 (40–62)	31 (17–50)	25 (13–44)	27 (9–57)	44 (35–54)	
- Medium risk	36 (30–41)	28 (19–39)	59 (41–75)	25 (13–44)	33 (13–63)	38 (29–47)	
- High risk	23 (18–28)	21 (14–32)	9 (3–27)	50 32–68)	40 17–68)	18 (12–26)	
Activity limitation[a]	61 (22, 87)	54 (17, 83)	61 (35, 87)	74 (14, 96)	72 (31, 91)	65 (22, 87)	<0.001
General health[a]	60 (26, 90)	65 (35, 90)	60 (19, 90)	50 (20, 86)	50 (16, 74)	65 (25, 90)	0.005

LBP low back pain
[a]Median (10%, 90% centiles)
[b]Proportion (95% CI)
[b]P-values for test of any differences across the four QTF categories

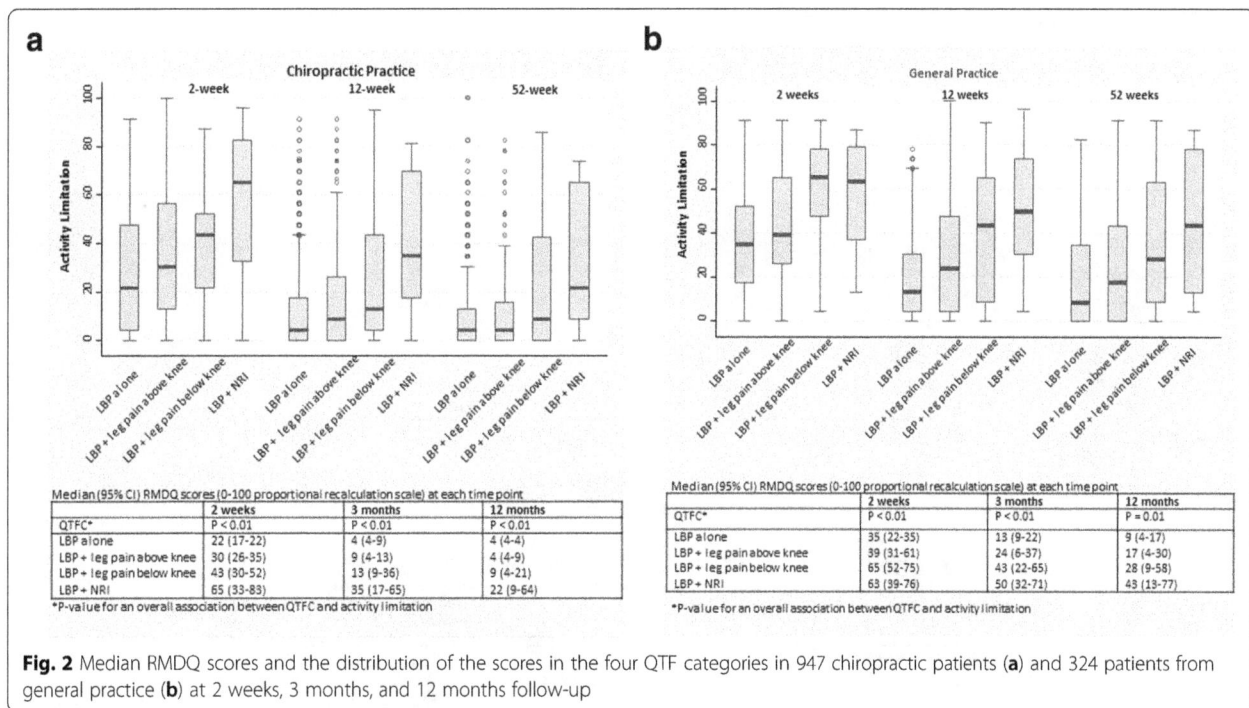

Fig. 2 Median RMDQ scores and the distribution of the scores in the four QTF categories in 947 chiropractic patients (**a**) and 324 patients from general practice (**b**) at 2 weeks, 3 months, and 12 months follow-up

Adjusted associations between QTF categories and outcomes (objective 3)

Adjusting simultaneously for age, sex and educational level did not change the statistical significance of the association between the QTF categories and outcomes except for the association with the recovery trajectory, which after adjusting was no longer statistically significant. The estimates did not change to a relevant degree (Additional file 1). The largest change in odds ratio occurred in the association between 'LBP + NRI' and the poor outcome trajectory, where the odds ratio changed from 5.53 to 4.27 in the chiropractic cohort. In the case of significant associations, the ordering of the effect estimates across the four categories did not change when adjusting.

Ranking of the four QTF categories (objective 4)

For nearly all outcomes with a statistically significant association with the QTF categories a ranking of increasing severity from the QTF category 1 to 4 could be observed although for some outcomes it was difficult to differentiate between 'LBP alone' and 'LBP + leg pain above the knee' and for others 'LBP + leg pain below the knee' was very similar to 'LBP + NRI' (Fig. 5). In the comparisons of the outcomes of neighbouring QTF categories, 'LBP + leg pain above the knee' had worse outcomes than 'LBP alone' in 11

Table 2 Relationship between QTF categories and global perceived effect (GPE)

QTF categories	2 weeks, proportion improved % (95% CI)		3 months, proportion improved % (95% CI)		12 months, proportion improved % (95% CI)	
	Chiropractic patients $P < 0.01$*	General practice patients $P < 0.01$*	Chiropractic patients $P = 0.2$*	General practice patients $P = 0.2$*	Chiropractic patients $P = 0.4$*	General practice patients $P = 0.5$*
All patients	74 (70–77)	36 (31–42)	82 (79–85)	60 (54–66)	73 (23–30)	54 (48–60)
'LBP alone'	77 (73–81)	49 (38–60)	82 (78–85)	69 (58–78)	74 (69–78)	53 (42–65)
'LBP + leg pain above the knee'	72 (64–79)	43 (28–60)	85 (79–90)	66 (49–80)	75 (67–81)	66 (48–80)
'LBP + leg pain below the knee'	61 (46–74)	19 (9–38)	73 (59–83)	46 (29–65)	63 (49–76)	54 (34–72)
'LBP + NRI'	40 (17–68)	20 (7–45)	87 (55–97)	56 (31–78)	73 (43–91)	44 (20–70)

Proportions improved after 2 weeks, 3 months and 12 months
LBP low back pain, *NRI* nerve root involvement
*P-value for an overall association between QTF categories and GPE

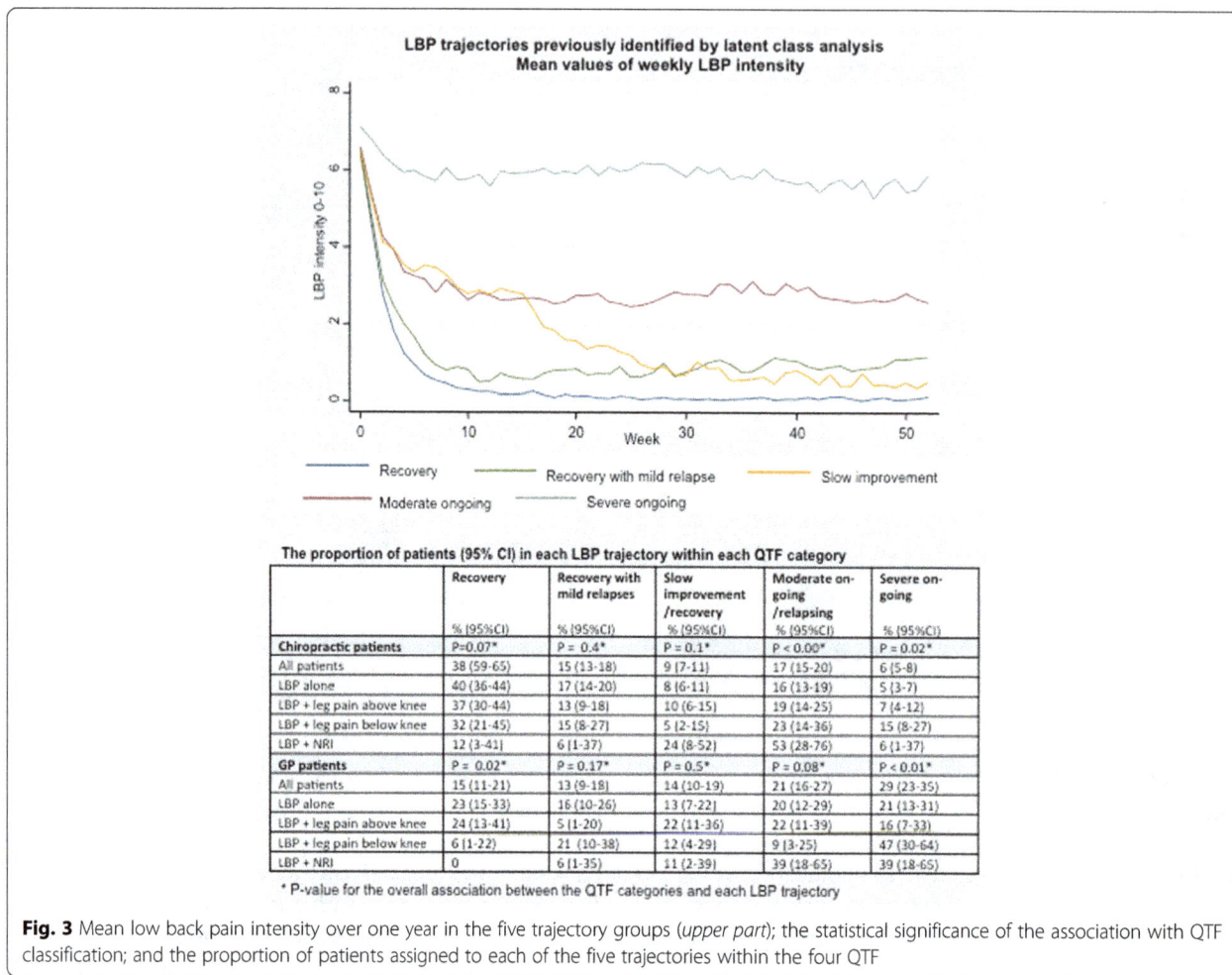

The proportion of patients (95% CI) in each LBP trajectory within each QTF category

	Recovery	Recovery with mild relapses	Slow improvement /recovery	Moderate on-going /relapsing	Severe on-going
	% (95%CI)	% (95%CI)	% (95%CI)	% (95%CI)	% (95%CI)
Chiropractic patients	P=0.07*	P = 0.4*	P = 0.1*	P < 0.00*	P = 0.02*
All patients	38 (59-65)	15 (13-18)	9 (7-11)	17 (15-20)	6 (5-8)
LBP alone	40 (36-44)	17 (14-20)	8 (6-11)	16 (13-19)	5 (3-7)
LBP + leg pain above knee	37 (30-44)	13 (9-18)	10 (6-15)	19 (14-25)	7 (4-12)
LBP + leg pain below knee	32 (21-45)	15 (8-27)	5 (2-15)	23 (14-36)	15 (8-27)
LBP + NRI	12 (3-41)	6 (1-37)	24 (8-52)	53 (28-76)	6 (1-37)
GP patients	P = 0.02*	P = 0.17*	P = 0.5*	P = 0.08*	P < 0.01*
All patients	15 (11-21)	13 (9-18)	14 (10-19)	21 (16-27)	29 (23-35)
LBP alone	23 (15-33)	16 (10-26)	13 (7-22)	20 (12-29)	21 (13-31)
LBP + leg pain above knee	24 (13-41)	5 (1-20)	22 (11-36)	22 (11-39)	16 (7-33)
LBP + leg pain below knee	6 (1-22)	21 (10-38)	12 (4-29)	9 (3-25)	47 (30-64)
LBP + NRI	0	6 (1-35)	11 (2-39)	39 (18-65)	39 (18-65)

* P-value for the overall association between the QTF categories and each LBP trajectory

Fig. 3 Mean low back pain intensity over one year in the five trajectory groups (*upper part*); the statistical significance of the association with QTF classification; and the proportion of patients assigned to each of the five trajectories within the four QTF

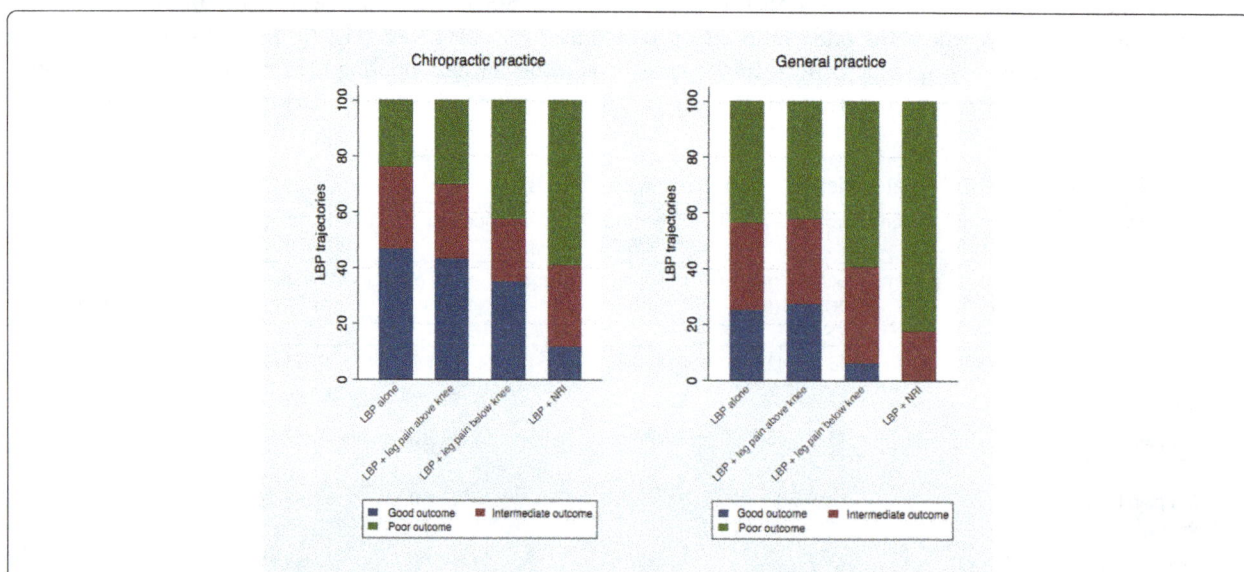

Fig. 4 Distribution of the three low back pain trajectories groups (good, intermediate, and poor outcome) within the four QTF categories. Based on 947 chiropractic patients and 324 patients from general practice

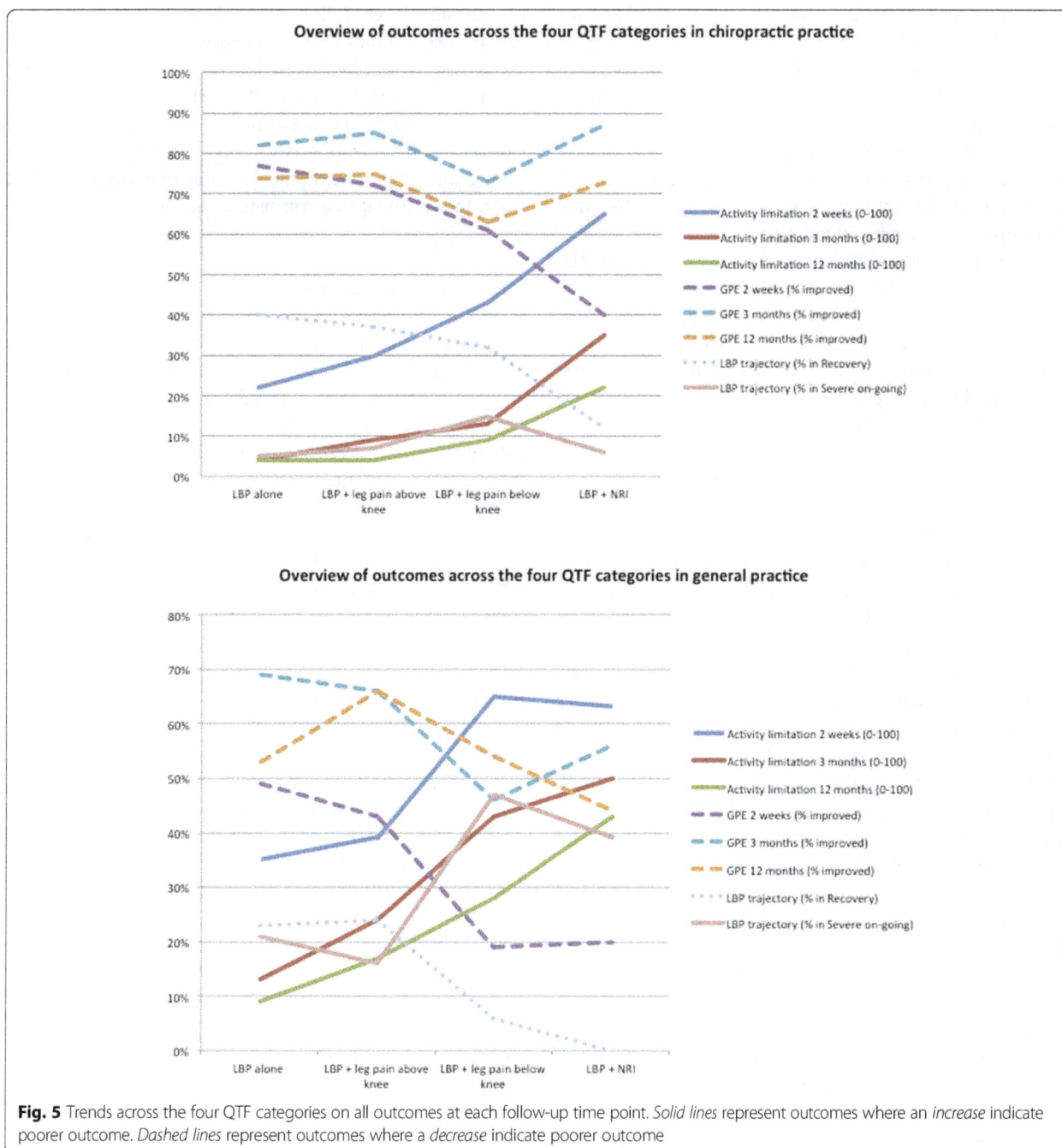

Fig. 5 Trends across the four QTF categories on all outcomes at each follow-up time point. *Solid lines* represent outcomes where an *increase* indicate poorer outcome. *Dashed lines* represent outcomes where a *decrease* indicate poorer outcome

out of 16 possible comparisons, 'LBP + leg pain below the knee' was associated with worse outcomes than 'LBP + leg pain above the knee' in 15 out of 16 comparisons, and 'LBP + NRI' had worse outcomes than 'LBP + leg pain below the knee' in 10 of 16 comparisons.

Discussion

Summary of main findings

To our knowledge, this is the first study in primary care in which the presence and extent of leg pain and NRI were determined by clinical assessment and the separative capacity of the four QTF categories was examined. We found that patients in the four QTF categories had different clinical presentations when seeking care, and that they also differed on outcomes. Pain and activity limitation were worse at all follow-up time points for patients with leg pain compared with patients with 'LBP alone', especially so for patients with pain below the knee and NRI. Importantly, our results suggest that patients with 'LBP + NRI' constitute a subgroup with its own characteristics and course and that the clinical examination thus is an important part of differentiating between categories of LBP-related leg pain. We also confirmed that in epidemiological studies when a clinical examination is not feasible the differentiation between pain above and below the knee does carry valuable information. The observed ranking of increasing severity in outcomes from the QTF category 1 to category 4 was similar for patients seen in chiropractic and general practice in spite of the fact that the type of care is not the same in chiropractic and general practice.

Consistent group differences demonstrated that the QTF categories do identify distinct LBP subgroups. The differences in expected outcomes between 'LBP alone' and 'LBP + NRI' in both cohorts and between 'LBP + leg pain below the knee' and 'LBP + NRI' in the chiropractic cohort reached a magnitude we regard as clinically relevant, i.e. provided a clinically relevant degree of separation [34]. Thus, the QTF classification is an easily applicable tool providing insight about the expected outcome of patients at a group level and it may be useful in the communication with patients. However, the variation within categories also implied that the QTF classification is not an accurate predictor of individuals' outcomes.

An earlier analysis of the same cohorts has shown that the patients in general practice were generally worse on a wide range of health parameters than the chiropractic patients at presentation [19]. The present study furthermore demonstrated that a considerably smaller proportion of chiropractic patients than general practice patients were categorized as having 'LBP + NRI'. This may be caused by symptoms of NRI triggering different care seeking behaviors than other back pain complaints, but might also be due to the collection of information on signs of NRI. According to the study protocol, the chiropractors had to do a thorough neurological examination whereas general practitioners were to answer a yes/no question on the presence of abnormal neurological findings. Thus, in chiropractic practice the classification of category 4 followed a standardized examination that may have resulted in a more precise diagnosis compared with general practice. This may in turn explain why the biggest difference between any of the four QTF categories in chiropractic patients was between patients with 'LBP + leg pain below the knee' and patients with 'LBP + NRI' whereas the difference between these two categories in general practice was less pronounced.

Comparison with existing literature

The results showing that LBP with leg pain below the knee with or without NRI is associated with a worse prognosis than LBP alone or LBP with leg pain above the knee is in line with previous studies from primary and secondary care in which absolute disability scores were about three times higher in patients having LBP with leg pain below the knee and 4–8 times higher in patients with LBP with NRI compared to patients with LBP alone at both 3-

months and 1-year follow-up [8, 9, 13, 15]. In contrast to one of these studies [13], we observed different outcomes for patients with LBP with leg pain above the knee as compared to patients with LBP with leg pain below the knee. This difference between the two studies may be caused by the previous study investigating LBP of very long duration in which pain location may become a less important element in a complex condition.

Strengths and limitations

A major strength of this study was the standardized clinical examination for signs of NRI conducted in the chiropractic cohort. Also the sample size was adequately large to result in relative precise estimates of group differences despite the limitation of some infrequent QTF categories. Data were collected prospectively and included both patient-reported information and clinical data, and to our knowledge this was the first study to include LBP trajectories derived from latent class analyses as an outcome measure.

LBP is a largely episodic/recurrent condition for most individuals manifesting itself on and off over the entire lifespan [35–37]. To establish a more detailed description of pain patterns, data collection by means of frequent text messaging on mobile phones has been introduced and different back pain trajectories have been identified and linked to clinical parameters in several other studies [38–41]. We used LBP trajectories as an outcome measure although the psychometric properties of this outcome measure have not been investigated. However these LBP trajectories represent patterns of LBP similar to those observed in other primary care cohorts [39, 42–44] and provided an opportunity to include a measure of the clinical course that does not assume that pain outcomes differ only in severity at certain time points but also in course pattern. It was reassuring that the general findings on this outcome variable reflected the same relationships as those on activity limitation.

Obviously, the study is limited by a lack of standardization of the clinical examination in general practice which may have caused less distinct differences between leg pain below the knee and NRI in that cohort than what is truly the case. Another limitation of the study was the incomplete follow-up in both cohorts and the fact that only two thirds of patients from general practice were classified according to the QTF categories. However, patients classified were similar to patients not classified and responders were similar to non-responders. It is therefore unlikely that the results are influenced by this incompleteness. Also, it is a limitation that pain location was not obtained from patients categorized with 'LBP + NRI'. It would be useful to know what proportion of this group actually reports pain below the knee.

The only outcome that was not associated with the QTF categories was GPE at the 3-months and 1-year follow-ups. This may imply that GPE is likely to be unsuitable as a long-term outcome. It has been suggested that patients have difficulty taking their baseline status into account when scoring the GPE, and that the GPE ratings are influenced by peoples current health status [29], which is likely to become increasingly problematic with longer follow-up periods.

It was outside the scope of this study to investigate the value of the QTF categories in comparison to or in addition to other classification tools or prognostic markers.

Implications for clinical practice and future research

This study demonstrated that the QTF categories provide a simple way for clinicians to classify patients with non-specific LBP into subgroups with expected different outcomes. The results from this study underpin the importance of establishing a diagnosis of NRI based on a clinical examination and not merely on self-reported symptoms and our results support that both localization of pain and NRI are relevant prognostic factors [9, 13, 15, 16]. Next it should be investigated if the QTF categories add information to existing LBP prediction models and if the QTF categories moderate the effect of recommended treatments for LBP. Generally, in the design of research projects it should be recognized that data from the clinical examination are needed when identification of relatively homogeneous groups of patients with LBP-related leg pain is required. Finally, the results imply that systematic reviews and meta-analyses should assess the consequences of combining leg pain categories and whenever possible report the different categories separately.

Conclusion

Our results confirm that the QTF categories do identify LBP subgroups differing in baseline characteristics as well as in expected outcomes. The latter appear to be of a clinically relevant degree and reflect a ranking in severity. Patient outcomes are best when pain is restricted to the low back, worse if the pain radiates down the leg (worst with pain below the knee), and most severe if there are neurological symptoms in the leg as well. To identify the latter group, a clinical examination is warranted. Clearly, the four QTF categories deserve more interest in relation to research into improvement of prediction tools and treatment decisions.

Abbreviations
FABQ: Fear-avoidance beliefs questionnaire; GPE: Global perceived effect; LBP: Low back pain; NRI: Nerve root involvement; NRS: Numeric rating scale; QTF: Quebec Task Force; QTFC: Quebec Task Force categories; RMDQ: Roland Morris Disability Questionnaire

Acknowledgements
Not applicable.

Funding
LHa received funding from The Danish Chiropractors' Foundation and the Region of Southern Denmark. The Nordic Institute of Chiropractic and Clinical Biomechanics and AK's position at the University of Southern Denmark are financially supported by the Danish Chiropractors' Foundation. The funding body had no role in the design of the study, collection, analysis, and interpretation of data and in writing the manuscript.

Authors' contributions
LHa, AK, LH, CLY and WV contributed to the design of the study. LHa carried out data analysis and drafting of the manuscript. AK, LH, CLY and WV provided advice on the statistical analyses, and critically revised the manuscript. All authors read and approved the final manuscript.

Competing interests
LH and AK are members of the Editorial Board of BMC Musculoskeletal Disorders; the other authors declare that they have no competing interests.

Consent for publication
Not applicable.

Author details
[1]Department of Sports Science and Clinical Biomechanics, University of Southern Denmark, Odense, Denmark. [2]Nordic Institute of Chiropractic and Clinical Biomechanics, Odense, Denmark. [3]Research Department, Spine Center of Southern Denmark, Hospital Lillebælt, Middelfart, Denmark. [4]Institute for Regional Health Research, University of Southern Denmark, Odense, Denmark. [5]Institute for Medical Biometry and Statistics, Faculty of Medicine and Medical Center, University of Freiburg, Freiburg, Germany.

References
1. Vos T, Flaxman AD, Naghavi M, Lozano R, Michaud C, Ezzati M, Shibuya K, Salomon JA, Abdalla S, Aboyans V, et al. Years lived with disability (YLDs) for 1160 sequelae of 289 diseases and injuries 1990–2010: a systematic analysis for the Global Burden of Disease Study 2010. Lancet. 2012;380(9859): 2163–96.
2. United States Bone and Joint Initiative. The Burden of Musculoskeletal Diseases in the United States (BMUS) TE, 2014. Rosemont, IL. Available at http://www.boneandjointburden.org. Accessed 3 May 2016.
3. Flachs EM EL, Koch MB, Ryd JT, Dibba E, Skov-Ettrup L, Juel K. Sygdomsbyrden i Danmark – sygdomme. In: Statens Institut for Folkesundhed, Syddansk Universitet. København: Sundhedsstyrelsen; 2015.
4. van Tulder M, Becker A, Bekkering T, Breen A, del Real MT, Hutchinson A, Koes B, Laerum E, Malmivaara A. Chapter 3. European guidelines for the management of acute nonspecific low back pain in primary care. Eur Spine J. 2006;15 Suppl 2:S169–191.
5. Karayannis NV, Jull GA, Hodges PW. Physiotherapy movement based classification approaches to low back pain: comparison of subgroups through review and developer/expert survey. BMC Musculoskelet Disord. 2012;13:24.
6. Fairbank J, Gwilym SE, France JC, Daffner SD, Dettori J, Hermsmeyer J, Andersson G. The role of classification of chronic low back pain. Spine. 2011;36(21 Suppl):S19–42.
7. O SW. Scientific approach to the assessment and management of activity-related spinal disorders. A monograph for clinicians. Report of the Quebec Task Force on Spinal Disorders. Spine. 1987;12(7 Suppl):S1-59.
8. Atlas SJ, Deyo RA, Patrick DL, Convery K, Keller RB, Singer DE. The Quebec Task Force classification for spinal disorders and the severity, treatment, and outcomes of sciatica and lumbar spinal stenosis. Spine. 1996;21(24):2885–92.
9. Loisel P, Vachon B, Lemaire J, Durand MJ, Poitras S, Stock S, Tremblay C. Discriminative and predictive validity assessment of the quebec task force classification. Spine. 2002;27(8):851–7.

10. Werneke MW, Hart DL. Categorizing patients with occupational low back pain by use of the Quebec Task Force Classification system versus pain pattern classification procedures: discriminant and predictive validity. Phys Ther. 2004;84(3):243–54.

11. Selim AJ, Ren XS, Fincke G, Deyo RA, Rogers W, Miller D, Linzer M, Kazis L. The importance of radiating leg pain in assessing health outcomes among patients with low back pain. Results from the Veterans Health Study. Spine. 1998;23(4):470–4.

12. Kongsted A, Kent P, Albert H, Jensen TS, Manniche C. Patients with low back pain differ from those who also have leg pain or signs of nerve root involvement - a cross-sectional study. BMC Musculoskelet Disord. 2012;13:236.

13. Kongsted A, Kent P, Jensen TS, Albert H, Manniche C. Prognostic implications of the Quebec Task Force classification of back-related leg pain: an analysis of longitudinal routine clinical data. BMC Musculoskelet Disord. 2013;14:171.

14. Hider SL, Whitehurst DG, Thomas E, Foster NE. Pain location matters: the impact of leg pain on health care use, work disability and quality of life in patients with low back pain. Eur Spine J. 2015;24(3):444–51.

15. Hill JC, Konstantinou K, Egbewale BE, Dunn KM, Lewis M, van der Windt D. Clinical outcomes among low back pain consulters with referred leg pain in primary care. Spine. 2011;36(25):2168–75.

16. Konstantinou K, Hider SL, Jordan JL, Lewis M, Dunn KM, Hay EM. The impact of low back-related leg pain on outcomes as compared with low back pain alone: a systematic review of the literature. Clin J Pain. 2013;29(7):644–54.

17. Ashworth J, Konstantinou K, Dunn KM. Prognostic factors in non-surgically treated sciatica: a systematic review. BMC Musculoskelet Disord. 2011;12:208.

18. Koes BW, van Tulder M, Lin CW, Macedo LG, McAuley J, Maher C. An updated overview of clinical guidelines for the management of non-specific low back pain in primary care. Eur Spine J. 2010;19(12):2075–94.

19. Hestbaek L, Munck A, Hartvigsen L, Jarbol DE, Sondergaard J, Kongsted A. Low back pain in primary care: a description of 1250 patients with low back pain in danish general and chiropractic practice. Int J Fam Med. 2014;2014:106102.

20. Kongsted A, Kent P, Hestbaek L, Vach W. Patients with low back pain had distinct clinical course patterns that were typically neither complete recovery nor constant pain. A latent class analysis of longitudinal data. Spine J. 2015;15(5):885–94.

21. Eirikstoft H, Kongsted A. Patient characteristics in low back pain subgroups based on an existing classification system. A descriptive cohort study in chiropractic practice. Man Ther. 2014;19(1):65–71.

22. Kent P, Lauridsen HH. Managing missing scores on the Roland Morris Disability Questionnaire. Spine. 2011;36(22):1878–84.

23. Jensen MP, Miller L, Fisher LD. Assessment of pain during medical procedures: a comparison of three scales. Clin J Pain. 1998;14(4):343–9.

24. Kongsted A, Vach W, Axo M, Bech RN, Hestbaek L. Expectation of recovery from low back pain: a longitudinal cohort study investigating patient characteristics related to expectations and the association between expectations and 3-month outcome. Spine. 2014;39(1):81–90.

25. Bech P, Rasmussen NA, Olsen LR, Noerholm V, Abildgaard W. The sensitivity and specificity of the Major Depression Inventory, using the Present State Examination as the index of diagnostic validity. J Affect Disord. 2001;66(2–3): 159–64.

26. Waddell G, Newton M, Henderson I, Somerville D, Main CJ. A Fear-Avoidance Beliefs Questionnaire (FABQ) and the role of fear-avoidance beliefs in chronic low back pain and disability. Pain. 1993;52(2):157–68.

27. Rabin R, de Charro F. EQ-5D: a measure of health status from the EuroQol Group. Ann Med. 2001;33(5):337–43.

28. Hill JC, Dunn KM, Lewis M, Mullis R, Main CJ, Foster NE, Hay EM. A primary care back pain screening tool: identifying patient subgroups for initial treatment. Arthritis Rheum. 2008;59(5):632–41.

29. Kamper SJ, Ostelo RW, Knol DL, Maher CG, de Vet HC, Hancock MJ. Global Perceived Effect scales provided reliable assessments of health transition in people with musculoskeletal disorders, but ratings are strongly influenced by current status. J Clin Epidemiol. 2010;63(7):760–6. e761.

30. Axen I, Bodin L, Bergstrom G, Halasz L, Lange F, Lovgren PW, Rosenbaum A, Leboeuf-Yde C, Jensen I. The use of weekly text messaging over 6 months was a feasible method for monitoring the clinical course of low back pain in patients seeking chiropractic care. J Clin Epidemiol. 2012;65(4):454–61.

31. Kongsted A, Kent P, Axen I, Downie AS, Dunn KM. What have we learned from ten years of trajectory research in low back pain? BMC Musculoskelet Disord. 2016;17:220.

32. Bombardier C, Hayden J, Beaton DE. Minimal clinically important difference. Low back pain: outcome measures. J Rheumatol. 2001;28(2):431–8.

33. Ostelo RW, Deyo RA, Stratford P, Waddell G, Croft P, Von Korff M, Bouter LM, de Vet HC. Interpreting change scores for pain and functional status in low back pain: towards international consensus regarding minimal important change. Spine. 2008;33(1):90–4.

34. Royston PSW. A new measure of prognostic separation in survival data. Stat Med. 2004;23(5):723–48.

35. Axen I, Leboeuf-Yde C. Trajectories of low back pain. Best Pract Res Clin Rheumatol. 2013;27(5):601–12.

36. Dunn KM, Hestbaek L, Cassidy JD. Low back pain across the life course. Best Pract Res Clin Rheumatol. 2013;27(5):591–600.

37. Lemeunier N, Leboeuf-Yde C, Gagey O. The natural course of low back pain: a systematic critical literature review. Chiropr Man Ther. 2012;20(1):33.

38. Leboeuf-Yde C, Lemeunier N, Wedderkopp N, Kjaer P. Evidence-based classification of low back pain in the general population: one-year data collected with SMS Track. Chiropr Man Ther. 2013;21:30.

39. Axen I, Bodin L, Bergstrom G, Halasz L, Lange F, Lovgren PW, Rosenbaum A, Leboeuf-Yde C, Jensen I. Clustering patients on the basis of their individual course of low back pain over a six month period. BMC Musculoskelet Disord. 2011;12:99.

40. Kongsted A, Leboeuf-Yde C. The Nordic back pain subpopulation program-individual patterns of low back pain established by means of text messaging: a longitudinal pilot study. Chiropr Osteopath. 2009;17:11.

41. Macedo LG, Maher CG, Latimer J, McAuley JH, Hodges PW, Rogers WT. Nature and determinants of the course of chronic low back pain over a 12-month period: a cluster analysis. Phys Ther. 2014;94(2):210–21.

42. Dunn KM, Jordan K, Croft PR. Characterizing the course of low back pain: a latent class analysis. Am J Epidemiol. 2006;163(8):754–61.

43. Downie AS, Hancock MJ, Rzewuska M, Williams CM, Lin CW, Maher CG. Trajectories of acute low back pain: a latent class growth analysis. Pain. 2016;157(1):225–34.

44. Deyo RA, Bryan M, Comstock BA, Turner JA, Heagerty P, Friedly J, Avins AL, Nedeljkovic SS, Nerenz DR, Jarvik JG. Trajectories of symptoms and function in older adults with low back disorders. Spine. 2015;40(17):1352–62.

9

Risk classification of patients referred to secondary care for low back pain

Monica Unsgaard-Tøndel[1,2*], Ingunn Gunnes Kregnes[3], Tom I. L. Nilsen[2,4], Gunn Hege Marchand[1,3] and Torunn Askim[1]

Abstract

Background: Nonspecific low back pain is characterized by a wide range of possible triggering and conserving factors, and initial screening needs to scope widely with multilevel addressment of possible factors contributing to the pain experience. Screening tools for classification of patients have been developed to support clinicians. The primary aim of this study was to assess the criterion validity of STarT Back Screening Tool (STarT Back) against the more comprehensive Örebro Musculoskeletal Pain Questionnaire (ÖMPSQ), in a Norwegian sample of patients referred to secondary care for low back pain. Secondary aims were to assess risk classification of the patients, as indicated by both instruments, and to compare pain and work characteristics between patients in the different STarT Back risk categories.

Methods: An observational, cross-sectional survey among patients with low back pain referred to outpatient secondary care assessment at Trondheim University Hospital, Norway. Cohen's Kappa coefficient, Pearson's r and a Bland-Altman plot were used to assess criterion validity of STarT Back against ÖMPSQ. Furthermore, linear regression was used to estimate mean differences with 95% CI in pain and work related variables between the risk groups defined by the STarT Back tool.

Results: A total of 182 persons participated in the study. The Pearsons correlation coefficient for correspondence between scores on ÖMPSQ and STarT Back was 0.76. The Kappa value for classification agreement between the instruments was 0.35. Risk group classification according to STarT Back allocated 34.1% of the patients in the low risk group, 42.3% in the medium risk, and 23.6% in the high risk group. According to ÖMPSQ, 24.7% of the participants were allocated in the low risk group, 28.6% in the medium risk, and 46.7% in the high risk group. Patients classified with high risk according to Start Back showed a higher score on pain and work related characteristics as measured by ÖMPSQ.

Conclusion: The correlation between score on the screening tools was good, while the classification agreement between the screening instruments was low. Screening for work factors may be important in patients referred to multidisciplinary management in secondary care.

Keywords: Primary care, Secondary care, Low back pain, Screening, Multidisciplinary, Work

Background

Low back pain is the leading cause of years lived with disability globally [1, 2]. In addition to a negative impact on the individual's health, it is associated with substantial financial costs, partly for management that is not supported by scientific evidence [3].

Management guidelines suggest that patients seeking care for nonspecific and uncomplicated low back pain should be offered treatment in primary care [4]. On the other hand, patients with possible indicators of serious pathology or with compound treatment needs due to complex psychosocial challenges should be referred to specialist health service for further investigation and treatment [5]. Specific causes for low back pain are uncommon, and for about 85% of patients, low back pain

* Correspondence: monica.unsgaard.tondel@ntnu.no
[1]Department of Neuromedicine and Movement Science (INB), NTNU, Faculty of Medicine and Health Sciences, N-7491 Trondheim, Norway
[2]Department of Public Health and Nursing, Norwegian University of Science and Technology, Faculty of Medicine and Health Sciences, Trondheim, Norway
Full list of author information is available at the end of the article

is defined as nonspecific since the pain does not seem to be connected to specific organic impairments [6]. Nonspecific low back pain is characterized by a wide range of possible triggering and conserving factors, including lifestyle, behavioral, biomechanical, and psychosocial influences [7, 8]. Therefore, initial screening needs to scope widely with multilevel addressment of possible factors contributing to the pain experience.

There are data suggesting that in general, previous management for patients with low back pain have failed to address its multifactorial nature and accordingly not contributed significantly to patients' improvement in the long term [8]. Part of the reason for this may be that multifactorial and knowledge based assessment tools have not been available. However, screening tools for classification of patients have been developed to support clinicians when identifying the specific needs of individual patients. The STarT Back screening tool (STarT Back) is one such screening tool [9]. It contains nine items covering eight domains, which were selected based on established prognostic factors suggested to affect probability of recovery. STarT Back was originally validated in England [9], and has been tested and adapted in a range of countries including Belgium [10], Denmark [11, 12], Finland [13], China [14], Germany [15], Norway [16] and Sweden [17]. Most of these studies have been performed in primary care. Another screening tool is the more comprehensive Örebro Musculoskeletal Pain Screening Questionnaire (ÖMPSQ), which was developed in Sweden for early identification of patients at risk for developing a persistent back problem [18]. ÖMPSQ has been considered an appropriate reference standard since it is an established tool to support clinicians in identifying patients in need of more comprehensive treatment for low back pain [19]. Since the performance of screening tools is highly context dependent, testing the tool in varied clinical settings is necessary. Therefore we wished to explore whether risk estimation by STarT Back is comparable to ÖMPSQ in a Norwegian multidisciplinary secondary care setting.

The primary aim of this study was to assess the criterion validity of the STarT Back Screening Tool against the Örebro Musculoskeletal Pain Screening Questionnaire in a Norwegian sample of patients with low back pain referred to assessment at a university hospital. Secondary aims were to assess risk classification of the patients, as indicated by both instruments, and to compare pain and work characteristics between patients in the different STarT Back risk categories.

Methods
Design
An observational, cross-sectional survey was performed in an outpatient multidisciplinary clinic for musculoskeletal pain in Trondheim University Hospital, Norway.

Participants
The study sample was patients referred for secondary line management because of low back pain. The inclusion criteria were as follows: Referred from their physician, manual therapist or chiropractor in the primary health care system with low back pain for more than 6 weeks. Exclusion criteria were age under 18, insufficient language capabilities, malignant disease, and unresolved social security or insurance problems.

Variables
Background variables
Background variables included age, gender, marital status, country of birth, educational level, and work status. Participants that were not out of work, sicklisted or on work assessment allowance were classified as employed. We defined people with any percentage of sickleave as sicklisted. Information on other diseases category was also collected, including headache, pulmonary disease, coronary disease, hypertension, diabetes and an open category for diseases specified by the participants.

Measures
STarT Back screening tool contains nine questions, and was developed based on prognostic factors for longstanding disability due to low back pain [9]. The questions cover the following eight constructs: bothersomeness, referred leg pain, comorbid pain, disability, catastrophizing, fear, anxiety, and depression. Based on dichotomizing responses patients were given an overall tool score and a psychosocial subscale score. Patients were allocated to the high risk group if the psychosocial subscale score was ≥4, to the low risk group if the overall score was ' 4, and to the medium risk group if the overall score was ≥4. Participants with missing items on STarT Back screening tool were excluded from the analysis if risk classification could not be established as described in the original study [9].

Örebro Musculoskeletal Pain Screening Questionnaire (ÖMPSQ) was developed to assist health care providers in assessing risk of developing a persistent back problem. Originally it was aiming at predicting risk for work absenteeism due to sickness [20]. The scoring system ranges from zero to 210, with higher scores indicating a higher risk of poor outcome. It has shown good psychometric properties [18, 21] and moderate predictive ability in identifying patients with spinal pain at risk of persisting pain and disability [22]. The questionnaire contains 25 items, and items 5–25 are scored [23]. Lower cut-off limits for ÖMPSQ were 89 for medium risk and 112 for high risk (corresponds to 42 and 53% of total score). Based on a recent study, we chose to omit the work questions in the ÖMPSQ total score for non-working patients [24]. Therefore the five work-related items no 6, 8, 16, 17, and 20) were excluded for participants out of work, and new scoring range and cut-off values were calculated based on the percentage of total score omitting five variables (i.e. 42 and 53% of 160). This gave cutoffs of 67 and 85 for medium and high risk classification among non-workers, respectively.

Analysis

To assess criterion validity of STarT Back, the agreement in risk classification (low, medium, and high) based on STarT Back and ÖMPSQ was assessed by Cohen's Kappa coefficient. The calculations were done for the overall study population, but since some of the items of the ÖMPSQ are work related, we also estimated the agreement in risk classification for patients who were classified as workers. We also calculated *the mean* ÖMPSQ score with 95% confidence interval (CI) according to *STarT Back* total score (Fig. 1). Since the two scores are measured on different scales, we converted both scores to percentage scores before we used Pearson's r to estimate the correlation between STarT Back and ÖMPSQ. The acceptability limits were defined as: poor ≤ 30; adequate $0.31-0.59$, and excellent ≥ 0.60 [25]. The percentage scores were also used in a Bland-Altman plot assessing the agreement between STarT Back and ÖMPSQ screening tools.

Risk classification of the patients, as indicated by both instruments was described by a classification table. Finally, we used linear regression to estimate mean differences with 95% CI in pain and work related variables between the three risk groups defined by the STarT Back tool. Non-normally distributed variables were analyzed using non-parametric Mann-Whitney U test and results presented as differences in median values between risk groups.

Results

A total of 300 patients received the study questionnaire, and 199 (66%) returned it. After excluding 17 persons due to incomplete answers or age below 18 years, 182 patients (61%) were available for statistical analysis. Among those, 73% were employed, mean age was 48 years (SD = 15), and 51% were men (Table 1).

The Kappa value for agreement between risk group classification was 0.35 (Table 2). Restricting the sample to only workers gave the same level of agreement (Kappa 0.36). Figure 1 shows that mean percentage of total ÖMPSQ-score increased monotonically with increasing STarT Back total score, and the two scores showed a high correlation ($r = 0.76$, p^{c}0.001). The Bland Altman plot (Fig. 2) display the difference between the two instruments according to the average percentage scores for both instruments, and suggests that the agreement between the instruments is highest for middle range scores. Mean bias is 1.6, but for patients scoring in the lower range on both scores there is tendency that STarT Back generates lower score than ÖMPSQ. On the other hand, in patients with higher average scores, STarT Back seems to generate higher scores than ÖMPSQ.

Start Back Screening tool allocated 34.1% of the participants in the low risk group, 42.3% in the medium risk group, and 23.6% in the high risk group. Corresponding values for ÖMPSQ was 24.7% of the participants in the

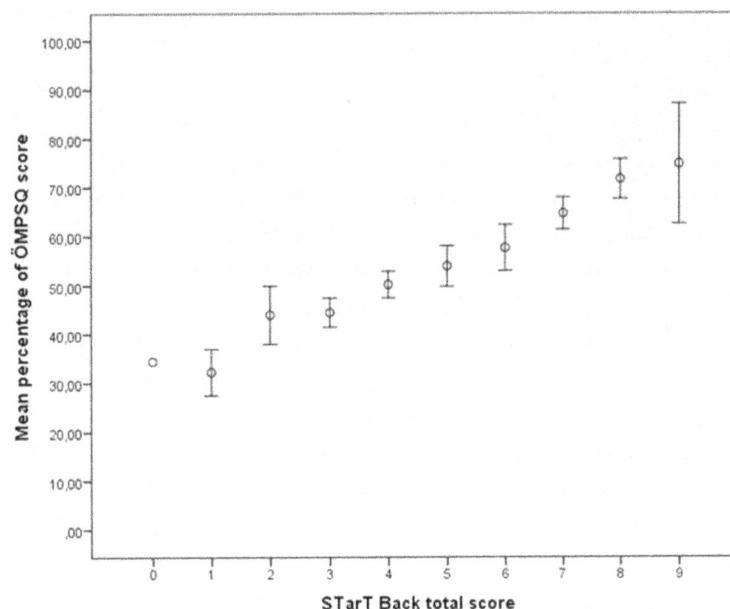

Fig. 1 Mean percent of Örebro Musculoskeletal Pain Score Questionnaire (ÖMPSQ) according to Start Back total score. Vertical bars represent 95% confidence interval. (Pearson's $r = 0.76$)

Table 1 Characteristics of study population

Variables	Total	STarT Back risk groups		
		Low	Medium	High
	N = 182	n = 62	n = 77	n = 43
Age[a]	48 (15)	47 (15)	50 (15)	47 (14)
Gender, men[b]	92 (51)	29 (47)	40 (52)	23 (54)
Other diseases[b]	127 (70)	39 (63)	57 (74)	31 (72)
Musculoskeletal comorbidity[b]	68 (37)	17 (27)	33 (43)	18 (42)
Married[b]	97 (53)	30 (48)	43 (56)	24 (56)
Born in Norway[b]	169 (93)	60 (97)	73 (95)	36 (84)
University / college education[b]	77 (42)	31 (50)	32 (42)	14 (33)
Employed[b]	133 (73)	51 (82)	55 (71)	27 (63)
Sicklisted[b]	58 (32)	16 (26)	26 (34)	16 (37)

[a]Mean, SD
[b]N, percent

low risk group, 28.6% in the medium risk group, and 46.7% in the high risk group (Table 2). In supplementary analyses restricted to workers only, 38.3% were allocated in the low risk group, 41.4% in the medium risk group, and 20.3% in the high risk group as defined by STarT Back.

There was a dose-dependent relation between scores on pain and work items on ÖMPSQ and STarT Back risk group (Table 3), except for the item on job satisfaction. Pain variables differed most between low and medium risk group, while work variables separated most clearly between the medium and high risk group as defined by STarT Back.

Discussion

This study indicated high correlation between instrument scores and low agreement between risk classification between StarT Back tool and ÖMPSQ for patients referred to secondary care because of low back pain. Risk group classification according to STarT Back allocated 23.6% in the high risk group. According to ÖMPSQ, 46.7% were allocated in the high risk group. Patients classified with high risk according to Start Back showed a higher score on pain and work related characteristics as measured by ÖMPSQ.

The Start Back total score highly correlated with ÖMPSQ total score, indicating good criterion validity for STarT Back in a Norwegian sample of low back pain patients referred to a multidisciplinary outpatient clinic in secondary care. This result is comparable with previous studies performed in other countries and settings. Bruyere and coworkers [10] addressed the correlation between the ÖMPSQ and STarT Back and found a Spearman correlation coefficient of 0.74. The latter study included patients in settings different from the present study; a rehabilitation center, a back school, a private physiotherapy unit as well as persons with low back pain at a fitness center [10]. ÖMPSQ has also been compared to STarT Back screening tool in England, including two hundred and forty-four consecutive non-specific low back pain consulters at general practitioners [19]. They found a correlation between STarT Back tool and ÖMPSQ of 0.80 and classification agreement Kappa 0.57. Significant differences between STarT Back and ÖMPSQ-registered threshold were observed in that STarT Back allocated fewer patients to high risk classification.

Despite very good correlation between the two scales, the findings from the risk classification in the present study showed that 22 out of the 52 patients classified as medium risk by ÖMPSQ were classified as low risk on Start Back. Additionally, 41 out of the 85 patients with high risk according to ÖMPSQ were classified with moderate risk according to Start Back, in line with the study from England [19]. One may ask whether these discrepancies were related to the fact that ÖMPSQ has five work-related questions and have been suggested to be a good predictor of future absenteeism [18], while Start Back does not include any work questions. Studies assessing the validity of the short-form ÖMPSQ that includes ten items, of which two covers work that is optional connected to the home or to paid work may support this hypothesis as it showed less discrepancies in classification when compared to STarT Back [17, 26]. Because STarT Back does not cover work, we hypothesized that STarT Back could underestimate risk for participants with work-related obstacles for recovery. Our results showed that patients classified with high risk

Table 2 Classification table showing agreement between risk group stratification as defined by STarT Back and Örebro screening tools

Start Back Screening tool risk group	Örebro Musculoskeletal Pain Questionnaire risk group				
	Low	Medium	High	Total	Percentage
Low	35	22	5	62	34.1
Medium	9	27	41	77	42.3
High	1	3	39	43	23.6
Total	45	52	85	182	
Percentage	24.7	28.6	46.7		

Kappa coefficient = 0.35

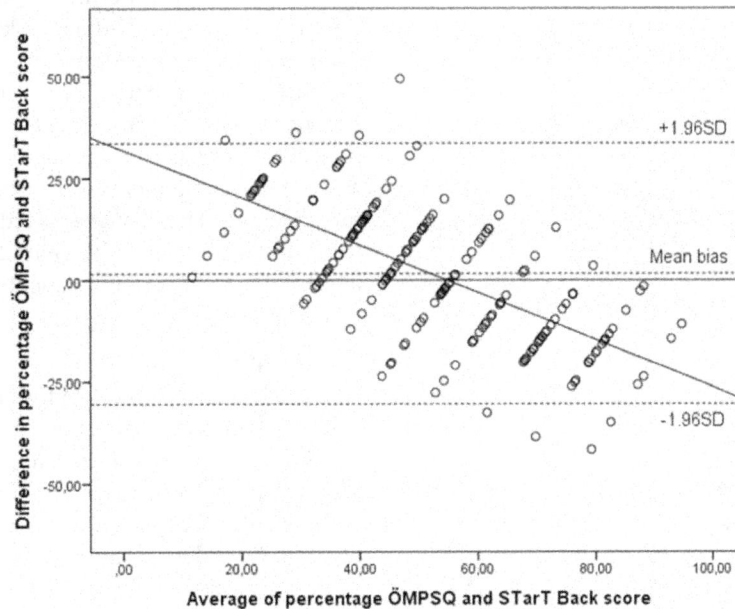

Fig. 2 Agreement between STarT Back screening tool and Örebro Musculoskeletal Pain Screening Questionnaire (ÖMPSQ). Dotted lines in the Bland-Altman plot represent mean bias with 95% limits of agreement. The solid diagonal line represent the difference between the screening tools regressed on the average of the two tools (slope = − 0.58). X-axis displays average percentage score between both instruments. Y-axis display differences in percentage score

according to Start Back showed a significantly higher score on work related characteristics as measured by ÖMPSQ, with one exception for the item on job satisfaction. These findings suggest that specifically screening for work factors is important in this group of patients. This is also indicated by the difference in ÖMPSQ-scores between workers and non-workers, in line with results from a recent factors analysis [27]. Further research is needed to confirm this relation, and to address the need for more knowledge regarding referral practice and the right candidates for multidisciplinary rehabilitation to restore employability [28].

Another finding was that the agreement for score was best for middle range scores, and that the compliance between tools were lower in both ends of the scoring scales. For the higher mean percentage scores, the tendency was that STarT Back tool allocated higher score. In spite of that, Örebro allocated a higher percentage of participants to the high risk group, again indicating a lack of correspondence between the cut-off limits for the instruments.

The results indicated that between 24.7 (ÖMPSQ) and 34.1 (STarT Back) percent of the respondents had low risk for longstanding disability due to low back pain. Clinical guidelines recommend secondary care referral when management needs are too complex for primary care management [4]. Given that, it is somewhat surprising that as much as 25–34% of the patients were classified low risk. Multidisciplinary management in

secondary care is the recommended treatment choice for patients with significant obstacles to recovery and / or when previous treatment have not been effective [5]. In general, secondary care referral may be due to complex psychosocially oriented treatment needs or to suspicion of organic disease from the primary care contact. The outpatient clinic in the present study offers multidisciplinary treatment targeting psychosocial needs as well as examination of potential pathoanatomic triggers. Therefore, screening tools designed for early addressing of psychosocial obstacles for recovery in primary care may not be sufficient or relevant to consider if a patient should be managed in secondary care.

To our knowledge, no studies have compared scores and classification by these two screening instruments in patients referred to secondary care. On the other hand, the predictive value of both instruments in secondary care has been evaluated. An Australian study concluded that the instruments add no further value over and above clinical judgement [29], and a Danish study concluded that the predictive ability of STarT Back is less good in secondary care compared to primary care [30]. Again, it is plausible to suggest that the most relevant screening items for primary and secondary care patients differ.

Strengths and limitations

This is a cross-sectional study, and it cannot evaluate the predictive value of the screening instruments. The

Table 3 Mean differences from linear regression analyses[a] of selected pain and work related variables between Start Back risk groups (work related variables analyzed only on people in work, and higher scores represent worse problems)

	STarT Back risk group		
	Low risk	Medium risk	High risk
Pain			
Intensity last week, 1–10 points			
Mean (SD)	3.8 (2.0)	5.1 (2.5)	5.7 (2.7)
Difference (95% CI)	0.0 (reference)	1.2 (0.3–2.1)	1.9 (0.8–2.9)
Intensity past 3 months, 1–10 points			
Mean (SD)	6.0 (1.5)	6.9 (1.5)	7.9 (1.5)
Difference (95% CI)	0.0 (reference)	1.0 (0.4–1.5)	1.9 (1.2–2.6)
Duration, weeks			
Median (IQR)	46 (20–52)	52 (33–52)	52 (47–52)
Difference (p-value)	0 (reference)	8 (0.007)	8 (0.004)
Work			
Missed days of work, passed 18 months			
Median (IQR)	11 (0–137)	30 (5–137)	137 (60–365)
Difference (p-value)	0 (reference)	19 (0.14)	126 (0.001)
Heavy / monotoneous work, 1–10 points			
Median (IQR)	5 (3–7)	7 (5–8)	8 (6–9)
Difference (p-value)	0 (reference)	2 (0.02)	3 (0.004)
Workable in six months, 1–10 points			
Median (IQR)	1 (0–5)	2 (0–5)	6 (2–9)
Difference (p-value)	0 (reference)	1 (0.13)	5 (< 0.001)
Job satisfaction, 1–10 points			
Median (IQR)	2 (1–4)	2 (1–5)	3 (1–5)
Difference (p-value)	0 (reference)	0 (0.23)	1 (0.17)
Should not work (fear), 1–10 points			
Median (IQR)	4 (0–6)	5 (3–9)	10 (6–10)
Difference (p-value)	0 (reference)	1 (0.01)	6 (< 0.001)

[a]Non-normally distributed variables were analyzed using non-parametric Mann-Whitney U test and results presented as differences in median values between risk groups

response rate was 66% and we cannot rule out that the study participants were different from the non-responders. Consequently, the results may not automatically be generalisable to the population of patients referred to the multidisciplinary clinic. Missing responses on some items may have introduced bias. To compensate for missing on the work items, supplementary analyses were performed to compare whole-sample results to results from analyses restricted to patients in work.

The results from the present study do not suggest that the risk classification by STarT Back is comparable to risk classification by ÖMPSQ for patients referred to secondary care for low back pain, though the instruments' scores correlated well. This study also suggests

that around one third of the patients referred to secondary care will be classified low risk according to these primary care screening tools. The results do not support the applicability of StarT Back screening tool as decision support in Norwegian secondary health care. This may be due to differences in timing of testing, clinical setting, and study sample compared to the original target group for screening. The results also indicated that the working items in ÖMPSQ may be central when addressing psychosocial load in working patients.

Conclusion

STarT Back scores correlated well to scores on ÖMPSQ, while classification agreement between the instruments was low in patients referred to multidisiplinary secondary care for low back pain. Patients classified as high risk by STarT Back reported more challenges connected to work on ÖMPSQ sub-items.

Abbreviations
CI: Confidence interval; ÖMPSQ: Örebro Musculoskeletal Pain Screening Questionnaire; STarT Back: STarT Back screening tool

Acknowledgements
The authors would like to thank the study participants for their contribution in the data collection.

Authors' contributions
IGK, MUT and TA designed the study. TILN and MUT analyzed the data. MUT wrote the paper. GHM, IGK, MUT, TA and TILN discussed the results, commented on the manuscript, and approved the final version.

Competing interests
The authors declare that they have no competing interests.

Author details
[1]Department of Neuromedicine and Movement Science (INB), NTNU, Faculty of Medicine and Health Sciences, N-7491 Trondheim, Norway. [2]Department of Public Health and Nursing, Norwegian University of Science and Technology, Faculty of Medicine and Health Sciences, Trondheim, Norway. [3]Department of Physical Medicine and Rehabilitation, St. Olav's Hospital, Trondheim University Hospital, Trondheim, Norway. [4]Clinic of Anaesthesia and Intensive Care, St Olavs Hospital, Trondheim University Hospital, Trondheim, Norway.

References
1. Hoy DG, Smith E, Cross M, Sanchez-Riera L, Blyth FM, Buchbinder R, Woolf AD, Driscoll T, Brooks P, March LM. Reflecting on the global burden of musculoskeletal conditions: lessons learnt from the global burden of disease 2010 study and the next steps forward. Ann Rheum Dis. 2015;74(1):4–7.
2. March L, Smith EU, Hoy DG, Cross MJ, Sanchez-Riera L, Blyth F, Buchbinder R, Vos T, Woolf AD. Burden of disability due to musculoskeletal (MSK) disorders. Best Pract Res Clin Rheumatol. 2014;28(3):353–66.
3. Srinivas SV, Deyo RA, Berger ZD. Application of "less is more" to low back pain. Arch Intern Med. 2012;172(13):1016–20.
4. Koes BW, van Tulder M, Lin CW, Macedo LG, McAuley J, Maher C. An updated overview of clinical guidelines for the management of non-specific low back pain in primary care. Eur Spine J. 2010;19(12):2075–94.

5. Bernstein IA, Malik Q, Carville S, Ward S. Low back pain and sciatica: summary of NICE guidance. BMJ. 2017;356:i6748.

6. van Tulder M, Becker A, Bekkering T, Breen A, del Real MT, Hutchinson A, Koes B, Laerum E, Malmivaara A, Care CBWGoGftMoALBPiP. Chapter 3. European guidelines for the management of acute nonspecific low back pain in primary care. Eur Spine J. 2006;15 Suppl 2:S169–91.

7. Christensen J, Fisker A, Mortensen EL, Olsen LR, Mortensen OS, Hartvigsen J, Langberg H. Comparison of mental distress in patients with low back pain and a population-based control group measured by symptoms check list–a case-referent study. Scand J Public Health. 2015;43(6):638–47.

8. O'Sullivan P, Caneiro JP, O'Keeffe M, O'Sullivan K. Unraveling the complexity of low back pain. J Orthop Sports Phys Ther. 2016;46(11):932–7.

9. Hill JC, Dunn KM, Lewis M, Mullis R, Main CJ, Foster NE, Hay EM. A primary care back pain screening tool: identifying patient subgroups for initial treatment. Arthritis Rheum. 2008;59(5):632–41.

10. Bruyere O, Demoulin M, Beaudart C, Hill JC, Maquet D, Genevay S, Mahieu G, Reginster JY, Crielaard JM, Demoulin C. Validity and reliability of the French version of the STarT back screening tool for patients with low back pain. Spine (Phila Pa 1976). 2014;39(2):E123–8.

11. Morso L, Albert H, Kent P, Manniche C, Hill J. Translation and discriminative validation of the STarT back screening tool into Danish. Eur Spine J. 2011; 20(12):2166–73.

12. Morso L, Kent P, Albert HB, Hill JC, Kongsted A, Manniche C. The predictive and external validity of the STarT back tool in Danish primary care. Eur Spine J. 2013;22(8):1859–67.

13. Piironen S, Paananen M, Haapea M, Hupli M, Zitting P, Ryynanen K, Takala EP, Korniloff K, Hill JC, Hakkinen A, et al. Transcultural adaption and psychometric properties of the STarT back screening tool among Finnish low back pain patients. Eur Spine J. 2016;25(1):287–95.

14. Luan S, Min Y, Li G, Lin C, Li X, Wu S, Ma C, Hill JC. Cross-cultural adaptation, reliability, and validity of the Chinese version of the STarT back screening tool in patients with low back pain. Spine (Phila Pa 1976). 2014;39(16):E974–9.

15. Karstens S, Krug K, Hill JC, Stock C, Steinhaeuser J, Szecsenyi J, Joos S. Validation of the German version of the STarT-back tool (STarT-G): a cohort study with patients from primary care practices. BMC Musculoskelet Disord. 2015;16:346.

16. Robinson HS, Dagfinrud H. Reliability and screening ability of the StarT back screening tool in patients with low back pain in physiotherapy practice, a cohort study. BMC Musculoskelet Disord. 2017;18(1):232.

17. Forsbrand M, Grahn B, Hill JC, Petersson IF, Sennehed CP, Stigmar K. Comparison of the Swedish STarT back screening tool and the short form of the Orebro musculoskeletal pain screening questionnaire in patients with acute or subacute back and neck pain. BMC Musculoskelet Disord. 2017; 18(1):89.

18. Linton SJ, Boersma K. Early identification of patients at risk of developing a persistent back problem: the predictive validity of the Orebro musculoskeletal pain questionnaire. Clin J Pain. 2003;19(2):80–6.

19. Hill JC, Dunn KM, Main CJ, Hay EM. Subgrouping low back pain: a comparison of the STarT back tool with the Orebro musculoskeletal pain screening questionnaire. Eur J Pain. 2010;14(1):83–9.

20. Linton SJ, Hallden K. Can we screen for problematic back pain? A screening questionnaire for predicting outcome in acute and subacute back pain. Clin J Pain. 1998;14(3):209–15.

21. Maher CG, Grotle M. Evaluation of the predictive validity of the Orebro musculoskeletal pain screening questionnaire. Clin J Pain. 2009;25(8):666–70.

22. Hockings RL, McAuley JH, Maher CG. A systematic review of the predictive ability of the Orebro musculoskeletal pain questionnaire. Spine (Phila Pa 1976). 2008;33(15):E494–500.

23. Ruokolainen O, Haapea M, Linton S, Korniloff K, Hakkinen A, Paananen M, Karppinen J. Construct validity and reliability of Finnish version of Orebro musculoskeletal pain screening questionnaire. Scand J Pain. 2016;13:148–53.

24. Soer R, Vroomen P, Stewart R, Coppes M, Stegeman P, Dijkstra P, Reneman M. Factor analyses for the Orebro musculoskeletal pain questionnaire for working and nonworking patients with chronic low back pain. Spine J. 2017;17(4):603–9.

25. Andresen EM. Criteria for assessing the tools of disability outcomes research. Arch Phys Med Rehabil. 2000;81(12 Suppl 2):S15–20.

26. Fuhro FF, Fagundes FR, Manzoni AC, Costa LO, Cabral CM. Orebro musculoskeletal pain screening questionnaire - short form and Start back screening tool: correlation and agreement analysis. Spine (Phila Pa 1976). 2016;41(15):E931–6.

27. Soegaard R, Christensen FB, Christiansen T, Bunger C. Costs and effects in lumbar spinal fusion. A follow-up study in 136 consecutive patients with chronic low back pain. Eur Spine J. 2007;16(5):657–68.

28. Pedersen P, Nielsen CV, Jensen OK, Jensen C, Labriola M. Employment status five years after a randomised controlled trial comparing multidisciplinary and brief intervention in employees on sick leave due to low back pain. Scand J Public Health. 2018;46(3):383–8.

29. Karran EL, Traeger AC, McAuley JH, Hillier SL, Yau YH, Moseley GL. The value of prognostic screening for patients with low back pain in secondary care. J Pain. 2017;18(6):673–86.

30. Morso L, Kent P, Manniche C, Albert HB. The predictive ability of the STarT back screening tool in a Danish secondary care setting. Eur Spine J. 2014; 23(1):120–8.

10

What is the association between the presence of comorbidities and the appropriateness of care for low back pain?

Shanthi Ramanathan[1,2,3*] (iD), Peter Hibbert[3,4,7], Louise Wiles[3,4], Christopher G. Maher[5,6] and William Runciman[3,4,7]

Abstract

Background: Although "non-specific" in 90% of cases, low back pain (LBP) is often treated as an independent entity, even though comorbidities are commonly associated with it. There is evidence that some LBP may be related to chronic conditions or be a symptom of poor health. The purpose of this study was to clarify the extent of comorbidities amongst a cohort of Australian adults with LBP and examine if having concurrent conditions has any association with appropriateness of care for LBP.

Methods: A population-based sample of patients with one or more of 22 common conditions was recruited by telephone; consents were obtained to review their medical records. Trained surveyors extracted information from their medical records to examine the care patients received for their LBP with respect to ten indicators of appropriate care, ratified by LBP experts. Using LBP as the index condition, lists of self-reported comorbidities and those that were documented in medical records were compared. Medical records were reviewed and analysed with respect to appropriateness of care to identify any significant differences in care received between patients with *LBP only* and those with LBP plus comorbidities.

Results: One hundred and sixty four LBP patients were included in the analysis. Over 60% of adults with LBP in Australia had one of 17 comorbidities documented, with females being more likely than males to have comorbid conditions (63% vs 37%, $p = 0.012$). The more comorbidities, the poorer their reported health status (63% vs 30%, $p = 0.006$). Patients with comorbidities were significantly less likely to receive appropriate LBP care on nine of the ten LBP indicators ($p < 0.05$).

Conclusions: This study established that the presence of comorbidities is associated with poorer care for LBP. Understanding why this is so is an important direction for future research. Further studies using a larger cohort are needed to explore the association between comorbidities and appropriateness of care for LBP, to better inform guidelines and practice in this area.

Keywords: Low back pain, Comorbidity, Appropriate care

* Correspondence: shanthi.ramanathan@hmri.org.au
[1]Hunter Medical Research Institute, Locked Bag 100, New Lambton Heights, Newcastle 2305, Australia
[2]Faculty of Health and Medicine, University of Newcastle, Newcastle, Australia
Full list of author information is available at the end of the article

Background

Low back pain (LBP) is the leading cause of activity limitation and absence from work, with over 70% of adults experiencing it at some stage in their lives [1, 2]. LBP is the health condition that has imposed the greatest disease burden globally since 1990 [3]. The direct costs of LBP have been estimated at AUD \$4.8 billion per year in Australia [4]. However, these are minor compared with the indirect costs, which have been estimated at over AUD \$8 billion per year in Australia [5].

Low back pain is often treated as an independent disorder with respect to the search for causes and cures. While the approach to LBP has, in recent years, moved from treating it as a purely anatomic-physiologic condition to a more complex multifaceted physical, neurochemical, biomechanical and psycho-social condition; the focus often continues to be on LBP as an isolated disorder [6]. However, comorbidities seem to be common with LBP [7–10], indicating that at least some back problems may not be distinct entities, but one of a number of symptoms of poor health in general.

In medicine, comorbidity is the presence of one or more additional diseases or disorders co-occurring with (that is, concurrent with) a primary disease or disorder and the rate of comorbidity and the number of chronic diseases experienced increases with age [11]. In Australia, almost 1 in 3 (29%) people aged 65 and over reported having three or more chronic diseases, compared with just 2.4% of those under 45 [10]. For a patient, comorbidities may have profound implications as the degree of physical and social disability rise with the number of co-existing conditions, which present several challenges in care [11–13]. Comorbidities are known to be associated with higher mortality and reduced quality of life and health providers need to take comorbid diseases into account when treating patients [6]. It is also suggested that future studies on consequences of comorbidity should investigate specific disease combinations [14].

As early as 1974, Gyntelberg showed significant relationships between LBP, angina pectoris, and various other diseases [15]; Biering-Sorensen (1984) found several physical conditions to be important indicators for future LBP [16]. Seferlis (2000) found a 4-fold increase in sick leave for other disorders in LBP patients [17] and Cote et al. (2007) noted that individuals seeking care for neck or back pain have worse health status than those who do not seek care [18]. A critical review of the LBP literature from the inception of Medline until the year 2000 found 23 separate studies that showed positive associations between LBP and the following disorders: headache/migraine, cardiovascular disease, respiratory disorders, neck pain, gynaecological disease, asthma, hay fever and other allergies, as well as general poor health

[6]. According to the authors *"the literature leaves no doubt that diseases cluster in some individuals and that low back pain is part of this pattern".* [6]

The National German Health Survey ($n = 7124$) found that all 31 physical diseases investigated were more common in subjects with LBP than those without LBP and that the most common were musculoskeletal disorders like rheumatoid arthritis, osteoarthritis and osteoporosis, followed by cardiovascular and cerebrovascular disease [8]. A Norwegian study found that LBP patients were significantly more likely to suffer from neck pain, upper back pain, pain in feet during exercise, headache, migraine, sleep problems, heat sensations, anxiety, and depression than patients without LBP [9]. In addition to physical disorders, both episodic and chronic LBP have also been shown to be significantly associated with mental illnesses such as depression, GI disease and anxiety [6, 19, 20] and increased healthcare utilization and costs [21]. Based on findings from the Australian Bureau of Statistic's 2014–2015 National Health Survey (ANHS), LBP is featured in the second and third most common comorbidities in Australian adults, based on eight selected chronic diseases (i.e. arthritis, asthma, LBP, cancer, cardiovascular disease, chronic obstructive pulmonary disease, diabetes, and mental health conditions) [10]. However, little is known about the consequences of such comorbidities with respect to appropriateness of care for LBP.

The CareTrack Australia study was designed to establish baseline estimates of the appropriateness of care delivered, at a population level, for 22 common conditions [22]. The study used retrospective medical record review to assess compliance against a set of ratified indicators of appropriate care for each condition of which LBP was one. The compliance results for LBP have been published at indicator level and show an overall compliance of 72%. [23]. The objective of this paper is to use the larger CareTrack dataset with contains information on concurrent conditions for each patient to identify:

1) comorbidities amongst patients with LBP in the CareTrack sample
2) the conditions most likely to be associated with LBP
3) any associations between comorbidities and other socio-demographic variables included in the study
4) any associations between comorbidities and the appropriateness of LBP care for the associated conditions in Australian adults.

Methods

The CareTrack methods have been described in detail elsewhere. [22, 24] Here, we describe some aspects of particular relevance to an examination of comorbidities in the context of LBP. A sample of adults designed to be representative of the Australian population was randomly selected from a telephone directory (the Australian Telstra White Pages) from defined regions within two states New South Wales and South Australia. [25] One adult was randomly selected from each household and recruited over the phone. Those who agreed were subsequently sent a mail package containing information about the study and a consent form to allow access to their medical records. Participants who provided consent were contacted by phone and asked if they had one or more of the 22 CareTrack conditions, and which healthcare providers they had seen for these in the years 2009 and 2010. Healthcare providers including GPs, chiropractors, physiotherapists, and specialist physicians were contacted and asked for consent for trained CareTrack surveyors to access the medical records of consenting participants. Only participants who had documented care for LBP during 2009 and 2010 were included in this analysis. Human Research Ethics Committee approval was obtained to undertake the data collection from the University of South Australia and all relevant bodies and sites. Figure 1 provides a summary of the various stages of the recruitment protocol, the inclusion criteria, and attrition at each stage to obtain the final LBP sample.

Details of comorbidities in the CareTrack sample were captured in two ways. First, participants who consented to having their medical records accessed as part of Care-Track were asked to identify the conditions that they were treated for in 2009/2010 during the second phone call (see Additional file 1 for details of the question). Second, consenting participants for whom access to medical records was granted also had any relevant conditions noted (where present) from their medical records. The data obtained from both these methods are presented in this paper to identify comorbidities in the CareTrack LBP sample, however, as there were differences in the patterns found using the two methods only data from the patient records were used in the analysis for associations with socio-demographic variables and indicators of appropriateness of LBP care. The levels of comorbidity associated with LBP were collapsed to three groups: those without any comorbidities, those with one or two other conditions on the CareTrack list, and those with three or more of these.

Chi-square tests were run to determine if there were any significant differences in the socio-demographic characteristics and the appropriateness of care received by these three groups of LBP patients. Significant differences were deemed to be those at the 95% level of confidence ($p > 0.05$).

Results

Level of comorbidity amongst LBP patients

In response to the question *In 2009 and 2010 have you been treated for [CareTrack condition]?* over 80% of LBP patients in the CareTrack sample reported receiving

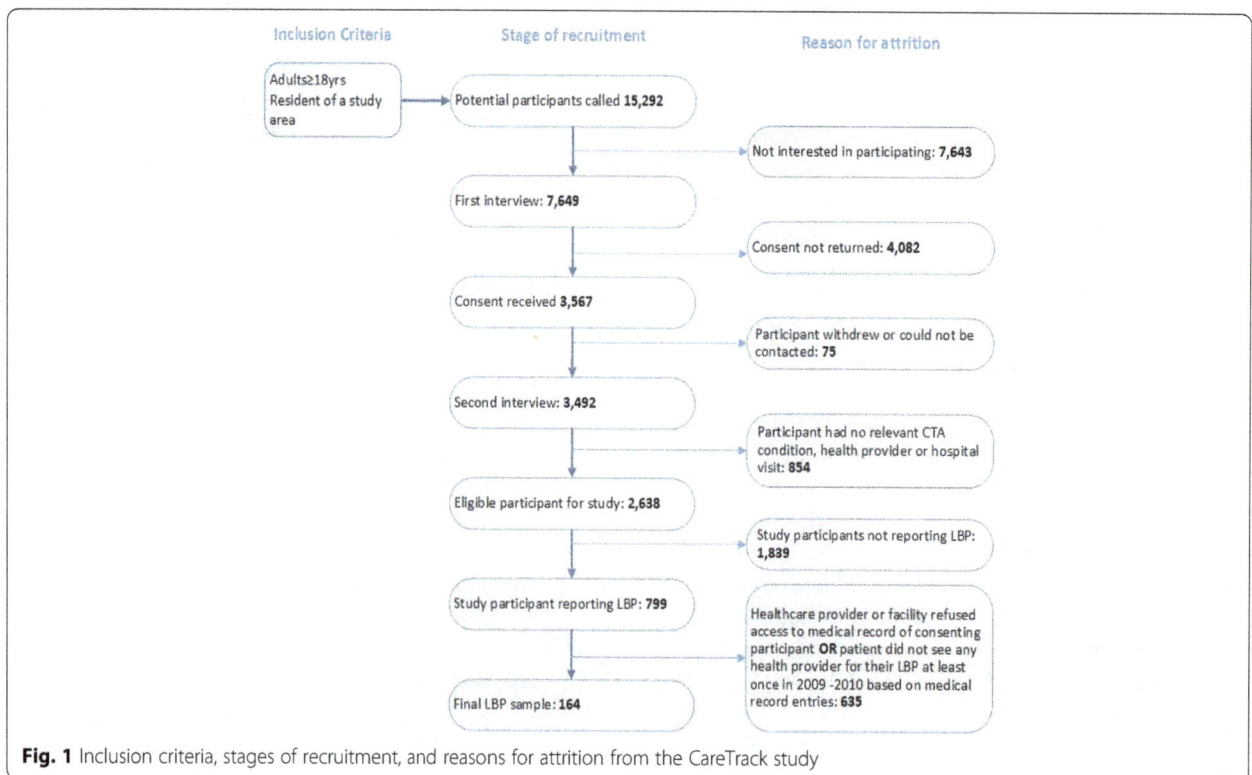

Fig. 1 Inclusion criteria, stages of recruitment, and reasons for attrition from the CareTrack study

treatment in 2009–2010 for at least one of the other 17 CareTrack conditions[1] during their second phone interview. Table 1 shows that the number of patient-reported conditions in the LBP CareTrack sample ranged between 1 and 10. The mean number of patient-reported conditions was 3.27 (including LBP), and the mode and median were both 3. However, in contrast, only 60% of LBP patients had been treated for at least one other Care-Track condition in the years 2009 and 2010 according to the evidence in their medical record. Thus, the level of comorbidity amongst LBP patients based on evidence in their medical record was lower than the level of comorbidity self-reported by patients. Whereas only 19% of LBP patients reported not having been treated for any of the other conditions covered by the CareTrack study, 40% were treated for only LBP in 2009–2010, based on the information in their medical records. The mean number of conditions based on medical record data was 2.46, the mode was 1 and the median was 2.

Conditions associated with LBP

The top ten specific comorbid conditions reported by LBP patients are presented in Table 2 with hypertension and hyperlipidaemia being the two most frequently reported (approximately two out of every five LBP patients reported having at least one of these conditions). Osteoarthritis and dyspepsia were the next most frequently reported conditions, with at least one in four LBP patients reporting that they had been treated for these conditions. The two most common comorbidities found in the medical records were hypertension (a condition for which approximately 29% of LBP patients had received treatment) and osteoarthritis (one in four LBP patients).

Table 1 Patients reporting other conditions in addition to their LBP, self-report vs medical record

Number of patient-reported conditions including LBP	Self-reported conditions		Conditions in medical record	
	Number n	Percentage %	Number n	Percentage %
LBP only	31	18.9	63	38.4
2	28	17.1	33	20.1
3	38	23.2	28	17.1
4	34	20.7	18	11.0
5	13	7.9	11	6.7
6	14	8.5	8	4.9
7	2	1.2	3	1.8
8	1	0.6		
9	1	0.6		
10	2	1.2		
Total	164	100	164	100

LBP low back pain

For all conditions, except for obesity which was not asked of patients during their phone interview, there were far more patients who reported being treated for those conditions than there was evidence for in the medical record.

Data from the medical records were used to undertake the analysis on the association between the levels of comorbidity and patient socio-demographic factors and appropriateness of LBP care. Table 3 shows the number of patients by comorbidity level and the percentage in each group based on evidence found in their medical records.

Comorbidity and patient socio-demographic variables

Table 4 presents the data for associations between the seven socio-demographic variables included in CareTrack and the level of comorbidity of LBP patients. Asterisks indicate statistically significant differences in sociodemographic variables by level of comorbidity. Patients with no comorbidities were significantly more likely to be *male* than *female* (60% versus 40%) and those with one or more comorbidities were more likely to be *female* (63% versus 37%). This result indicates that in the CareTrack sample, females with LBP were more likely to have other chronic conditions than males.

The second significant difference was that LBP patients who had three or more comorbidities were significantly more likely to report *poor to fair* health (63%) compared with those who had 1–2 other conditions (35%) and those who had *LBP only* (30%). Similarly, those with *LBP only* were significantly more likely to report *very good to excellent* health (37%) compared with only 11% of those with three or more comorbidities. There were no significant associations between level of comorbidity and age, educational attainment, work status, accessibility of healthcare or medical literacy.

Comorbidity and appropriate LBP care

Compliance with CareTrack indicators for appropriateness of care is shown in Table 5. Analyses revealed statistically significant differences in rates of compliance by number of comorbidities for nine of the ten LBP indicators for appropriateness of care assessed as part of the CareTrack study (see Table 5).

For the first six indicators, a clear pattern is evident. Patients who had been treated for one or more "other" conditions besides LBP in 2009–10 were significantly less likely to have had (i) their medical history documented, (ii) a physical or neurological examination, or (iii) assessments for infection, (iv) assessment for cancer or (v) assessment for fractures than patients who had *LBP only*. In addition, compared with patients with *LBP only* and *those with fewer than three comorbidities* those patients with *three or more comorbid conditions* were

Table 2 Top ten comorbid conditions associated with LBP, based upon self-report and medical records

| Top ten | Self-report | | Medical record | |
Conditions on the CareTrack list	Number of LBP patients with condition	Percentage of LBP patients with condition	Number of LBP patients with condition	Percentage of LBP patients with condition
Hypertension	67	40.9	47	28.7
Osteoarthritis	50	30.5	42	25.6
Hyperlipidaemia	66	40.2	26	15.9
Dyspepsia	42	25.6	22	13.4
Depression	36	22.0	16	9.8
Osteoporosis	25	15.2	13	7.9
Coronary Artery Disease	16	9.8	12	7.3
Diabetes	20	12.2	9	5.5
Asthma	23	14	8	4.9
Obesity ([a])			15	9.1
Atrial Fibrillation	13	7.9		

Legend: ([a]) Not asked for during phone interviews, *LBP* low back pain

also significantly less likely to be assessed for cauda equina syndrome, more likely to be prescribed dexamethasone, other oral steroids, colchicine or antidepressants and more likely to not be advised against resting in bed. The only indicator that was not associated with comorbidity was the one relating to NOT receiving transcutaneous electrical nerve stimulation (TENS), lumbar corsets and support belts or spinal traction ($p = 0.933$).

Discussion

Understanding more about comorbidities can provide vital information for prevention, management and treatment of diseases including LBP. This study found that at least 62% of the 164 LBP patients in the CareTrack study had at least one other chronic condition. Comparisons with data from the 2014–15 ANHS [10] and the first German National Health Survey [9] are summarised in the bottom half of Table 6 (results). The CareTrack proportion of LBP sufferers with comorbidities obtained from their medical record was similar to the ANHS findings (62% versus 65%) but was significantly higher when using their survey data (81% vs 65%). In contrast, the German national study sample [8] had significantly higher rates of comorbidity compared with both the

Table 3 Recoding of LBP patients into three groups by number of comorbid conditions

| Number of comorbidities | Found in medical records for 2009/2010 | |
	Number	Percentage(%)
LBP only	63	38.4
1–2 additional conditions	61	37.2
3 or more other conditions	40	24.4
Total	164	100.0

Legend: *LBP* low back pain

CareTrack medical record (62%) and survey (81%) proportions. Rather than reflect an inconsistency in the findings, these discrepancies are most likely a consequence of the different methods used in each study, as summarised in the top half of Table 6. The two most significant of these in terms of impact on comparability are: (1) the way LBP and other conditions were defined and (2) the number of conditions included in each study. Both the ANHS and the German study asked participants if they had "ever" had a range of conditions whereas the CareTrack study asked them if they had "*been treated for* [condition] *in the years 2009/2010.*" In addition, definitions of LBP ranged from having LBP within a 7-day period to having it for over 6 months. Second, the number of conditions covered by the three studies varied from eight to 31. These differences made comparability of prevalence of comorbidity problematic.

In contrast, the most prevalent conditions to be associated with LBP showed similarity across all three studies, despite some definitional issues. Hypertension, osteoarthritis and hyperlipidaemia were the three most prevalent conditions for LBP patients in the CareTrack study and the first two were also ranked top three in the other studies, confirming that LBP is most closely associated with cardiovascular and musculoskeletal conditions.

Hypertension and hyperlipidaemia were also consistent with more than 23 other studies that clearly illustrate that LBP is associated with cardiovascular disease and poor health overall [8]. A potential reason for this association may be that these diseases share some common risk factors such as physical inactivity and overweight/obesity. Together these findings support the theory by Hestbaek and colleagues [6] that LBP is often clustered with other conditions and poorer overall health. This clustering of conditions (with LBP as the index condition) is more

Table 4 Patient comorbidities associated with other LBP patient variables

Demographic variable	Categories	LBP only (n = 63)	1–2 comorbidities (n = 61)	3 or more comorbidities (n = 40)	p value
Gender*	Male	60%	37%	37%	0.012*
	Female	40%	63%	63%	
Age	18–39	10%	8%	5%	0.574
	40–54	30%	29%	18%	
	55–74	52%	48%	58%	
	75+	8%	16%	18%	
Educational attainment	Year 10 & under	25%	25%	45%	0.421
	HSC	16%	14%	16%	
	Trade Cert/Diploma	40%	43%	26%	
	University	19%	17%	13%	
Work status	Employed	44%	31%	34%	0.186
	Unemployed	2%	0%	3%	
	Retired	48%	52%	58%	
	Student/other	6%	18%	5%	
Health status*	Poor to fair	30%	35%	63%	0.006*
	Average	33%	40%	26%	
	Good to excellent	37%	25%	11%	
Accessibility of healthcare	Difficult to very difficult	14%	14%	21%	0.575
	Neither	8%	11%	16%	
	Easy to very easy	78%	75%	63%	
Medical literacy	Low	3%	3%	8%	0.669
	Moderate	16%	13%	18%	
	High	81%	84%	74%	

Legend: * = statistically significant difference, $p < 0.05$, *LBP* low back pain

Table 5 Compliance by comorbidities, medical record data

Indicator	Overall Compliance % (95% CI)	LBP Only (%)	1–2 comor-bidities (%)	3 or more comor-bidities (%)	p value
Medical history documented at presentation	94 (92–96)	96.9	90.1	87.2	< 0.001*
Physical examination performed and documented at presentation	87% (84–90)	95.0	76.5	64.4	< 0.001*
Assessed for spine fractures (trauma, history of previous fracture, prolonged use of steroids)	81% (77–84)	86.1	71.2	75.0	< 0.001*
Assessed for cancer (history of cancer, unexplained weight loss, immunosuppression)	75% (71–79)	81.2	64.9	65.8	< 0.001*
Assessed for infection (fever, IV drug use)	41% (37–46)	48.8	26.5	34.9	< 0.001*
Neurological examination performed – (strength, sensation and reflexes in lower limbs)	63% (58–67)	66.9	55.9	43.9	< 0.001*
Assessed for cauda equina syndrome	50% (45–54)	53.2	49.8	31.8	< 0.001*
NOT prescribed any of the following medications: dexamethasone, other oral steroids, colchicine or antidepressants	83% (75–92)	97.1	83.9	67.6	0.005*
DID NOT receive any of the following treatments: transcutaneous electrical nerve stimulation (TENS), lumbar corsets and support belts, spinal traction	94% (89–99)	95.0	93.4	94.4	0.933
NOT advised to rest in bed.	98% (89–100)	100.0	100.0	91.4	0.003*

Legend: * = statistically significant difference, $p < 0.05$, *LBP* low back pain

Table 6 Comparability of CareTrack findings and methodological features with the ANHS and the German National Survey

		CareTrack Medical Records	CareTrack Survey	National Health Survey [10]	German Health Survey [8]
Methods	Based on self-report	N	Y	Y	Y
	Country	Australia	Australia	Australia	Germany
	Year data collected	2011	2011	2016	1997–1999
	Inclusion criteria (LBP)	Treated for condition in 2009–10	Condition lasted less than 6 months (acute)	Lifetime prevalence and had condition for more than 6 months (chronic)	Suffered from LBP in past 7-days – 7 day prevalence
	Inclusion criteria (other)	Treated for condition in 2009–10	Treated for condition in 2009–10	Lifetime prevalence and had condition for more than 6 months (chronic)	Ever been diagnosed - lifetime prevalence
	No. of comorbid conditions included	17	17	8	31
Results	LBP only	38%	19%	35%	8%
	LBP plus 1 condition	20%	17%	30%	13%
	LBP plus 2 or more conditions	42%	64%	35%	77%
	Proportion with comorbidities	62%	81%	65%	92%
	Highest comorbid condition	Hypertension (28.7%)	Hypertension (40.9%)	Osteoarthritis (31.4%)	Osteoarthritis (50%)
	2nd highest	Osteoarthritis (25.6%)	Hyperlipidaemia (40.2%)	Circulatory system disease (30.9%)	Gastritis (30%)
	3rd highest	Hyperlipidaemia (15.9%)	Osteoarthritis (30.5%)	Mental and Behavioural disorder (29.8%)	Hypertension (26%)

Legend: 10 = Australian Institute of Health and Welfare. Australia's health 2016. Australia's Health Series No 15. Catalogue No AUS 199. AIHW. Canberra; 2016.
8 = Schneider S, Mohnen SM, Schiltenwolf M, Rau C. Comorbidity of low back pain: Representative outcomes of a national health study in the Federal Republic of Germany. European Journal of Pain. 2007;11(4):387–97

prevalent amongst females, a finding consistent with the ANHS data and the German study – both found that females (with or without LBP) had significantly more health problems than their male counterparts [8, 10]. Patients with three or more comorbidities were also more likely to report *poor to fair* health compared with those who had 1–2 other conditions or those without comorbidities, confirming previous findings that LBP is associated with a person's health status which would be expected to deteriorate with each additional chronic condition.

A significant finding from this CareTrack study sub-analysis was that LBP patients who had comorbid conditions were at greater risk of receiving care of a lower quality than those who only had LBP. This is the first time that this type of analysis has ever been undertaken for LBP patients. Even having one additional condition meant that LBP patients were significantly less likely to be adequately examined and assessed for a range of conditions such as fractures, cancer and infection and those with three or more comorbid conditions were at further risk of being prescribed unnecessary medication and not being given appropriate advice for managing their LBP. This finding has important implications for managing patients with LBP. Healthcare providers treating LBP need to

ensure that patients with comorbidities are adequately examined, assessed and managed. This issue of appropriateness of care also needs to be examined in detail using a larger cohort to explore why patients with more co-morbidities are less likely to receive appropriate LBP care and to determine if particular disease combinations are at greater risk of sub-standard care. While current LBP guidelines appear generic enough to apply to all patients they should be tested on a range of patients with various comorbidities. [26]

Further studies should also examine continuity of care and patient satisfaction, important areas for patients with more than one disease who are likely to be treated by several healthcare providers simultaneously. Such studies can also focus on determining the nature of the relationship between LBP and other comorbidities – does LBP cause other diseases or vice versa; do these conditions simply co-exist or do they have a common cause or risk factors?

Strengths and limitations
The key strength of the CareTrack methods is in the random selection of patients (a population-based rather than a convenience-based sample). However, an unavoidable

consequence of this strategy, compounded by limited research funds, was that the number of participants with LBP was low ($n = 164$), especially when compared with similar studies. The approach used was also associated with a high rate of attrition of potential participants (see Fig. 1) and several sources of potential bias, particularly in favour of recruiting older Australians. Another potential limitation is the possibility that care had been provided but was not recorded, an issue estimated to affect about 5% but no more than 10% of instances. [27]. A final limitation is the number of conditions included in the study and confinement to conditions that were treated in 2009–10, both of which were likely to have reduced the overall level of comorbidity amongst the CareTrack LBP cohort. Within the scope of this study, it was not possible to definitively assess the accuracy of both patient self-reports and medical records. It is possible that patients may have had some of these other conditions they identified at some point in their lifetime (particularly in the period between 2010 and when they were interviewed) but not have received any treatment for them in 2009–2010, hence their absence from parts of the medical records reviewed. Equally plausible explanations for the discrepancy could be incomplete medical records and/or inaccurate patient recall.

Conclusion

Findings from this sub-study of CareTrack data indicate that there is a moderate to high level of comorbidity amongst LBP patients in Australia and that comorbidity is more prevalent in females, consistent with previous studies. The findings also confirm prior evidence that LBP is associated with cardiovascular illness, other musculoskeletal conditions and poorer general health. The most significant finding from this study was that LBP patients with comorbidities were significantly less likely to receive appropriate care for LBP. Future studies using a larger cohort are needed to explore this association between comorbidity and appropriate care for LBP to better inform clinical guidelines and practice in this area.

Endnotes

[1]Some other conditions such as cancer, venous thromboembolism and surgical site infections, whilst part of the CareTrack study, were not assessed as part of the self-reporting component of the research.

Abbreviations
ANHS: Australian National Health Survey; AUD: Australian Dollar; CareTrack: Care Track Australia Study; GI: Glycaemic index; LBP: Low back pain

Acknowledgements
The authors thank the participants, healthcare providers, practice managers, medical record staff, and expert reviewers who generously gave their time and the six surveyors who undertook the medical record extraction. In particular, the authors acknowledge the work of Tamara Hooper who coordinated data collection from medical records, Natalie Hannaford who coordinated the development of the LBP indicators, Russ Redford who assisted with the coding and provided statistical advice and Claire Gardiner for assistance with Fig. 1. The authors also acknowledge the contribution of the other CareTrack Chief investigators to the overall Care-Track study including its conception: Jeffrey Braithwaite, Johanna Westbrook, and Enrico Coiera.

Funding
The Australian National Health and Medical Research Council (Program Grant No 568612) funds were received in support of this work through a national competitive grant application process. The funder played no role in the design, execution or dissemination of this research.

Authors' contributions
As part of her PhD, SR conceptualised the sub-study, undertook the relevant analysis and wrote the first draft of the manuscript. WR conceptualised the CareTrack study and provided critical input and direction during the conceptual phases of this sub-study. PH was the CareTrack Program Manager and data custodian who made substantial contributions to the acquisition of the data used in this manuscript, LW assisted with sourcing and reviewing the literature for the background to this paper and CM provided expert input to the interpretation of the findings. All authors reviewed several versions of the draft manuscript and approved the final version prior to submission.

Consent for publication
Not applicable.

Competing interests
None of the authors have any competing interests to declare.

Author details
[1]Hunter Medical Research Institute, Locked Bag 100, New Lambton Heights, Newcastle 2305, Australia. [2]Faculty of Health and Medicine, University of Newcastle, Newcastle, Australia. [3]Centre for Healthcare Resilience and Implementation Science, Australian Institute of Health Innovation, Macquarie University, Sydney, Australia. [4]Centre for Population Health Research, Sansom Institute for Health Research, The University of South Australia, Adelaide, Australia. [5]Institute for Musculoskeletal Health, Sydney, Australia. [6]Sydney School of Public Health, Sydney Medical School, University of Sydney, Sydney, Australia. [7]Australian Patient Safety Foundation, Adelaide, Australia.

References
1. Oliveira CB, Maher CG, Pinto RZ, Traeger AC, Lin C-WC, Chenot J-F, et al. Clinical practice guidelines for the management of non-specific low back pain in primary care: an updated overview. Eur Spine J. 2018. https://doi.org/10.1007/s00586-018-5673-2.
2. Walker BF, Muller R, Grant WD. Low back pain in Australian adults. Prevalence and associated disability. J Manip Physiol Ther. 2004;27(4):238–44.
3. Vos T, Abajobir AA, Abate KH, Abbafati C, Abbas KM, Abd-Allah F, et al. Global, regional, and national incidence, prevalence, and years lived with disability for 328 diseases and injuries for 195 countries, 1990-2016: a systematic analysis for the global burden of disease study 2016. Lancet. 2017;390(10100):1211–59.
4. Arthritis and Osteoporosis Victoria and Deloittes Access Economics. A problem worth solving: The rising cost of musculoskeletal conditions in Australia. In. Elsternwick: Arthritis and Osteoporosis. Victoria; 2013.
5. Crow WT, Willis DR. Estimating cost of care for patients with acute low back pain: a retrospective review of patient records. J Am Osteopath Assoc. 2009;109(4):229–33.
6. Hestbaek L, Leboeuf-Yde C, Manniche C. Is low back pain part of a general health pattern or is it a separate and distinctive entity? A critical literature review of comorbidity with low back pain. J Manip Physiol Ther. 2003;26(4):243–52.

7.   Beales DJ, Smith AJ, O'Sullivan PB, Straker LM. Low Back pain and comorbidity clusters at 17 years of age: a cross-sectional examination of health-related quality of life and specific low Back pain impacts. J Adolesc Health. 2012;50(5):509–16.

8.   Schneider S, Mohnen SM, Schiltenwolf M, Rau C. Comorbidity of low back pain: representative outcomes of a national health study in the Federal Republic of Germany. Eur J Pain. 2007;11(4):387–97.

9.   Hagen EM, Svensen E, Eriksen HR, Ihlebæk CM, Ursin H. Comorbid subjective health complaints in low Back pain. Spine. 2006;31(13):1491–5.

10. Australian Institute of Health and Welfare. Australia's. Health 2016. In: AIHW, editor. Australia's Health Series No 15. Catalogue No AUS 199, Australia's Health Series No 15. Canberra; 2016.

11. Newman AB. Comorbidity and multimorbidity. Dordrecht: Springer; 2012.

12. Søndergaard E, Willadsen TG, Guassora AD, Vestergaard M, Tomasdottir MO, Borgquist L, et al. Problems and challenges in relation to the treatment of patients with multimorbidity: general practitioners' views and attitudes. Scand J Prim Health Care. 2015;33(2):121–6.

13. Gijsen R, Hoeymans N, Schellevis FG, Ruwaard D, Satariano WA, van den Bos GAM. Causes and consequences of comorbidity: a review. J Clin Epidemiol. 2001;54(7):661–74.

14. Gijsen R, Hoeymans N, Schellevis F, Ruwaard D, Satariano W, van den Bos G. Causes and consequences of comorbidity. J Clin Epidemiol. 2001;54(7):661–74.

15. Gyntelberg F. One year incidence of low back pain among male residents of Copenhagen aged 40-59. Dan Med Bull. 1974;21(1):30–6.

16. Biering-Sorensen F. Physical measurements as risk indicators for low-Back trouble over a one-year period. Spine. 1984;9(2):106–19.

17. Seferlis T, Németh G, Carlsson A-M. Prediction of functional disability, recurrences, and chronicity after 1 year in 180 patients who required sick leave for acute low-Back pain. J Spinal Disord Tech. 2000;13(6):470–7.

18. Coté M, Rossignol M, Dionne C, Truchon M, Arsenault B, Poitras S, et al. An interdisciplinary guideline development process: the clinic on low-back pain in interdisciplinary practice (CLIP) low-back pain guidelines, vol. 2. BioMed Central Ltd: England; 2007.

19. Nordin M, Hiebert R, Pietrek M, Alexander M, Crane M, Lewis S. Association of comorbidity and outcome in episodes of nonspecific low back pain in occupational populations. J Occup Environ Med. 2002;44(7):677–84.

20. Gore M, Sadosky A, Stacey BR, Tai K-S, Leslie D. The burden of chronic low Back pain: clinical comorbidities, treatment patterns, and health care costs in usual care settings. Spine. 2012;37(11):E668–E77.

21. Ritzwoller D, Crounse L, Shetterly S, Rublee D. The association of comorbidities, utilization and costs for patients identified with low back pain. BMC Musculoskelet Disord. 2006;7(1):72.

22. Runciman W, Hunt T, Hannaford N, Hibbert P, Westbrook J, Coiera E, et al. CareTrack: assessing the appropriateness of health care delivery in Australia. Med J Aust. 2012;197(2):100–5.

23. Ramanathan SA, Hibbert PD, Maher CG, Day RO, Hindmarsh DM, Hooper TD, et al. CareTrack: toward appropriate Care for low Back Pain. Spine. 2017;42(13):E802–E9.

24. Hunt TD, Ramanathan SA, Hannaford NA, Hibbert PD, Braithwaite J, Coiera E, et al. CareTrack Australia: assessing the appropriateness of adult healthcare: protocol for a retrospective medical record review. BMJ Open. 2012;2(1).

25. Telstra Corporation Limited. Telstra White Pages. Adelaide, South East, Eyre Peninsula, Sydney, Newcastle, Broken Hill: Telstra; 2010.

26. Uhlig K, Leff B, Kent D, Dy S, Brunnhuber K, Burgers JS, et al. A framework for crafting clinical practice guidelines that are relevant to the care and management of people with multimorbidity. J Gen Intern Med. 2014;29(4):670–9.

27. McGlynn EA, Asch SM, Adams J, Keesey J, Hicks J, DeCristofaro A, et al. The quality of health care delivered to adults in the United States. N Engl J Med. 2003;348(26):2635–45.

11

Assessment of potential risk factors for new onset disabling low back pain in Japanese workers: findings from the CUPID (cultural and psychosocial influences on disability) study

Mika Kawaguchi[1*], Ko Matsudaira[2], Takayuki Sawada[1], Tadashi Koga[1,3], Akiko Ishizuka[1], Tatsuya Isomura[1,4] and David Coggon[5,6]

Abstract

Background: Most studies of risk factors for new low back pain (LBP) have been conducted in Western populations, but because of cultural and environmental differences, the impact of causal factors may not be the same in other countries. We used longitudinal data from the Cultural and Psychosocial Influences on Disability (CUPID) study to assess risk factors for new onset of disabling LBP among Japanese workers.

Methods: Data came from a 1-year prospective follow-up of nurses, office workers, sales/marketing personnel, and transportation workers, initially aged 20–59 years, who were employed in or near Tokyo. A baseline questionnaire included items on past history of LBP, personal characteristics, ergonomic work demands, and work-related psychosocial factors. Further information about LBP was collected at follow-up. Analysis was restricted to participants who had been free from LBP during the 12 months before baseline. Logistic regression was used to assess baseline risk factors for new onset of disabling LBP (i.e. LBP that had interfered with work) during the 12 months of follow-up.

Results: Among 955 participants free from LBP during the 12 months before baseline, 58 (6.1%) reported a new episode of disabling LBP during the 12-month follow-up period. After mutual adjustment in a multivariate logistic regression analysis, which included the four factors that showed associations individually ($p < 0.1$) in analyses adjusted only for gender and age, the highest odds ratio (OR) was for past history of LBP (2.8, 95% [confidence interval {CI}]: 1.6–4.9), followed by working ≥60 h per week (1.8, 95% CI: 1.0–3.5) and lifting weights ≥25 kg by hand (1.6, 95% CI: 0.9–3.0). When past history of LBP was excluded from the model, ORs for the remaining risk factors were virtually unchanged.

Conclusions: Our findings suggest that among Japanese workers, as elsewhere, past history of LBP is a major risk factor for the development of new episodes of disabling back pain. They give limited support to the association with occupational lifting that has been observed in earlier research, both in Japan and in Western countries. In addition, they suggest a possible role of long working hours, which merits further investigation.

Keywords: New onset, Disabling low back pain, Prospective study, Risk factors, Japanese workers, Symptom-free

* Correspondence: mika_kawaguchi@jp-css.com
[1]Clinical Study Support, Inc., 2F Daiei Bldg., 1-11-20 Nishiki, Naka-ku, Nagoya 460-0003, Japan
Full list of author information is available at the end of the article

Background

Low back pain (LBP) affects most adults at some point in their lives, some 85–95% of cases being classed as 'non-specific' (i.e. without identifiable underlying pathology) [1, 2]. In recent decades, it has consistently been the leading cause globally of years lived with disability [3], and in Japan, it is one of the most common causes of disability, with a reported lifetime prevalence of more than 80% [4]. In the workplace, it is a costly problem, not only impairing the health of employees, but also reducing productivity [5]. The largest societal costs arise from cases in which the pain is disabling [6].

Various risk factors for the development of LBP have been identified previously, including mechanical stress from occupational activities such as lifting, bending, twisting and manual handling [7], and also psychosocial factors such as low mood, somatizing tendency (a tendency to worry about common somatic symptoms), job dissatisfaction, and adverse health beliefs about the causes and prognosis of back disorders [7–12]. Moreover, epidemiological studies indicate that most people with a history of LBP experience a recurrence within a year [13–16]. Thus, the occurrence of LBP is an important predictor of future episodes [7, 8, 17–20].

Most of the research on these risk factors has been conducted in Western populations, but it is possible that because of cultural and environmental differences, their impacts are not the same in other countries [21]. In an earlier prospective cohort study of Japanese workers who had been symptom-free for at least 1 year, we found that, in accordance with observations in Western populations [7, 22–24], past history of LBP, interpersonal stress at work, and frequent occupational lifting were all important predictors of disabling LBP [25]. Before that study, risk factors for new onset LBP, and in particular the role of psychosocial aspects of work, had not been properly assessed through prospective epidemiological research in Japan, and there remains a need for further investigation to confirm its findings.

We therefore conducted a new longitudinal study, as part of an international investigation of risk factors for musculoskeletal pain and associated disability, the Cultural and Psychosocial Influences on Disability (CUPID) study, which focused on workers aged 20–59 years from 47 occupational groups in 18 countries [26–30]. Using data from the CUPID study, we again assessed risk factors for new onset of disabling LBP among Japanese workers.

Methods

Study design

Our target population for the present study was Japanese workers. We used data from a 1-year prospective follow-up of Japanese participants in the CUPID study, which were collected from four groups of workers employed in or near Tokyo: nurses from a university hospital; office workers in administrative and clerical jobs at the same hospital, four pharmaceutical companies and a privately-owned trading company; sales/marketing personnel from six pharmaceutical companies; and transportation workers (mainly lorry drivers and loaders) from two courier companies transporting baggage and mail.

Data collection

At each participating organization, a self-administered questionnaire with a covering letter from the study team was distributed to all employees in specified jobs. Workers were asked to return the completed questionnaire by post directly to the study administration office, including their name and mailing address for the purpose of follow-up. During 2009, a total of 3187 baseline questionnaires were distributed (nurses: 1074; office workers: 425; sales/marketing personnel: 380; transportation operatives: 1308), and of these, 2651 (83.2%) were completed and returned. After approximately 1 year, a follow-up questionnaire was sent to those participants who had returned the baseline questionnaire and consented to further contact. Of the 2651 participants who completed the baseline questionnaire, 1809 (68.2%) returned satisfactory follow-up questionnaires.

Baseline questionnaire

The baseline questionnaire comprised a Japanese translation of the original CUPID questionnaire [26], supplemented with additional questions for Japanese workers. Accuracy of translation was checked by independent back-translation into English.

Among other things, the questionnaire assessed the occurrence of LBP during the past 12 months, experience of LBP more than 12 months earlier (past history of LBP), and various individual and work-related risk factors [6]. LBP was defined as occurring in an area between the costal margin and inferior gluteal folds that was depicted in a diagram [26]. Severity of LBP was classified to four grades, based on a scheme devised by Von Korff: grade 0 (no LBP), grade 1 (LBP not interfering with work), grade 2 (LBP interfering with work), and grade 3 (LBP interfering with work and leading to sick-leave) [31].

The baseline questionnaire also assessed various personal characteristics (age, gender, age at which full-time education was finished, marital status, obesity [body mass index {BMI} $\geq$ 25 kg/m^2], smoking habits, habitual exercise), tenure of current job, hours worked per week, whether an average working day entailed lifting weights of $\geq$25 kg by hand, work-related psychosocial factors (interpersonal stress at work, inadequate breaks, job control, support from others when at work, job satisfaction), mental health, emotional trauma in childhood, awareness of colleagues and family members with LBP, somatizing tendency, and adverse beliefs about LBP.

Smoking was quantified in terms of the Brinkman Index (calculated as the product of the total number of cigarettes smoked per day and the duration of smoking in years) [32]. Individuals with a Brinkman Index of ≥400 were classed as heavy smokers, and the remainder (including non-smokers) as non-heavy smokers.

Work-related psychosocial factors were each assessed through a single question. Questions on interpersonal stress and inadequate breaks were supplementary to the original English version of the CUPID questionnaire, and allowed for two possible answers – yes or no. Job control was defined as lacking when participants reported "seldom" or "never/almost never" having choice in deciding how to work. Support at work was classed as lacking in those who said that they "seldom" or "never" received help or support from colleagues when they encountered difficulties in their work. Job dissatisfaction was deemed to occur when in response a question about the extent to which they had been satisfied with their job as whole taking everything into consideration, participants answered "dissatisfied" or "very dissatisfied".

To assess mental health, relevant items from the MOS 36-item short-form health survey (SF-36) ver.1.2 were used [33, 34]. A score of 52 or lower on the SF-36 ver.1.2 mental health summary was taken to indicate depressed mood, 52 being the cut-point for diagnosing depression in Japanese adults [35].

Somatizing tendency was assessed using questions from the Brief Symptom Inventory [36], and was graded according to the number of symptoms (0, 1, ≥2) from a total of five (faintness or dizziness, pains in the heart or chest, nausea or upset stomach, trouble getting breath, hot or cold spells) that were reported as at least moderately distressing in the past week.

Adverse beliefs about LBP were assessed through questions derived from the Fear Avoidance Beliefs Questionnaire [37]. Participants were classed as having adverse beliefs about physical activity if they completely agreed that for someone with LBP, physical activity should be avoided as it might cause harm and that rest is needed to get better. They were deemed to have adverse beliefs about work-relatedness if they completely agreed that LBP is commonly caused by work. And they were considered to have adverse beliefs about prognosis if they completely agreed that neglecting LBP can cause permanent health problems and completely disagreed that such problems usually get better within 3 months.

Follow-up questionnaire
The follow-up questionnaire included items on any change of job since baseline, and the presence and severity of LBP in the past 12 months. The severity of LBP was graded in the same way as at baseline.

Eligibility criteria
In our analysis for this report, we restricted our attention to participants who had been free from LBP for the past 12 months at baseline, and who did not change their job during the follow-up period.

Outcome
The outcome of interest was any new onset of disabling LBP during the 12 months of follow-up, where pain was defined as disabling if it had interfered with work (grade 2 or 3).

Statistical methods
Descriptive statistics were calculated, and then logistic regression was used to explore associations with risk factors. These were summarised by odds ratios (ORs) with 95% confidence intervals (CIs). First, each risk factor was analysed separately: a) with adjustment only for age and gender; and b) with adjustment also for past history of LBP, which had been identified as an important risk factor in earlier research including our own [7, 25]. Risk factors with p-values <0.1 when adjusted only for age and gender were then taken forward for inclusion in a single multivariate model with mutual adjustment. The software package SAS Release 9.3 (SAS Institute, Cary, NC) was used for all statistical analyses.

Ethical approval
Ethical approval for the study was obtained from the ethics committees of the University of Tokyo Hospital and review board of the Japan Labour Health and Welfare Organization. All participants provided written informed consent.

Results
Baseline characteristics of the study participants
Of the 1809 participants who responded to the 1-year follow-up questionnaire, 955 had reported no LBP during the previous 12 months at baseline, and were included in subsequent analyses (Fig. 1). Their mean (standard deviation: SD) age at baseline was 36.7 (9.9) years, most were male (n = 651; 68.3%), and they had a mean (SD) BMI at baseline of 22.2 (3.0) kg/m^2. The proportions by occupational group were: transportation operatives (38.1%), nurses (23.8%), sales/marketing personnel (21.1%), and office workers (16.7%).

Incidence of new onset disabling low back pain
Among the 955 eligible participants, 58 (6.1%) reported a new episode of disabling LBP during the 12-month follow-up period. Their mean (SD) age at baseline was 34.4 (8.7) years, and most were male (62.1%). In most cases the severity was graded 2 (n = 43, 74.1%), but 15 (25.9%) had grade 3 LBP. Among the latter, total sick-leave during the 12 months was mostly 1–5 days (73.3%), while the rest had been absent for 6–30 days (26.7%).

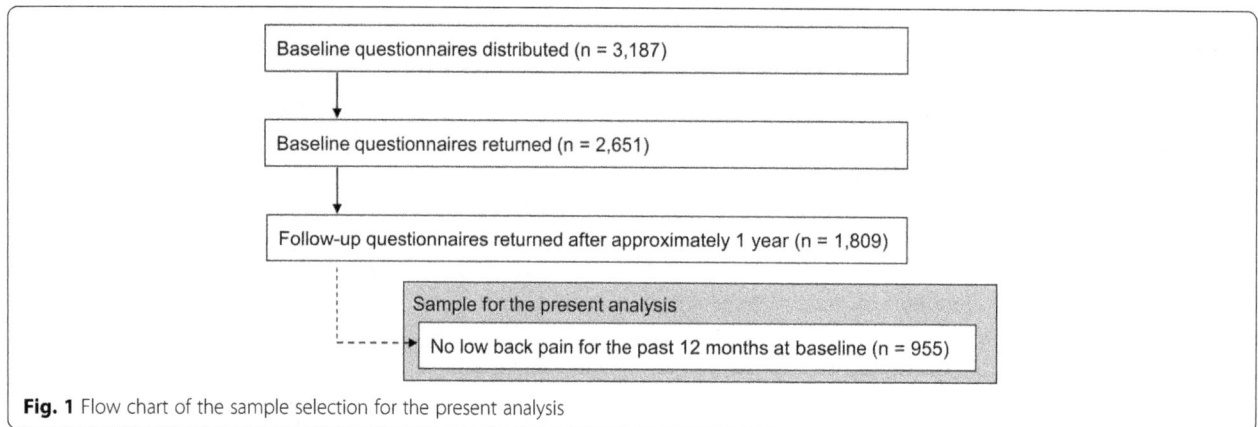

Fig. 1 Flow chart of the sample selection for the present analysis

Association of new onset disabling low back pain with risk factors

Table 1 shows ORs for the onset of disabling LBP, after adjustment for age and gender, and then also for past history of LBP. In the analyses adjusted only for gender and age, four factors were associated with p-values <0.1, and thus met the criterion for inclusion in subsequent multivariate analysis. These were: past history of LBP (OR: 2.6, 95% CI: 1.5–4.6), working ≥60 h per week (OR: 2.1, 95% CI: 1.1–4.0), lifting weights of ≥25 kg by hand (OR: 1.9, 95% CI: 1.1–3.3), and inadequate breaks (OR: 1.8, 95% CI: 1.0–3.1). When associations were adjusted also for past history of LBP, working ≥60 h per week (OR: 2.0, 95% CI: 1.1–3.9) and lifting weights ≥25 kg by hand (OR: 1.9, 95% CI: 1.1–3.3) remained the strongest risk factors.

After mutual adjustment in multivariate logistic regression analysis, the ORs were a little lower overall, but with a similar pattern to that in the earlier analyses (Table 2). The highest OR was for past history of LBP (OR: 2.8, 95% CI: 1.6–4.9), followed by working ≥60 h per week (OR: 1.8, 95% CI: 1.0–3.5) and lifting weights ≥25 kg by hand (OR: 1.6, 95% CI: 0.9–3.0). When past history of LBP was excluded from the model, ORs were virtually unchanged.

Discussion

These results indicate that past history of LBP and working long hours were risk factors for the new onset of disabling LBP among Japanese workers who had been symptom-free during the 12 months before baseline. In addition, risk was increased in participants who reported occupational lifting, although not significantly at a 5% level.

In the present investigation, the incidence of disabling LBP was relatively low (6.1%) which may reflect our strict definition of disability (interference with work), as well as the requirement for a long symptom-free period before baseline. It has previously been proposed that an episode of LBP can be classed as new if it occurs after a

period of at least 1–3 months without symptoms [38]. However, LBP is commonly recurrent within a year [13–16]. Moreover, a recent systematic review indicated that only 33% of patients in a primary care setting have recovered from non-specific LBP at a year after onset, whereas approximately 65% still experience pain [39]. Give these findings, we felt justified in requiring a 12-month symptom-free period at baseline, when exploring risk factors for new episodes, although we recognize that the criteria are to some extent arbitrary. In our earlier study, the incidence of new disabling LBP during 2 years of follow-up in workers who had been without LBP for more than 12 months before baseline was 3.9%, which is a little lower than in the current investigation [25].

We found that past history of LBP was the strongest and most significant risk factor for new disabling LBP, with an OR of almost three. This accords with our earlier study in Japan [25], and also with observations in Western populations [7, 8, 17–20]. It may be that the occurrence of a back problem renders an individual more vulnerable to future episodes of LBP (e.g. through changes in spinal structure and function or in the central processing of pain). Alternatively, the association might reflect continuing exposure to risk factors that were responsible for the initial development of the back problem. In our analysis, the association with past history of LBP was present after adjustment for other risk factors, but there may have been other important determinants of LBP that we did not assess.

In addition to past history of LBP, working ≥60 h per week and lifting weights of ≥25 kg by hand carried significantly elevated risk in analyses that adjusted for age and gender, the association with occupational lifting falling just short of significance when risk estimates were mutually adjusted. Biomechanical loading of the spine from manual handling tasks such as lifting, has been found experimentally to be greater in the presence of demands for mental processing that induce stress [24, 40]. Moreover, working overtime has been reported to increase

Table 1 Associations of risk factors at baseline with new onset of disabling low back pain

Risk factor	[a]n (%)	[b]OR	(95% CI)	[c]OR	(95% CI)
Age					
< 40 years	618 (65.2)				
40–49 years	200 (21.1)				
≥ 50 years	130 (13.7)				
Female gender	302 (31.7)				
Past history of LBP	313 (33.8)	2.6	(1.5–4.6)*		
Finished full-time education before age 19 years	304 (31.9)	1.4	(0.8–2.6)	1.4	(0.7–2.7)
BMI ≥ 25 kg/m² (obesity)	133 (14.2)	1.1	(0.5–2.5)	0.9	(0.4–2.1)
< 5 h sleep per day	82 (8.7)	1.8	(0.8–3.9)	1.5	(0.6–3.4)
Not married	445 (46.9)	0.8	(0.4–1.4)	0.8	(0.4–1.4)
Heavy smoker	133 (13.9)	0.8	(0.4–1.5)	0.6	(0.2–1.9)
Employed in current job for <1 year	96 (10.1)	1.2	(0.5–2.7)	1.3	(0.6–3.1)
Work ≥60 h per week	364 (38.8)	2.1	(1.1–4.0)*	2.0	(1.1–3.9)*
Lift weights ≥25 kg by hand	452 (47.3)	1.9	(1.1–3.3)*	1.9	(1.1–3.3)*
Aware of colleague(s) with LBP	687 (72.5)	1.2	(0.6–2.2)	1.1	(0.6–2.2)
Aware of family member(s) with LBP	301 (31.5)	1.2	(0.7–2.2)	1.1	(0.6–2.0)
Irregular work shifts	304 (31.9)	1.1	(0.6–2.0)	1.1	(0.6–1.9)
Interpersonal stress at work	458 (48.0)	1.3	(0.7–2.2)	1.1	(0.6–1.9)
Inadequate breaks at work	507 (53.1)	1.8	(1.0–3.1)	1.6	(0.9–2.9)
Lack of job control	347 (36.4)	0.9	(0.5–1.5)	0.8	(0.5–1.5)
Lack of support at work	72 (7.7)	2.0	(0.8–4.6)	1.9	(0.8–4.6)
Dissatisfied with job	378 (39.7)	0.8	(0.4–1.4)	0.7	(0.4–1.3)
Low mood	265 (28.0)	1.0	(0.6–1.9)	1.0	(0.5–1.8)
Regular exercise < once per week	652 (69.3)	1.0	(0.6–1.8)	0.9	(0.5–1.7)
Emotional trauma in childhood	66 (7.1)	2.0	(0.9–4.7)	1.7	(0.7–3.9)
Number distressing somatic symptoms					
0	760 (80.3)	1.0		1.0	
1	132 (13.9)	1.3	(0.6–2.6)	1.4	(0.7–2.9)
≥ 2	55 (5.8)	0.3	(0.0–1.9)	0.3	(0.0–2.0)
Adverse beliefs about LBP					
Work relatedness	306 (32.3)	1.3	(0.8–2.3)	1.3	(0.8–2.3)
Physical activity	208 (22.0)	1.0	(0.5–1.9)	1.1	(0.5–2.0)
Prognosis	155 (16.4)	0.8	(0.4–1.7)	0.9	(0.4–1.9)

Totals may not sum to 100% due to rounding

OR odds ratio; CI confidence interval; LBP low back pain

[a]Data on individual risk factors were missing for up to 29 participants. Each logistic regression analysis was limited to participants with complete information on all of the risk factors included in the relevant model

[b]Odds ratios (with 95% confidence intervals) adjusted for age and gender

[c]Odds ratios (with 95% confidence intervals) adjusted for age, gender and past history of LBP

*P < 0.05. A cut-point of P < 0.1 was adopted to select risk factors for inclusion in a subsequent multivariate model (see Table 2)

risk of musculoskeletal disorders such as LBP [41]. While excessive working hours, perhaps entailing physical exhaustion as well as mental strain, could of itself lead to LBP, it might also act by potentiating the risks from spinal strain as a consequence of heavy lifting.

Long working hours may also reflect an element of "workaholism" in which an employee, whether for personal reasons or in response to an over-demanding job, spends excessive time at work to the detriment of his or her personal life [42]. This too is a previously reported risk factor for disabling LBP [43].

An association with long working hours was not apparent in our earlier study [25]. On the other hand, that investigation found new incidence of disabling LBP

Table 2 Mutually adjusted associations of risk factors at baseline with new onset of disabling low back pain

Risk factor	[a]OR	(95% CI)	[b]OR	(95% CI)
Age				
< 40 years	1.0		1.0	
40–49 years	0.8	0.4–1.8	1.0	0.5–2.0
≥ 50 years	0.7	0.2–1.9	0.7	0.2–2.1
Female gender	1.4	0.7–2.8	1.5	0.8–3.0
Work ≥60 h per week	1.8	1.0–3.5	1.9	1.0–3.6
Lift weights ≥25 kg by hand	1.6	0.9–3.0	1.5	0.8–2.8
Inadequate break time at work	1.4	0.7–2.6	1.4	0.8–2.7
Past history of LBP	2.8	1.6–4.9	–	–

Participants with missing data for any of the variables in the model were excluded
[a]Mutually adjusted odds ratios (with 95% confidence intervals) derived from a logistic regression model which included all of the variables for which results are presented
[b]Mutually adjusted odds ratios (with 95% confidence intervals) derived from a logistic regression model which included all of the variables for which results are presented but did not adjust for past history of LBP

aside was significantly related to interpersonal stress at work, a finding that was not replicated in the current analysis. These differences may reflect differing characteristics of the populations studied. For example, in the earlier investigation, the participants were mostly male (88.3%) and office workers (76.1%). Alternatively, they could have occurred by chance. They underline the need for replication of results, especially when multiple risk factors are examined without strong prior expectations, and there is therefore greater potential for false positive results.

That said, the findings of the present study are not clearly different from those in Western populations. Divergence from other countries in the factors affecting new onset of disabling LBP might perhaps have been expected as a consequence of cultural differences. However, a trend to westernization in Japan may have reduced those differences. Alternatively, our questionnaire may not have covered risk factors that would differ from those in other countries or cultures.

Some limitations of our investigation should be noted. First, the generalizability of the results may be limited because the study sample was not fully representative. For example, the proportion of female participants was small in comparison with that in the national workforce of Japan. Second, because information about exposures and symptoms was obtained by self-report, some degree of misclassification is likely. Physical exposures, such as heavy lifting, might be assessed better using objective measures. Because of constraints on the total length of the questionnaire, the ascertainment of interpersonal stress

was based on a single question rather than the longer Brief Job Stress Questionnaire [44] that we had used to assess psychosocial factors including interpersonal stress in our earlier study. In addition, there is a possibility of recall bias, given that the presence and severity of LBP, both at baseline and follow-up, were ascertained retrospectively. For example, participants with physically demanding jobs may have been more likely to recall symptoms and difficulty with work. Third, because the outcome was relatively infrequent, statistical power was limited. Lastly, although the present analysis included most of the well-established risk factors for new onset LBP, as well as other potential risk factors that have been suggested by earlier studies, it is possible that some important determinants, perhaps distributed differentially by occupational group, were overlooked, leading to unrecognized residual confounding. Given these limitations, our results should be interpreted with caution.

Conclusion

In conclusion, our findings suggest that among Japanese workers, as elsewhere, past history of LBP is a major risk factor for the development of new episodes of disabling back pain. They give limited support to the association with occupational lifting that has been observed in earlier research, both in Japan and in Western countries. In addition, they suggest a possible role of long working hours, which merits further investigation.

Abbreviations
BMI: Body mass index; CI: Confidence interval; CUPID: Cultural and Psychosocial Influences on Disability; LBP: Low back pain; OR: Odds ratio; SD: Standard deviation; SF-36: MOS 36-item short-form health survey

Acknowledgements
We thank the CUPID collaborators, especially Dr. Keith T. Palmer and Dr. Noriko Yoshimura, for all their dedications to the study and also thank Sasakawa Foundation for supporting the further collaboration.

Funding
The study was a part of clinical research projects funded by the Japan Labour Health and Welfare Organization. The research projects aimed to resolve occupational health issues and disseminate the research findings. This organization did not have any role in the design of the study, collection, analysis, and interpretation of data, and writing of the manuscript.

Authors' contributions
KM designed the study. TI translated the questionnaires into Japanese. MK, TI, KM, and DC wrote the first draft of the manuscript and revised drafts. AI managed data. TK and DC contributed to statistical analyses and interpretation of data. TS analysed the data. KM and DC reviewed the final version of the manuscript for its intellectual content. All authors read and approved the final version manuscript.

Consent for publication

Not applicable.

Competing interests

KM received grant support including an endowed chair from AYUMI Pharmaceutical Corporation, Nippon Zoki Pharmaceutical Co., Ltd., ONO PHARMACEUTICAL CO., LTD., Eli Lilly Japan K.K., Sumitomo Dainippon Pharma Co., Ltd., Astellas Pharma Inc., TOTO LTD., OKAMURA CORPORATION, and Eisai Co., Ltd.; honoraria for lecturing from AYUMI Pharmaceutical Corporation, Nippon Zoki Pharmaceutical Co., Ltd., ONO PHARMACEUTICAL CO., LTD., Pfizer Japan Inc., Shionogi & Co., Ltd., Eli Lilly Japan K.K., Astellas Pharma Inc., HISAMITSU PHARMACEUTICAL CO., INC., Janssen Pharmaceutical K.K., KAKEN PHARMACEUTICAL CO., LTD., TEIJIN PHARMA LIMITED., Eisai Co., Ltd., and TOTO LTD.; and advisory fees from Shionogi & Co., Ltd., outside this study. These entities did not have any role in the study design; data collection, analysis, and interpretation; manuscript writing; and/or decision to submit for publication. MK, TS, TK, AI, TI, and DC have no competing interests to declare.

Author details

[1]Clinical Study Support, Inc., 2F Daiei Bldg., 1-11-20 Nishiki, Naka-ku, Nagoya 460-0003, Japan. [2]Department of Medical Research and Management for Musculoskeletal Pain, 22nd Century Medical and Research Center, Faculty of Medicine, The University of Tokyo, Tokyo, Japan. [3]Shin Nippon Biomedical Laboratories, Ltd., Kagoshima, Japan. [4]Institute of Medical Science, Tokyo Medical University, Tokyo, Japan. [5]MRC Lifecourse Epidemiology Unit, Southampton General Hospital, University of Southampton, Southampton, UK. [6]Arthritis Research UK/MRC Centre for Musculoskeletal Health and Work, University of Southampton, Southampton, UK.

References

1. Krismer M, van Tulder M. Low back pain (non-specific). Best Pract Res Clin Rheumatol. 2007;21:77–91.
2. Deyo RA, Rainville J, Kent DL. What can the history and physical examination tell us about low back pain? JAMA. 1992;268:760–5.
3. Vos T, Flaxman AD, Naghavi M, Lozano R, Michaud C, Ezzati M, et al. Years lived with disability (YLDs) for 1160 sequelae of 289 diseases and injuries 1990-2010: a systematic analysis for the global burden of disease study 2010. Lancet. 2012;380:2163–96.
4. Fujii T, Matsudaira K. Prevalence of low back pain and factors associated with chronic disabling back pain in Japan. Eur Spine J. 2013;22:432–8.
5. Feldman JB. The prevention of occupational low back pain disability: evidence-based reviews point in a new direction. J Surg Orthop Adv. 2004;13:1–14.
6. Snook SH. Work-related low back pain: secondary intervention. J Electromyogr Kinesiol. 2004;14:153–60.
7. Waddell G, Burton AK. Occupational health guidelines for the management of low back pain at work: evidence review. Occup Med. 2001;51:124–35.
8. Papageorgiou AC, Croft PR, Thomas E, Ferry S, Jayson MI, Silman AJ. Influence of previous pain experience on the episode incident of low back pain: results the South Manchester back pain study. Pain. 1996;66:181–5.
9. Pincus T, Burton AK, Vogel S, Field AP. A systematic review of psychological factors as predictors of chronicity/disability in prospective cohorts of low back pain. Spine (Phila Pa 1976). 2002;27(5):E109–20.
10. Hoogendoorn WE, van Poppel MN, Bongers PM, Koes BW, Bouter LM. Systematic review of psychosocial factors at work and private life as risk factors for back pain. Spine (Phila Pa 1976). 2000;25(16):2114–25.
11. Linton SJ. Occupational psychological factors increase the risk for back pain: a systematic review. J Occup Rehabil. 2001;11(1):53–66.
12. Farioli A, Mattioli S, Quaglieri A, Curti S, Violante FS, Coggon D. Musculoskeletal pain in Europe: the role of personal, occupational, and social risk factors. Scand J Work Environ Health. 2014;40(1):36–46.
13. Carey TS, Garrett JM, Jackman A, Hadler N. Recurrence and care seeking after acute back pain: results of a long-term follow-up study. North Carolina back pain project. Med Care. 1999;37:157–64.
14. Pengel L, Herbert R, Maher CG, Refshauge KM. Acute low back pain: a systematic review of its prognosis. BMJ. 2003;327:323–7.
15. Von Korff M. Studying the natural history of back pain. Spine. 1994;19(18 Suppl):2041S–6S.
16. Von Korff M, Deyo RA, Cherkin DC, Barlow W. Back pain in primary care: outcomes at 1 year. Spine. 1993;18:855–62.
17. Burton AK, Balagué F, Cardon G, Eriksen HR, Henrotin Y, Lahad A, COST B13 Working Group on European Guidelines for Prevention in Low Back Pain et al. How to prevent low back pain. Best Pract Res Clin Rheumatol 2005;19:541–555.
18. Hestbaek L, Leboeuf-Yde C, Kyvik KO. Is comorbidity in adolescence a predictor for adult low back pain? A prospective study of a young population. BMC Musculoskelet Disord. 2006;7:29–35.
19. Harreby M, Kjer J, Hesselsøe G, Neergaard K. Epidemiological aspects and risk factors for low back pain in 38-year-old men and woman: a 25-year prospective cohort study of 640 school children. Eur Spine J. 1996;5:312–8.
20. Smedley J, Egger P, Cooper C, Coggon D. Prospective cohort study of predictors of incident low back pain in nurses. BMJ. 1997;314(7089):122–58.
21. Waddell G. Social interactions. In: Waddell G, editor. The back pain revolution. 2nd ed. Edinburgh: Chuechill-Livingstone; 2004. p. 241–63.
22. Linton SJ. Psychological risk factors for neck and back pain. In: Nachemson AJ, Jonsson E, editors. Neck and back pain: the scientific evidence of causes, diagnosis and treatment. Philadelphia: Lippincot Williams & Wilkins; 2000. p. 57–78.
23. Harkness EF, Macfarlane GJ, Nahit ES, Silman AJ, McBeth J. Risk factors for new-onset low back pain amongst cohorts of newly employed workers. Rheumatology. 2003;42:959–68.
24. Davis KG, Marras WS, Heaney CA, Waters TR, Gupta P. The impact of mental processing and pacing on spine loading. Spine. 2002;27:2645–53.
25. Matsudaira K, Konishi H, Miyoshi K, Isomura T, Takeshita K, Hara N, et al. Potential risk factors for new onset of back pain disability in Japanese workers: findings from the Japan epidemiological research of occupation-related back pain study. Spine. 2012;37:1324–33.
26. Coggon D, Ntani G, Palmer KT, Felli VE, Harari R, Barrero LH, et al. The CUPID (cultural and psychosocial influences on disability) study: methods of data collection and characteristics of study sample. PLoS One. 2012;7:e39820.
27. Coggon D, Ntani G, Vargas-Prada S, Martinez JM, Serra C, Benavides FG, Members of CUPID Collaboration, et al. International variation in absence from work attributed to musculoskeletal illness: findings from the CUPID study. Occup Environ Med. 2013;70:575–84.
28. Matsudaira K, Palmer KT, Reading I, Hirai M, Yoshimura N, Coggon D. Prevalence and correlates of regional pain and associated disability in Japanese workers. Occup Environ Med. 2011;68:191–6.
29. Coggon D, Ntani G, Palmer KT, Felli VE, Harari R, Barrero LH. Patterns of multisite pain and associations with risk factors. Pain. 2013;154:1769–77.
30. Fujii T, Matsudaira K, Yoshimura N, Hirai M, Tanaka S. Associations between neck and shoulder discomfort (Katakori) and job demand, job control, and worksite support. Mod Rheumatol. 2013;23:1198–204.
31. Von Korff M, Ormel J, Keefe FJ, Dworkin SF. Grading the severity of chronic pain. Pain. 1992;50:133–49.
32. Brinkman GL, Coates O. The effect of bronchitis, smoking and occupation on ventilation. Ann Rev Respir Dis. 1963;87:684–93.
33. Fukuhara S, Bito S, Green J, Hsiao A, Kurokawa K. Translation, adaptation, and validation of the SF-36 health survey for use in Japan. J Clin Epidemiol. 1998;51:1037–44.
34. Fukuhara S, Ware JE Jr, Kosinski M, Wada S, Gandek B. Psychometric and clinical tests of validity of the Japanese SF-36 health survey. J Clin Epidemiol. 1998;51:1045–53.
35. Yamazaki S, Fukuhara S, Green J. Usefulness of five-item and three-item mental health inventories to screen for depressive symptoms in the general population of Japan. Health Qual Life Outcomes. 2005;3:48.
36. Waddell G, Newton M, Henderson I, Somerville D, Main CJ. A fear-avoidance beliefs questionnaire (FABQ) and the role of fear-avoidance beliefs in chronic low back pain and disability. Pain. 1993;52(2):157–68.
37. Derogatis LR, Melisaratos N. The brief symptom inventory: an introductory report. Psychol Med. 1983;13(3):595–605.
38. de Vet HCW, Heymans MW, Dunn KM, Pope DP, van der Beek AJ, Macfarlane GJ, et al. Episode of low back pain. A proposal for uniform definition to be used in research. Spine. 2002;27:2409–16.
39. Itz CJ, Geurts JW, van Kleef M, Nelemans P. Clinical course of non-specific low back pain: a systematic review of prospective cohort studies set in primary care. Eur J Pain. 2013;17:5–15.

40. Katsuhira J, Matsudaira K, Iwakiri K, Kimura Y, Ohashi T, Ono R, et al. Effect of mental processing on low back load while lifting an object. Spine. 2013;38:E832–9.

41. Koda S, Yasuda N, Sugihara Y, Ohara H, Udo H, Otani T, et al. Analyses of work-relatedness of health problems among truck drivers by questionnaire survey. Sangyo Eiseigaku Zasshi. 2000;42:6–16. (in Japanese)

42. Scott KS, Moore KS, Miceli MP. An exploration of the meaning and consequences of Workaholism. Human Relations. 1997;50:287–314.

43. Matsudaira K, Shimazu A, Fujii T, Kubota K, Sawada T, Kikuchi N, et al. Workaholism as a risk factor for depressive mood, disabling back pain, and sickness absence. PLoS One. 2013;8:e75140.

44. Shimomitsu T, Yokoyama K, Ono Y, Maruta T, Tanigawa T. Development of a novel brief job stress questionnaire. In: Kato S, editor. Report of the research grant for the prevention of work-related diseases from the Ministry of Labour. Tokyo: Ministry of Labour; 1998. p. 107–15.

12

Development of the Japanese Core Outcome Measures Index (COMI): cross-cultural adaptation and psychometric validation

Ko Matsudaira[1,2]*, Hiroyuki Oka[1], Yasushi Oshima[3], Hirotaka Chikuda[3,4], Yuki Taniguchi[3], Yoshitaka Matsubayashi[3], Mika Kawaguchi[5], Emiko Sato[5], Haruka Murano[5], Thomas Laurent[5], Sakae Tanaka[3] and Anne F. Mannion[6]

Abstract

Background: The patient-rated Core Outcome Measures Index (COMI) assesses the multidimensional impact of back problems on the sufferer. The brevity and comprehensibility of the tool make it practical for use in clinical and research settings. Although the COMI has been cross-culturally adapted in various languages worldwide, there is currently no Japanese version. The aim of this study was to develop a Japanese version of the COMI by: (1) performing a cross-cultural adaptation of the English version and (2) evaluating the psychometric properties of the Japanese version of the COMI in Japanese volunteers with chronic back problems.

Methods: The English version of the COMI was cross-culturally adapted for the Japanese language using established guidelines. The pre-final version was pilot-tested in five Japanese-speaking patients with low back pain (LBP) and a history of spine surgery. The psychometric properties of the Japanese COMI were tested in a group of 1052 individuals with chronic LBP (LBP ≥3 months), aged 20–69 years, who were recruited through a web-based survey. The psychometric properties that were evaluated included convergent and known-group validity, using the following reference questionnaires: EuroQol 5 Dimension, Roland Morris Disability Questionnaire, Short Form 8™ Health Survey, and the Keele STarT Back Screening Tool.

Results: The pre-final version of the cross-culturally adapted Japanese COMI was completed without any major problems of understanding or acceptability. For the evaluation of its psychometric properties, tests for convergent validity showed moderate correlations between COMI items and the respective reference questionnaires for symptom-specific well-being [− 0.33–−0.48] and disability domains [0.48] and strong correlations (> 0.5) for the other domains and the COMI summary score. The analysis of known-group validity showed a linear trend for the COMI score in relation to prognostic risk ($P < 0.001$).

Conclusions: The Japanese COMI retained conceptual equivalence to the original using comprehensible and acceptable Japanese expressions. We developed a Japanese version of the COMI that displayed qualities that support its convergent and known-group validity. The availability of a Japanese version of the COMI should allow for improved documentation of the care provided to patients with back problems.

Keywords: Cross cultural adaptation, Psychometric validation, Core outcome measures index, Low back pain, Degenerative disorders of the lumbar spine

* Correspondence: kohart801@gmail.com
[1]Department of Medical Research and Management for Musculoskeletal Pain, 22nd Century Medical and Research Center, Faculty of Medicine, The University of Tokyo, Tokyo, Bunkyo-ku, Japan
[2]Department of Pain Medicine, Fukushima Medical University School of Medicine, Fukushima, Japan
Full list of author information is available at the end of the article

Background

Low back pain (LBP) is a common, disabling health problem. Although its prognosis is mostly benign [1], 2–7% of patients develop chronic LBP [2]. Since chronic LBP affects patients' lives beyond physical pain and disability, assessments that encompass multidimensional self-reported outcomes are required for documenting the impact of LBP and the response to treatment.

The Core Outcome Measures Index (COMI) was developed to evaluate the multidimensional impact of LBP. It was based on a set of single questions (concerned with pain symptoms, function, symptom-specific well-being, and disability) that had been recommended for use by an expert group [3]. These items, and an additional question on general quality of life, were subsequently put together and validated as an index [4]. With established reliability, validity, and responsiveness [4–7], the brief but comprehensive coverage of the COMI alleviates response burden on patients, rendering the COMI a practical tool in clinical and research settings.

Since its initial development, the availability and use of the COMI has expanded: it has been cross-culturally adapted for an array of different languages, and these language versions have displayed good psychometric properties [4–6, 8–11]. It has also been modified for use in patients with neck problems [7, 12]). To date, however, no Japanese version has been developed. In order to apply this parsimonious and practical tool in Japanese clinical settings, a need was seen for the COMI to be cross-culturally adapted for use in Japanese patients. The availability of a Japanese version of the COMI would promote the wider use of the questionnaire and allow for improved documentation of care in Japanese patients with back problems.

The aim of this study was to develop a Japanese version of the COMI by: (1) performing a cross-cultural adaptation of the English version and (2) evaluating the psychometric properties of the Japanese version of the COMI in volunteers with chronic back problems, resident in Japan.

Methods

The English version of the COMI was cross-culturally adapted for the Japanese language, in accordance with previously published guidelines [13, 14], and its psychometric properties were evaluated in data collected in a cross-sectional survey. Ethical approval was obtained from the ethical committee of The University of Tokyo [Approval number: 10665-(1)]. All participants in the survey gave their consent electronically and were compensated with vouchers (e.g., shopping points). No personally identifiable information was collected.

COMI

COMI comprises seven items: back pain, leg/buttock pain, function, symptom-specific well-being, general quality of life, social disability, and work disability. All items refer to the last week, except for the two disability items (past 4 weeks). Back and leg/buttock pain are rated on separate 10-point graphic rating scales; the other items are responded to using a 5-point scale. A higher score indicates a worse status.

Scores are calculated for each domain and for the summary score [15]. For the latter, the higher score of the back or leg/buttock pain is first taken as the pain domain score. Then, the other item scores are converted from their 5-point scales into a 0 to 10-point range using increments of 2.5 (0, 2.5, 5.0, 7.5, 10.0). Social and work disability scores are averaged to form one disability domain score. Averaging the five domain scores (now each scored 0–10) — pain, function, symptom-specific well-being, general quality of life, and disability — yields a summary score ranging from 0 to 10 (best to worst health status) [4, 6].

The Japanese COMI questions were supplemented with another question to identify the predominant problem [16], using an item from the Spine Tango patient self-assessment form [17]. This independent item is not included in the COMI scoring [16]. The item enquires as to which problem is the most troublesome (back pain, leg pain, sensory disturbances, or other).

Cross-cultural adaptation
Translation and synthesis

Two native Japanese speakers (an expert in the measured concept and clinical contents of the questionnaire and a layperson not familiar with the concept) independently translated the original version into Japanese. Their different profiles and backgrounds were expected to enhance conceptual and semantic equivalence. The two translations were compared with each other and with the original. After any discrepancies were resolved by discussion and consensus, the two translations were synthesized into one Japanese consensus version.

Back-translation

Two native English speakers blinded to the original English version and not familiar with the concepts independently back-translated the Japanese consensus version into English.

Expert committee

Two forward-translators, one methodologist (a researcher with experience in cross-cultural adaptations), and one clinician constituted an expert committee to produce a pre-final version of the Japanese COMI by consolidating all the translated versions in close contact with the developer of the COMI and the back translators. The committee members reviewed and discussed all the translations to assure semantic and conceptual equivalence between the original and translated versions. All the processes and rationales involved prior to reaching a consensus were documented in written form.

Pilot-test

Five Japanese-speaking patients with LBP and a history of spine surgery completed the pre-final version. After completion, the patients were debriefed regarding their general comments on the instrument and their understanding of the questions, to confirm comprehensibility and conceptual equivalence. Debriefing results were reviewed and the findings were used in producing the final version of the Japanese COMI.

Psychometric validation

Participants

Evaluation of the psychometric properties of the Japanese COMI was carried out in individuals with chronic LBP, aged 20–69 years. We recruited participants through a web-based survey outsourced to the Internet research company, IDEA PROGGET Co., Ltd. (Tokyo, Japan). Any individual residing in Japan who is aged ≥15 years and is interested in online surveys can register themselves with the research company and can freely choose whether they wish to participate in a given survey, based on the invitation emails distributed by the research company. Figure 1 depicts the recruitment flow of the participants; 630,000 in the eligible age range were randomly selected from the registered individuals and invited to participate in the initial screening survey. Those individuals interested in the survey ($n = 100,149$) were screened for age and the presence of chronic LBP (defined as LBP lasting for ≥3 months) with severity graded as follows: I, no interference with everyday activities; II, interference with everyday activities but no absence from social activities including work, housework, and school; or III, interference with social activities, leading to absence from social activities [18]. Patients with LBP caused by cancer, inflammation, aneurysm, urolithiasis, or fracture were excluded. The screening yielded 37,015 participants satisfying the admission criteria.

After the screening, eligible participants were randomly selected based on computer-generated randomization sequences, stratified by sex and LBP severity, in order to obtain an equal number of males and females in each severity group. A total of 1787 eligible participants who were registered at the time of our survey were invited to take part in the study; 13 patients who withdrew registration to the panel after the screening were not invited. Those who were interested in the invitation responded to the questionnaire battery of their own free will.

Questionnaire battery

The questionnaire battery included questions regarding sociodemographic and clinical characteristics, the Japanese COMI, the EuroQol 5 Dimension (EQ-5D) [19], the Roland Morris Disability Questionnaire (RDQ) [20], the Short Form 8™ Health Survey (SF-8) [21], and the Keele STarT Back Screening Tool (STarT) [22] [Table 1].

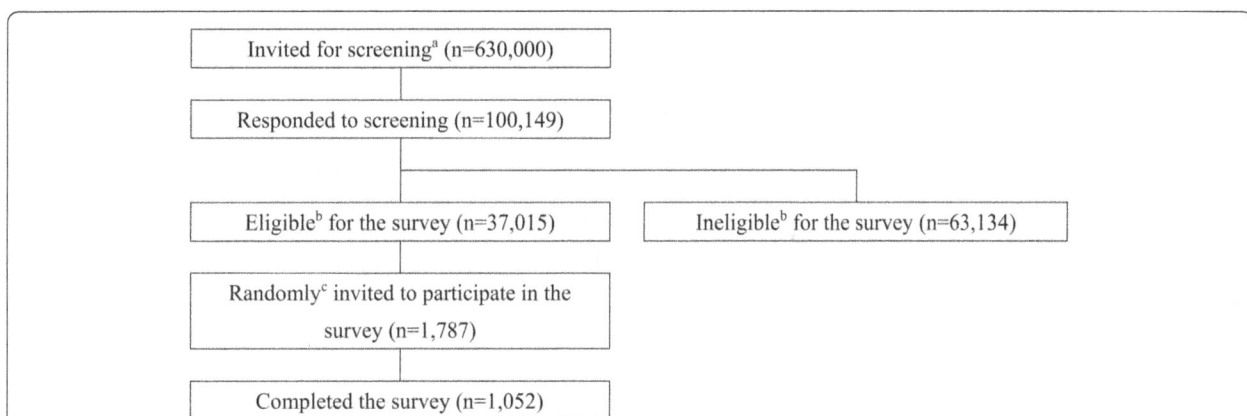

Fig. 1 Participant recruitment flow for the Japanese COMI validation study. *a* Of the whole registrants to the Internet research company, 630,000 in the eligible age range (20–69 years) were randomly invited to participate in the screening survey. *b* Screening respondents were considered eligible for the survey if they had chronic LBP (LBP lasting for ≥3 months) with severity graded as follows: I, no interference with everyday activities; II, interference with everyday activities but no absence from social activities including work, housework, and school; or III, interference with social activities, leading to absence from social activities [18]; but without LBP caused by cancer, inflammation, aneurysm, urolithiasis, or fracture. *c* Eligible participants were randomly selected based on computer-generated randomization sequences, stratified by sex and LBP severity, in order to obtain an equal number of males and females in each severity group. A total of 1787 eligible participants who were registered at the time of our survey were invited to take part in the study; 13 patients who withdrew registration to the panel after the screening were not invited

Table 1 Reference questionnaires

Questionnaire	Content	Scale	Item number	Score range	COMI domains expected to correlate strongly
EQ-5D [18]	General health status				Summary, QOL
The descriptive system	Mobility, self-care, usual activities, pain/discomfort, and anxiety/depression	3-point Likert	5	−0.111–1.000[a]	
EQ-VAS		VAS	1	0–100[b]	
RDQ [19]	Physical disability due to low back pain	Dichotomous (yes or no)	24	0–24[c]	Summary, Function, Disability
SF-8 [20]	General health-related quality of life	5- or 6-point Likert	8		
PCS				5.32–70.69[d]	Summary, Pain, Function, Symptom-specific well-being, QOL
MCS				10.11–74.51[d]	Symptom-specific well-being, QOL
STarT [21]	Potentially modifiable prognostic indicators Five questions related to the psychological factors constitute the sub-score	5-point Likert and Dichotomous (agree or disagree)	9	0–9[e]	Summary, Pain, Function, Disability

[a]Calculated using the value set for the Japanese population [34]. The score of 1 denotes "full health" and 0 "death"
[b]The score of 0 indicates worst imaginable health state and 100 best possible health state
[c]A higher score indicates greater disability
[d]Calculated based on a norm-based scoring method given in the instrument guidelines [21]. A higher score indicates better health
[e]A total score of 0–3 indicates low prognostic risk; a total score of ≥4 with sub score of ≤3, medium prognostic risk; sub score of ≥4, high prognostic risk
EQ-5D: the EuroQol 5 Dimension; VAS: visual analogue scale; RDQ: Roland Morris Disability Questionnaire; SF-8: Short Form 8™ Health Survey; PCS: physical component summary; MCS: mental component summary; STarT: the Keele STarT Back Screening Tool

Statistical analysis

The sociodemographic and clinical characteristics of the participants were summarized descriptively. To evaluate the ability of the Japanese COMI to capture the full range of the impact of LBP, we assessed floor and ceiling effects (percentage of individuals reporting worst and best status, respectively) for each COMI item and domain, for the COMI summary score, and also for the other questionnaires. Floor effects were considered present if > 15% of the participants achieved the worst status, and ceiling effects were considered present if > 15% of the participants achieved the best status [23].

The validity of the Japanese COMI was evaluated in terms of convergent validity and known-group validity. For convergent validity, the degree of correlation between each COMI domain or the COMI summary score with the reference questionnaire measuring the same or similar traits was measured using Spearman rank correlation coefficients. We considered a correlation coefficient of 0.1 as weak, 0.3, moderate, and 0.5, strong [24]. The correlation between the COMI and the corresponding reference questionnaires was expected to be strong [Table 1].

Known-group validity was evaluated by examining whether the COMI scores differed among the STarT prognostic risk groups. Participants were stratified into three risk groups based on the total score of the 9 questions and on the sub-score for the 5 psychological questions of the STarT: low risk (total score of 0–3), medium risk (total score of ≥4 with sub-score of ≤3), and high risk (sub score of ≥4) groups [22]. We used the Jonckheere-Terpstra test [25, 26] to test for a trend in the COMI summary score in association with the prognostic risk level. The non-parametric Jonckheere-Terpstra test evaluates the difference between the scores for a continuous variable among defined groups, taking the ordering of the groups (prognostic risk levels, in this study) into account.

Although not typically considered appropriate for multidimensional indexes [27], for the purposes of comparison with other language versions we assessed internal consistency of the Japanese COMI using the standardized Cronbach's alpha, whereby coefficients above 0.7 are usually considered acceptable [28].

The Jonckheere-Terpstra test was one-sided and the other tests were two-sided. The significance level was set at 0.05. Data were analyzed using SAS software version 9.4 (SAS Institute, Inc., Cary, NC, USA).

Results

Cross-cultural adaptation

Translation

The following few items required modification in the forward translations: "pins and needles" (in the questionnaire instruction and "location of the main problem" item), "recreational activities" (social disability), "moderately" (response option of function), and "none" (response option of social and work disability). The concepts of "pins and needles" and "recreational activities" do not fully correspond to any concise Japanese expressions. For "moderately" and "none", the literal forward-translations to reflect the equivalent order and intervals between the original response options were considered to make the translations unnatural to the respondents. We sought expressions that would retain the original concepts and at the same time be familiar to Japanese speakers. The former two were back-translated as follows: "pins and needles" as "prickling sensation", and "recreational activities" as "engaging in hobbies, and recreation" or "vocational activities, or amusement activities". For each of the response options ("moderately" and "none"), we left two tentative translations (back-translations: "moderately" and "somewhat" for "moderately"; and "none" and "0 days" for "none"), with the aim of selecting the most natural expression based on the pilot-test results (see below).

Pilot-test

All five Japanese LBP patients answered the pre-final version of the Japanese COMI without major problems in relation to comprehensibility and acceptability. Of the tentative options for "moderately" and "none", we adopted expressions that back-translated as "moderately" and "none", respectively, for the final version, based on the participants' preferences and the conceptual equivalence to the original [Additional file 1].

Psychometric validation

A total of 1052 participants completed the questionnaires (Fig. 1). Completion of the web survey required answers to all questions and thus there were no missing data. The mean (standard deviation [SD]) age of the participants was 48.3 (12.6) years [Table 2]; 63.5% were male and 67.9% had non-specific LBP. LBP severity was evenly distributed among the three grades, I to III (about 33% each), as intended. In total, 79.4% individuals had had LBP for more than 18 months, but 60.8% had not taken any sick leave and 75.2% were not currently receiving any treatment for LBP.

Floor and ceiling effects

Table 3 shows the floor effects (worst status) and ceiling effects (best status) for the COMI and the reference questionnaires. The social and work disability items showed particularly high percentages for ceiling effects (72.5% and 82.9%, respectively).

Validity and internal consistency

Convergent validity was evaluated by assessing the correlations between the Japanese COMI scores and the scores on the relevant reference questionnaires that

measure the same or similar constructs. All the COMI domain scores and the COMI summary score correlated significantly with the respective reference questionnaires [Table 4]. Correlation coefficients met the expectation of indicating strong correlations (≥ 0.5) for all except for symptom-specific well-being (– 0.48 and – 0.33 with SF-8 physical component summary and mental component summary, respectively) and the disability domains (0.48 with STarT total), which indicated just moderate correlations. Correlations between the COMI summary scores and all the reference questionnaires were the strongest (– 0.52 to – 0.72).

The known-group validity was evaluated by comparing the COMI summary score among the low, middle, and high risk groups as measured with the STarT. The median COMI summary score was higher in the groups with higher prognostic risk (median [25th–75th percentile]: 3.1 [2.0–3.9], 4.6 [4.0–5.5], and 6.2 [5.2–7.1] in low, middle, and high prognostic risk groups, respectively) and demonstrated a significant, positive linear relationship with the prognostic risk level [Fig. 2] ($P < 0.001$, Jonckheere-Terpstra test).

Cronbach's alpha for the Japanese version of the COMI was 0.82.

Discussion

This study aimed to develop a Japanese version of the COMI. The cross-cultural adaptation process generated a Japanese version of the COMI that retained conceptual equivalence to the original, using comprehensible and acceptable Japanese expressions. Using a very large sample obtained from the general Japanese population, analyses of the psychometric properties of the Japanese COMI substantiated its validity.

We translated and linguistically validated the Japanese COMI based on published guidelines [13, 14], which facilitate a cross-cultural adaptation that retains equivalence to the original version. In the pilot test, all patients answered the Japanese COMI without any major problems regarding understanding or acceptability of the instrument. This suggests that the content of the Japanese COMI is equivalent to that of the original English version and uses expressions that are acceptable for Japanese patients.

Particularly high percentages for ceiling effects were observed for the social and work disability items. Other language versions [4, 5, 8–10] have also reported high percentages for ceiling effects for the disability domain or its items, although in none of these studies were the effects as pronounced as in the present study. The high percentages for ceiling effects that we documented may reflect the relatively low severity of LBP of the volunteers involved in the present study compared with those in previous studies: the proportion of individuals with

Table 2 Demographic and clinical characteristics of the participants ($n = 1052$)

Characteristics	n (%)
Sex	
Male	668 (63.5)
Age, year (mean ± SD)	48.3 ± 12.6
LBP before this episode	
Yes	869 (82.7)
Duration of current episode	
≥3–< 6 months	62 (5.9)
≥6–< 12 months	79 (7.5)
≥12–< 18 months	76 (7.2)
≥18 months	835 (79.4)
Severity of LBP	
Grade I[a]	351 (33.4)
Grade II[b]	353 (33.6)
Grade III[c]	348 (33.1)
Normal work	
Regular employee	405 (38.5)
Contract employee	171 (16.3)
Temporary employee	27 (2.6)
Business owner	76 (7.2)
Helping family business	8 (0.8)
Home worker	22 (2.1)
Student	3 (0.3)
Homemaker	136 (12.9)
Unemployed	178 (16.9)
Other	26 (2.5)
Length of current sick leave	
Not on sick leave	640 (60.8)
< 1 month	289 (27.5)
≥1–< 3 months	42 (4.0)
≥3–< 6 months	20 (1.9)
≥6–< 12 months	12 (1.1)
≥12–< 18 months	5 (0.5)
≥18 months	44 (4.2)
Educational level	
Junior High school	31 (2.9)
Secondary education	545 (51.8)
University education	427 (40.6)
Higher degree	46 (4.4)
Others	3 (0.3)
Type of work	
Sedentary	477 (45.3)
Physical	198 (18.8)
Others	377 (35.8)

Table 2 Demographic and clinical characteristics of the participants ($n = 1052$) *(Continued)*

Characteristics	n (%)
Current treatment for LBP	
Yes	261 (24.8)
Radiation of current pain	
To the buttock or thigh but not to the knee	182 (17.3)
To the buttock, thigh, shin and feet	156 (14.8)
No	714 (67.9)
Non-specific/Specific LBP	
Non-specific	714 (67.9)
Disc herniation, spinal stenosis or both	121 (11.5)
Other cause of radiation of pain	217 (20.6)
Pain location (COMI)	
Low back pain and back pain	499 (47.4)
Leg/buttock pain	133 (12.6)
Sensory disturbances (back, leg or buttocks)	163 (15.5)
Other	257 (24.4)

Data are presented as n (%), unless otherwise specified
There were no missing data since the survey completion required answers to all questions
[a]No interference with everyday activities
[b]Interference with everyday activities but not with social activities including work, housework, and school
[c]Interference with social activities including work, housework, and school
SD: standard deviation; LBP: low back pain; COMI: core outcome measure index

no sick leave was 40% and 32.9% in Italian [10] and French [9] studies, respectively; and the mean (SD) RDQ scores were 13.5 (5.6), 11.7 (5.7), 10.5 (6.3), and 11.6 (5.1) in German [4], Brazilian-Portuguese [8], Italian [10], and French [9] studies, respectively. In the present study, recruitment did not take place in hospitals or clinics, but was done online and included more individuals with less severe LBP that did not require treatment or sickness leave. The potential consequences of high floor and ceiling effects are that they can render an instrument unresponsive, since transitions to even more extreme statuses are not measurable. However, both German [4] and Spanish versions [5] of the COMI have been shown to be responsive (effect size: 0.95 (for the response 6 months after surgical or conservative treatment) in German [4] and 1.04 (for the response after surgery) in Spanish versions [5]), despite relatively large floor/ceiling effects of > 15% (floor effects for symptom-specific well-being (49.6%) and disability (18.5%) in the German version [4], and for back function (40.3%), symptom-specific well-being (64.9%), and disability (38.3%) in the Spanish version [5]; and ceiling effects for back function (31.2%) and disability (29.8%) in the German version [4]). Hence, the influence of large ceiling effects on the responsiveness of the Japanese COMI summary score might also be expected to be limited.

Table 3 Scores and distribution of the Japanese COMI and reference questionnaires

Scale/Domain	mean (SD)	Median	Range Min–Max	Floor effect (worst status) (%)	Ceiling effect (best status) (%)
COMI[a]					
Back Pain	3.7 (2.6)	3.0	0–10	1.5	12.4
Leg Pain	2.6 (2.7)	2.0	0–10	1.1	33.3
Pain	4.0 (2.7)	4.0	0–10	1.8	10.7
Back Function	2.5 (2.5)	2.5	0–10	2.6	36.5
Symptom-specific well-being	6.6 (3.1)	7.5	0–10	28.8	8.1
QOL	5.0 (2.4)	5.0	0–10	6.1	5.9
Social Disability	1.1 (2.3)	0.0	0–10	3.3	72.5
Work Disability	0.8 (2.0)	0.0	0–10	2.6	82.9
Summary Score	3.7 (1.8)	3.6	0–8.8	0.0	2.9
EQ-5D					
Summary Score	0.8 (0.2)	0.8	−0.111–1.000	0.3	34.7
VAS	66.8 (22.8)	70.0	0–100	0.1	2.5
RDQ[a]	4.0 (5.5)	2.0	0–24	0.8	35.5
SF-8					
PCS	45.1 (8.7)	46.1	11.97–63.53	0.0	0.0
MCS	46.0 (8.6)	47.5	11.53–65.09	0.0	0.0
STarT[a]	2.7 (2.4)	2.0	0–9	2.7	21.9
Total					
Sub score (psychological)	1.5 (1.5)	1.0	0–5	5.5	35.5

COMI: Core Outcome Measures Index; SD: standard deviation; QOL: quality of life; EQ-5D: the EuroQol 5 Dimension; VAS: visual analogue scale; RDQ: Roland Morris Disability Questionnaire; SF-8: Short Form 8™ Health Survey; PCS: physical component summary; MCS: mental component summary; STarT: the Keele STarT Back Screening Tool
[a]Higher score indicates worse status; lower score indicates better status

In the assessment of convergent validity, consistent with previous validation studies [4, 5, 8–11] the Japanese COMI correlated strongly with the relevant reference questionnaires that measure the same or similar constructs. The disability domain correlated strongly with RDQ, which specifically reflects physical disability, but less strongly with STarT total. This corroborates the convergent validity of the COMI disability domain as a measure specifically targeting physical disability and

correlating only moderately with STarT, which incorporates both physical disability and psychological factors. Despite the only moderate correlation with the COMI disability domain, the STarT total score (i.e., covering both physical and psychological aspects) correlated strongly with the COMI summary score, which reflects the influence of the back problem on many domains, substantiating the multidimensionality of the COMI. Finally, the scores for symptom-specific well-being

Table 4 Correlations[a] between the COMI and the related questionnaires and domains

	COMI					
	Pain	Function	Symptom-specific well-being	QOL	Disability	Summary
EQ-5D Summary index	−0.60	−0.58	−0.54	−0.60	−0.48	−0.72
RDQ	0.64	0.63	0.52	0.52	0.54	0.71
SF-8 PCS	−0.55	−0.62	−0.48	−0.50	−0.43	−0.66
SF-8 MCS	−0.36	−0.46	−0.33	−0.54	−0.34	−0.52
STarT Total	0.63	0.60	0.53	0.57	0.48	0.71
STarT Sub score (psychological)	0.56	0.56	0.50	0.55	0.43	0.67

All the correlations were significant ($P < 0.001$)
[a]Spearman Rank correlation coefficients
COMI: Core Outcome Measures Index; QOL: quality of life; EQ-5D: the EuroQol 5 Dimension; RDQ: Roland Morris Disability Questionnaire; SF-8: Short Form 8™ Health Survey; PCS: physical component summary; MCS: mental component summary; STarT: the Keele STarT Back Screening Tool

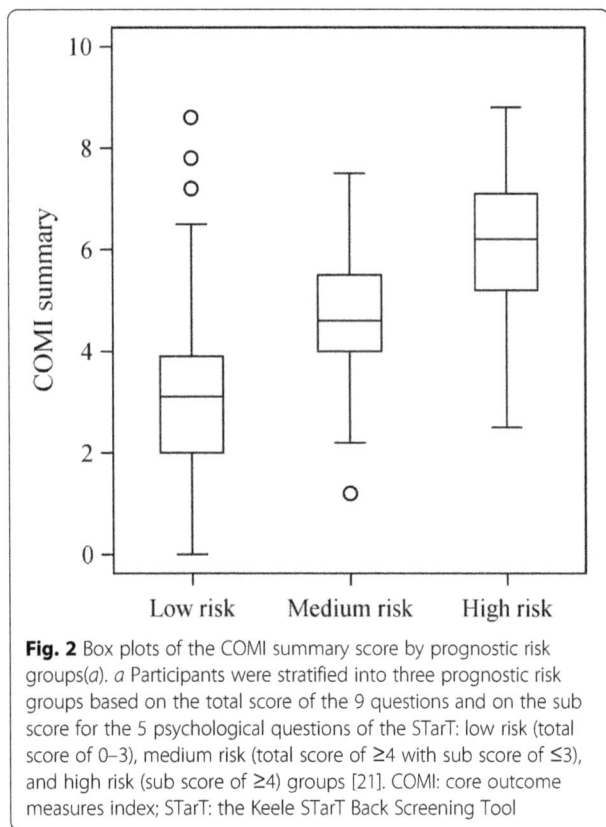

Fig. 2 Box plots of the COMI summary score by prognostic risk groups(*a*). *a* Participants were stratified into three prognostic risk groups based on the total score of the 9 questions and on the sub score for the 5 psychological questions of the STarT: low risk (total score of 0–3), medium risk (total score of ≥4 with sub score of ≤3), and high risk (sub score of ≥4) groups [21]. COMI: core outcome measures index; STarT: the Keele STarT Back Screening Tool

correlated only moderately with the SF-8 physical component summary (PCS) and mental component summary (MCS) scores. Other language versions also reported relatively weak correlations between symptom-specific well-being and quality-of-life reference scales [5, 9, 10]. It was considered that this item may measure a particularly unique concept that differs from "quality of life".

A previous study reported a linear increase in the number of LBP-related absences across the STarT risk groups [29]. Assuming that the number of absences reflects the impact of the back problem, in the same way that the multidimensional COMI score does, we also expected the COMI score to differ across the STarT prognostic risk levels. We hence evaluated known-group validity by examining the COMI scores for each of the prognostic risk levels. The result demonstrated a clear trend for a risk-associated increase in the COMI summary score. The trend suggests that the Japanese COMI is sensitive enough to reflect the level of prognostic risk.

For the purposes of comparing with other language versions, we calculated Cronbach's alpha (internal consistency) for the Japanese version of the COMI. With a value of 0.82 it was similar to the values (0.75–0.92) reported for other language versions [4, 5, 11]. However, given that the COMI was originally designed as a

multidimensional index (rather than a unidimensional scale), it is not actually considered necessary or even appropriate to determine its internal consistency [27].

There are some limitations to be considered when interpreting our findings. First, the number of subjects included in the pilot test of the pre-final version of the Japanese COMI may be considered small. However, 5–8 patients can probably be considered sufficient for pilot testing to assess issues and concerns regarding comprehensibility and conceptual equivalence, based on the recommendations of International Society for Pharmacoeconomics and Outcomes Research (ISPOR) to conduct cognitive debriefing in 5–8 persons [30]. Further, in usability studies it has been shown that testing in 5 persons gives you a grasp of problems, whereas much new is not observed after the 5th person [31–33]. We had intended to add more patients for further interview if major problems arose in the small group, which seemed not to be the case for this study. Second, the generalizability of the present results may be limited. Due to the nature of the online recruitment, some groups of individuals may be under-represented (e.g., those without access to the Internet) and others over-represented (e.g., those with a greater motivation to participate). Moreover, the present validation study limited participation to individuals aged 20–69 years with chronic LBP (≥3 months). Third, the study did not validate the "worst problem" item from the Spine Tango patient-assessment form, incorporated into our questionnaire battery. There may remain a need for future validation of the Japanese version of this single item, which is independent of the COMI summary score calculation. Finally, this study did not evaluate the test-retest reliability of the Japanese COMI. We first wanted to ensure that the Japanese COMI would measure what it was intended to measure, i.e. showed construct validity, to consolidate the ground for future examinations of its consistency and test-retest reliability. Further assessments of reliability are warranted prior to the use of the Japanese COMI in actual clinical or research settings.

Conclusions

We developed a Japanese version of the COMI that displayed qualities that support its convergent and known-group validity. The Japanese COMI represents a practical tool to capture the multidimensional impact of chronic LBP in Japanese patients. The availability of a Japanese version should facilitate the widespread use of the COMI and promote the standardization and accumulation of data, allowing improved documentation of the care received by patients with chronic LBP.

Abbreviations

COMI: Core Outcome Measures Index; EQ-5D: EuroQol 5 Dimension; LBP: Low back pain; MCS: Mental component summary; PCS: Physical component summary; RDQ: Roland Morris Disability Questionnaire; STarT: Keele STarT Back Screening Tool

Acknowledgments

Not applicable

Funding

This study was supported by a grant from the Ministry of Health, Labour and Welfare (14020301–01). This organization did not have any role in the design of the study, collection, analysis, and interpretation of data, or writing of the manuscript.

Authors' contributions

KM and HO contributed to the conception and design of the study and the acquisition and interpretation of the data, and critically revised the drafted manuscript for important intellectual content. YO, HC, YT, YM, ST, and AFM contributed to the interpretation of the data and critically revised the drafted manuscript for important intellectual content. MK and ES made substantial contributions to the conception of the study and drafted the manuscript. HM contributed to the analysis of the data and critically revised the drafted manuscript for important intellectual content. TL contributed to the analysis of the data and drafted the manuscript. All authors approved the final version of the manuscript to be published and agreed to be accountable for all aspects of the work in ensuring that questions related to the accuracy or integrity of any part of the work are appropriately investigated and resolved.

Consent for publication

Not applicable

Competing interests

KM received the research grant from Ministry of Health, Labour and Welfare for the submitted work; grant support including an endowed chair from Sumitomo Dainippon Pharma Co., Ltd. and OKAMURA CORPORATION; grant support including an endowed chair and lecture fees from AYUMI Pharmaceutical Corporation, Nippon Zoki Pharmaceutical Co., Ltd., ONO PHARMACEUTICAL CO., LTD., Eli Lilly Japan K.K., Astellas Pharma Inc., TOTO LTD., and Eisai Co., Ltd.; lecture fees from Pfizer Japan Inc., HISAMITSU PHARMACEUTICAL CO., INC., Janssen Pharmaceutical K.K., KAKEN PHARMACEUTICAL CO., LTD., TEIJIN PHARMA LIMITED; and lecture fees and advisory fees from Shionogi & Co., Ltd., outside the submitted work. HO, YO, HC, YT, YM, and AFM have nothing to disclose. MK, ES, HM, and TL are employed by Clinical Study Support, Inc.. ST received personal fees for expert testimony from Amgen inc., ASAHI KASEI PHARMA CORPORATION, Amgen Astellas BioPharma K.K., ONO PHARMACEUTICAL CO., LTD., KYOCERA Medical Corporation, DAIICHI SANKYO COMPANY, LIMITED, TEIJIN PHARMA LIMITED., Eli Lilly Japan K.K., and Pfizer Japan inc.; endowments from Astellas Pharma Inc., AYUMI Pharmaceutical Corporation, Pfizer Japan inc., Bristol-Myers Squibb, DAIICHI SANKYO COMPANY, LIMITED, and Chugai Pharmaceutical Co., Ltd.; and grants from The Japan Agency for Medical Research and Development (AMED), Japan -Society for the Promotion of Science (JSPS)/ Grant-in-Aid for Scientific Research (A), and Japan Society for the Promotion of Science (JSPS)/ Grant-in-Aid for Exploratory Research outside the submitted work.

Author details

[1]Department of Medical Research and Management for Musculoskeletal Pain, 22nd Century Medical and Research Center, Faculty of Medicine, The University of Tokyo, Tokyo, Bunkyo-ku, Japan. [2]Department of Pain Medicine, Fukushima Medical University School of Medicine, Fukushima, Japan. [3]Department of Orthopaedic Surgery, The University of Tokyo, Tokyo, Bunkyo-ku, Japan. [4]Department of Orthopedic Surgery, Gumma University Graduate School of Medicine, Maebashi, Japan. [5]Clinical Study Support, Inc., Nagoya, Japan. [6]Spine Center Division, Department of Teaching, Research and Development, Schulthess Klinik, Zürich, Switzerland.

References

1. Pengel LH, Herbert RD, Maher CG, Refshauge KM. Acute low back pain: systematic review of its prognosis. BMJ. 2003;327:323.
2. van Tulder M, Becker A, Bekkering T, Breen A, del Real MT, Hutchinson A, Koes B, Laerum E, Malmivaara A. COST B13 working group on guidelines for the Management of Acute low Back Pain in primary care. Chapter 3. European guidelines for the management of acute nonspecific low back pain in primary care. Eur Spine J. 2006;15(Suppl 2):S169–91.
3. Deyo RA, Battie M, Beurskens AJ, Bombardier C, Croft P, Koes B, Malmivaara A, Roland M, Von Korff M, Waddell G. Outcome measures for low back pain research. A proposal for standardized use. Spine (Phila Pa 1976) 1998;15. 23:2003–13.
4. Mannion AF, Elfering A, Staerkle R, Junge A, Grob D, Semmer NK, Jacobshagen N, Dvorak J, Boos N. Outcome assessment in low back pain: how low can you go? Eur Spine J. 2005;14:1014–26.
5. Ferrer M, Pellisé F, Escudero O, Alvarez L, Pont A, Alonso J, Deyo R. Validation of a minimum outcome core set in the evaluation of patients with back pain. Spine (Phila Pa 1976). 2006;31:1372–9.
6. Mannion AF, Porchet F, Kleinstück FS, Lattig F, Jeszenszky D, Bartanusz V, Dvorak J, Grob D. The quality of spine surgery from the patient's perspective. Part 1: the Core outcome measures index in clinical practice. Eur Spine J. 2009; 18(Suppl 3):367–73.
7. White P, Lewith G, Prescott P. The core outcomes for neck pain: validation of a new outcome measure. Spine (Phila Pa 1976) 2004;1. 29:1923–30.
8. Damasceno LH, Rocha PA, Barbosa ES, Barros CA, Canto FT, Defino HL, Mannion AF. Cross-cultural adaptation and assessment of the reliability and validity of the Core outcome measures index (COMI) for the Brazilian-Portuguese language. Eur Spine J. 2012;21:1273–82.
9. Genevay S, Cedraschi C, Marty M, Rozenberg S, De Goumoëns P, Faundez A, Balagué F, Porchet F, Mannion AF. Reliability and validity of the cross-culturally adapted French version of the Core outcome measures index (COMI) in patients with low back pain. Eur Spine J. 2012;21:130–7.
10. Mannion AF, Boneschi M, Teli M, Luca A, Zaina F, Negrini S, Schulz PJ. Reliability and validity of the cross-culturally adapted Italian version of the Core outcome measures index. Eur Spine J. 2012;21(Suppl 6):S737–49.
11. Nakhostin Ansari N, Naghdi S, Eskandari Z, Salsabili N, Kordi R, Hasson S. Reliability and validity of the Persian adaptation of the Core outcome measure index in patients with chronic low back pain. J Orthop Sci. 2016;21:723–6.
12. Fankhauser CD, Mutter U, Aghayev E, Mannion AF. Validity and responsiveness of the Core outcome measures index (COMI) for the neck. Eur Spine J. 2012;21:101–14.
13. Beaton DE, Bombardier C, Guillemin F, Ferraz MB. Guidelines for the process of cross-cultural adaptation of self-report measures. Spine (Phila Pa 1976) 2000;15. 25:3186–91.
14. Guillemin F, Bombardier C, Beaton D. Cross-cultural adaptation of health-related quality of life measures: literature review and proposed guidelines. J Clin Epidemiol. 1993;46:1417–32.
15. Pochon L, Kleinstück FS, Porchet F, Mannion AF. Influence of gender on patient-oriented outcomes in spine surgery. Eur Spine J. 2016;25:235–46.
16. Mannion AF, Mutter UM, Fekete TF, Porchet F, Jeszenszky D, Kleinstück FS. Validity of a single-item measure to assess leg or back pain as the predominant symptom in patients with degenerative disorders of the lumbar spine. Eur Spine J. 2014;23:882–7.
17. Spine Tango forms. http://www.eurospine.org/forms.htm. Accessed at November 8, 2016.
18. Von Korff M, Ormel J, Keefe FJ, Dworkin SF. Grading the severity of chronic pain. Pain. 1992;50:133–49.
19. Rabin R, Charro FD. EQ-5D: a measure of health status from the EuroQol group. Ann Med. 2001;33:337–43.
20. Roland M, Morris RA. Study of the natural history of back pain. Part I: development of a reliable and sensitive measure of disability in low-back pain. Spine (Phila Pa 1976). 1983;8:141–4.
21. Fukuhara S, Suzukamo Y. Manual of the SF-8 Japanese version, (in Japanese). Kyoto: Institute for Health Outcomes and Process Evaluation Research, 2004.
22. Hill JC, Dunn KM, Lewis M, Mullis R, Main CJ, Foster NE, Hay EM. A primary care back pain screening tool: identifying patient subgroups for initial treatment. Arthritis Rheum. 2008;59:632–41.
23. McHorney CA, Tarlov AR. Individual-patient monitoring in clinical practice: are available health status surveys adequate? Qual Life Res. 1995;4:293–307.

24. Cohen J. Statistical power analysis for the behavioral sciences. 2nd ed. Hillsdale: Lawrence Erlbaum Associates; 1988.

25. Jonckheere ARA. Distribution-free k-sample test against ordered alternatives. Biometrika. 1954;41(1/2):133–45.

26. Terpstra TJ. The asymptotic normality and consistency of Kendall's test against trend, when ties are present in one ranking. Indag Math. 1952;14:327–33.

27. Streiner DL, Norman GR, Cairney J. Health measurement scales: a practical guide to their development and use. 5th ed. Oxford: Oxford University Press; 2015.

28. Nunnally JC. Psychometric theory. New York: McGraw Hill; 1978.

29. Matsudaira K, Oka H, Kikuchi N, Haga Y, Sawada T, Tanaka S. Psychometric properties of the Japanese version of the STarT back tool in patients with low back pain. PLoS One. 2016;11:e0152019.

30. Wild D, Grove A, Martin M, Eremenco S, McElroy S, Verjee-Lorenz A, et al. ISPOR task force for translation and cultural adaptation. Principles of good practice for the translation and cultural adaptation process for patient-reported outcomes (PRO) measures: report of the ISPOR task force for translation and cultural adaptation. Value Health. 2005;8:94–104.

31. Jakob N, Landauer TK. A mathematical model of the finding of usability problems. Proceedings of the INTERACT'93 and CHI'93 conference on human factors in computing systems. ACM. 1993:206–13.

32. Nielsen Norman Group. Why You Only Need to Test with 5 Users. Nielsen Norman Group. https://www.nngroup.com/articles/why-you-only-need-to-test-with-5-users/ Accessed 13 September 2017.

33. Nielsen Norman Group. Heow Many Test Users in a Usability Study? Nielsen Norman Group. https://www.nngroup.com/articles/how-many-test-users/ Accessed 13 September 2017.

34. Ikeda S, Ikegami N. Preference-based measure (focus on EQ-5D). Igaku-Shoin: Tokyo; 2002.

13

Low back pain and limitations of daily living in Asia: longitudinal findings in the Thai cohort study

Vasoontara Yiengprugsawan[1]* [iD], Damian Hoy[2], Rachelle Buchbinder[3,4], Chris Bain[5], Sam-ang Seubsman[6] and Adrian C. Sleigh[7]

Abstract

Background: Low back pain (LBP) is a major cause of disability throughout the world. However, longitudinal evidence to relate low back pain and functional limitations is mostly confined to Western countries. In this study, we investigate the associations between low back pain and functional limitations in a prospective cohort of Thai adults.

Methods: We analysed information from the Thai Cohort Study of adult Open University adults which included 42,785 participants in both 2009 and 2013, with the majority aged 30 to 65 years and residing nationwide. We used multivariate logistic regression to explore the longitudinal associations between LBP in 2009 and 2013 ('never': no LBP in 2009 or 2013; 'reverting': LBP in 2009 but not in 2013; 'incident': no LBP in 2009 but LBP in 2013; and 'chronic': reporting LBP at both time points) and the outcome of functional limitations relating to Activities of Daily Living (ADL) in 2013.

Results: Low back pain was common with 30% of cohort members reporting low back pain in both 2009 and 2013 ('chronic LBP'). The 'chronic LBP' group was more likely than the 'never' back pain group to report functional limitations in 2013: adjusted odds ratios 1.60 [95% Confidence Interval: 1.38–1.85] for difficulties getting dressed; 1.98 [1.71–2.30] for walking; 2.02 [1.71–2.39] for climbing stairs; and 3.80 [3.38–4.27] for bending/kneeling. Those with 'incident LBP' or 'reverting LBP' both had increased odds of functional limitations in 2013 but the odds were not generally as high.

Conclusions: Our nationwide data from Thailand suggests that LBP is a frequent public health problem among economically productive age groups with adverse effects on the activities of daily living. This study adds to the limited longitudinal evidence on the substantial impact of low back pain in Southeast Asia.

Keywords: Low back pain, Functional limitations, Activities of daily living, Cohort study, Thailand

Background

Across the adult lifespan, low back pain (LBP) is very common [1, 2]. In Western settings, evidence suggests LBP affects 40 to 60% of working adults and adversely impacts quality of life, frequently on a daily basis [3, 4]. Low back pain can lead to severe and long term impairment.

The Global Burden of Disease Study listed LBP as a major cause of disability among musculoskeletal conditions and ranked LBP in the top five conditions contributing to loss of disability-adjusted life years [5, 6].

In the past decade, with its impact on productivity and activities of daily living, LBP has gained increasing attention in developing countries worldwide [2, 7]. These include, for example, a study among rural Tibetans noted LBP prevalence of 34% [8] and another study across occupation groups in Shanghai reported LBP prevalence ranging from 40% among teachers to 74% among garment workers [9]. LBP has a tendency to become chronic and a

* Correspondence: vasoontara.yieng@anu.edu.au; vasoontara.yieng@gmail.com
[1]Centre for Research on Ageing, Health and Wellbeing and Department of Global Health, Research School of Population Health, The Australian National University, Canberra, Australia
Full list of author information is available at the end of the article

systematic review of prospective cohort studies for LBP in office workers noted previous low back pain was a key factor for subsequent pain [10]. However, longitudinal evidence relating to causes and consequences of LBP remains limited, especially in low and middle-income countries.

In this paper, we focus on LBP in a large nationwide prospective cohort of Thai adults. We investigate longitudinal associations of LBP and functional limitations of daily living. We provide an estimate of the magnitude of LBP in working adults and its consequences 4 years later, thus adding to the evidence base of low back pain globally, and in middle-income countries such as Thailand.

Methods

This research is part of an overarching study of the health-risk transition underway in Thailand as maternal and child mortality and infectious diseases recede and chronic non-communicable diseases emerge [11]. To analyse the transition, we have developed a Thai Cohort Study enrolling 87,151 Sukhothai Thammathirat Open University distance learning adult students with a baseline 20-page comprehensive health and socio-physical-environment questionnaire in 2005. These cohort members share key sociodemographic characteristics with the general Thai population such as geographical distribution, modest median income, sex ratio, religion and ethnicity [12]. They were successfully followed up 4 and 8 years later (approximately 70% response rate in each wave; $n = 60,569$ in 2009 and $n = 42,785$ in 2013). The cohort from 2009 to 2013 is the population reported here.

Low back pain exposure and functional limitation outcomes

In both 2009 and 2013, cohort members were asked standardised questions about LBP and if it was bad enough to limit usual activities or change daily routines for more than one day [13]. The English version of the questions and the standard diagram in 2013 are as shown in Additional file 1. It should be noted that the Thai interpretation of the standard LBP diagram initially did not cover the whole lower buttock area, but this was resolved in 2013. The age stratified crude prevalence of LBP in 2013 was slightly higher compared with 2009; among other things, this could be explained by the larger anatomical area included in the 2013 diagram.

We separately classified LBP and 'severe' LBP across the 4 years as longitudinal categories: 'never' ('no' in 2009 and in 2013), 'reverting' ('yes' in 2009 and 'no' in 2013); 'incident' ('no' in 2009 and 'yes' in 2013); and 'chronic' ('yes' in 2009 and in 2013).

In 2013, cohort members were asked about their functional limitations related to Activities of Daily Living (ADL) in the past 4 weeks [14]: 1) climbing stairs; 2) walking 100 metres; 3) bending, kneeling or stooping;

and 4) dressing. Possible responses were: 'not at all'; 'a little'; 'a lot'. The ADL questions were not connected to low back pain questions.

Potential confounders

We collected a range of sociodemographic, behavioural and health information from cohort members at 2009 and 2013 follow-up. We also noted various other characteristics as reported in 2009 that could influence activities of daily living, including age, sex, urban-rural residence, and household monthly income (Thai Baht; 1$US ~ 30Baht). Occupation and work hours, available in the 2013 follow-up data, were used in the analyses. The average 2009–2013 values of four other covariates were used as follows: hours of standing and hours of sitting per day; physical activity (combined number of moderate or vigorous sessions per week); and body mass index (based on self-reported weight and height measurements) using recommended Asian cut-offs for overweight and obesity [15–17].

Statistical analyses

We analyse associations between 4-year low back pain and each of the four activity of daily living outcomes as measured in 2013 (ie climbing stairs, walking 100 metres, bending/kneeling, and getting dressed). Each functional limitation model included the longitudinal 2009–2013 LBP category (never-reverting-incident-chronic) as the independent variable of interest. Multivariate logistic regression was used for analyses reporting Odds Ratios and 95% Confidence Intervals, adjusting for the potential confounders. Individuals with missing data for any given analysis were excluded (<5% for each variable), thus totals could vary slightly due to available information.

Results

Cohort characteristics are summarised in Table 1: 45% were males; close to 80% were aged between 30 and 50 years; 55% resided in urban areas; and about 70% were managers, professionals or office workers. Table 1 also shows the prevalence of LBP and severe LBP by longitudinal categories (never, reverting, incident, chronic). For LBP, 37% were classified as 'never'; 20% as 'reverting'; 13% as 'incident'; and 30% as 'chronic'. For severe LBP, the corresponding prevalences were 95.3%, 1.7%. 2.3% and 0.7%. Notably, cohort members who had a high prevalence of 'chronic LBP' in both 2009 and 2013 were physical (skilled or elementary) workers (35%), with lower household income (36%), 9 h + standing daily (40%), and a body mass index of 30+ (34%).

Table 2 describes functional limitations among cohort members in 2013: approximately 6% of the cohort reported difficulty bending, 3.1% walking 100 metres, 2.2% climbing stairs, and 2.9% dressing oneself. There was a

Table 1 Cohort attributes by prevalence of low back pain (N = 42785), Thai Cohort Study

Low back pain status and cohort attributes in 2013 (%)	Longitudinal 2009–2013 low back pain dynamics[a]			
	Never 'No' 2009 & 'No' 2013	Reverting 'Yes' 2009 & 'No' 2013	Incident 'No' 2009 & 'Yes' 2013	Chronic 'Yes' 2009 & 'Yes' 2013
Low back pain	36.8 [14768]	20.0 [8055]	13.0 [5235]	30.0 [12042]
Severe low back pain restricting activities[b]	95.3 [38260]	1.7 [701]	2.3 [922]	0.7 [271]
Sex				
Male (45.1%)	38.1	19.1	13.4	29.5
Female (54.8%)	35.8	20.9	12.8	30.5
Age group, years				
< 35 (28.4%)	36.3	20.6	13.3	29.9
35–44 (45.5%)	35.8	20.5	13.2	30.4
45+ (30.2%)	38.8	19.0	12.6	29.7
Residence				
Urban (55.3%)	35.6	19.6	13.3	31.4
Rural (44.7%)	37.7	20.5	12.8	28.9
Occupation				
Professional and managers (40.3%)	38.5	20.0	13.3	27.9
Office assistant (30.5%)	36.4	20.9	12.6	30.2
Skilled worker/elementary (18.7%)	32.5	19.1	13.6	34.9
Others/not working (10.4%)	38.4	19.8	13.5	29.4
Work hours per week				
< 25 (7.2%)	34.8	19.8	13.5	31.8
25–40 (34.2%)	38.6	20.4	13.1	27.8
40+ (43.9%)	35.6	19.8	13.1	31.4
Not working (14.5%)	36.9	20.2	12.4	30.4
Household monthly income				
≤ 10,000 Baht (12.4%)	32.8	18.9	12.6	35.7
> 10,000 to 30,000 Baht (41.6%)	34.9	20.5	13.1	31.6
> 30,000 Baht (45.8%)	39.6	20.0	13.2	27.2
Hours sitting per day				
0–4 (25.4%)	36.6	20.1	12.6	30.7
5–8 (46.6%)	37.4	20.2	13.1	29.3
> 8 (27.8%)	36.1	19.9	13.4	30.6
Hours standing per day				
0–4 (70.9%)	37.4	20.0	13.3	29.3
5–8 (22.9%)	35.7	20.7	12.2	31.4
> 8 (6.1%)	33.7	19.2	13.2	33.9
Physical activity sessions per week[c]				
< 3 (50.2%)	35.7	19.9	13.5	30.9
3–6 (37.5%)	38.2	20.5	12.9	28.5
7+ (12.2%)	37.5	19.7	11.8	31.0
Body mass index (Asian cut offs)				
Underweight: BMI < 18.5 (5.7%)	37.6	21.6	12.1	28.7

Table 1 Cohort attributes by prevalence of low back pain (N = 42785), Thai Cohort Study *(Continued)*

Normal: BMI 18.5 to <23 (43.7%)	38.0	19.8	12.9	29.4
Overweight: BMI 23 to <25 (21.7%)	36.2	20.4	13.6	29.8
Obese I: BMI 25 to <30 (23.4%)	34.9	19.5	13.7	31.9
Obese II: BMI 30+ (5.3%)	32.4	20.7	13.0	34.0

[a]Based on status in 2009 and 2013 as follows: never, reverting, incident, and chronic
[b]'Severe' defined as low back pain bad enough to limit usual activities for more than one day
[c]Combined number of moderate or vigorous session (≥20 min per session)

gradient of increasing functional limitation across all activities as LBP status became increasingly proximate in time ('never' to 'reverting' to 'incident' to 'chronic').

Table 3 shows the associations between 2013 functional limitations and 2009–2013 longitudinal categories of LBP (never, reverting, incident and chronic), adjusting for the potential confounders listed in Table 1. 'Chronic' LBP was associated with the highest odds of functional limitations: Adjusted Odds Ratios and 95% CI were 1.60 [1.38–1.85] for difficulties getting dressed; 1.98 [1.71–2.30] for walking; 2.02 [1.71–2.39] for climbing stairs; and 3.80 [3.38–4.27] for bending or kneeling. 'Incident' LBP had similar OR patterns but the odds were not as high - corresponding AORs for each ADL limitations were 1.49 [1.28–1.80], 1.76 [1.46–2.12], 1.53 [1.22–1.91], and 2.65 [2.29–3.06], respectively. Notable among the behavioural variables with significant associations with all ADL limitations were hours of standing (except

for difficulty walking) and overweight to obese body mass index.

Those with 'severe' low back pain showed similar patterns but with higher odds of functional limitations; this is not explored further due to the relative rarity of severe LBP resulting in a small sample for statistical inference.

Discussion and conclusions

Low back pain was common in our cohort and approximately one third of participants reported LBP in both 2009 and 2013. We found an association between low back pain status from 2009 to 2013 and functional limitations for ADL in 2013, with increased limitations among those with severe low back pain. As well, ADL limitation was high among those with 'chronic' LBP (in both 2009 and 2013) and that limitation was greater than for those with 'incident' LBP, which in turn was

Table 2 Low back pain dynamics in the Thai Cohort Study (2009–2013) by functional limitations

Functional limitations	2013%	Longitudinal 2009–2013 low back pain dynamics by functional limitations, % (n)			
		Never 'No' 2009 & 'No' 2013	Reverting 'Yes' 2009 & 'No' 2013	Incident 'No' 2009 & Yes 2013	Chronic 'Yes' 2009 & 'Yes' 2013
Climbing stairs					
Never	84.5	89.9 (13225)	87.1 (6985)	81.9 (4246)	77.8 (9256)
A little	13.2	8.4 (1240)	11.0 (886)	15.6 (813)	18.9 (2257)
A lot	2.2	1.6 (236)	1.7 (140)	2.4 (126)	3.2 (383)
Walking 100 metres					
Never	81.3	87.6 (12855)	84.6 (6764)	78.1 (4050)	73.0 (8679)
A little	15.7	10.3 (1515)	13.0 (1041)	18.2 (946)	22.7 (2702)
A lot	3.1	2.1 (304)	2.3 (187)	3.5 (186)	4.1 (497)
Bending/stooping					
Never	56.7	71.5 (10519)	64.3 (5153)	45.9 (2397)	37.8 (4524)
A little	37.4	27.2 (4708)	31.6 (2537)	46.7 (2438)	51.7 (6192)
A lot	5.9	2.8 (410)	3.9 (318)	7.2 (378)	10.3 (1239)
Dressing self					
Never	82.8	88.4 (12978)	85.5 (6829)	79.1 (4105)	75.7 (8977)
A little	14.2	9.3 (1374)	11.7 (941)	17.3 (901)	20.4 (2428)
A lot	2.9	2.2 (327)	2.7 (216)	3.4 (178)	3.8 (451)

Table 3 Association between 2009 and 2013 longitudinal low back pain dynamics and 2013 functional limitations adjusting for potential covariates, Thai cohort study

Exposure variables	Outcomes - adjusted odds ratios [95% Confidence Intervals][a]			
Low back pain category (2009 to 2013)	Climbing stairs	Walking 100 m	Bending/kneeling	Getting dressed
Never - 'No' in 2009 & 'No' in 2013	Reference	Reference	Reference	Reference
Reverting - 'Yes' in 2009 & 'No' in 2013	1.10 [0.89–1.36]	1.14 [0.95–1.38]	**1.41** [1.21–1.64]	1.18 [0.99–1.41]
Incident - 'No in 2009 & 'Yes' in 2013	**1.53** [1.22–1.91]	**1.76** [1.46–2.12]	**2.65** [2.29–3.06]	**1.49** [1.28–1.80]
Chronic - 'Yes' in 2009 & 'Yes' in 2013	**2.02** [1.71–2.39]	**1.98** [1.71–2.30]	**3.80** [3.38–4.27]	**1.60** [1.38–1.85]
Covariates (2009, except[b] and[c])				
Sex				
Females (male - ref)	**1.19** [1.02–1.37]	1.03 [0.90–1.16]	**1.36** [1.24–1.50]	**1.39** [1.23–1.59]
Age groups (years)				
< 35	Reference			
35–44	0.91 [0.76–1.07]	0.93 [0.80–1.07]	0.98 [0.88–1.10]	**0.71** [0.61–0.81]
45+	0.95 [0.78–1.15]	0.96 [0.81–1.13]	**1.35** [1.20–1.52]	**0.56** [0.47–0.66]
Residence				
Urban (rural - ref)	0.97 [0.84–1.12]	0.93 [0.82–1.05]	0.95 [0.87–1.04]	1.02 [0.90–1.15]
Occupation[b]				
Professionals and managers	Reference			
Office assistant	1.08 [0.91–1.27]	1.11 [0.96–1.29]	1.00 [0.90–1.12]	0.97 [0.84–1.13]
Skilled or elementary workers	0.79 [0.64–0.98]	1.05 [0.88–1.24]	1.13 [0.99–1.28]	0.86 [0.72–1.03]
Others/ not working	1.02 [0.73–1.41]	0.94 [0.71–1.25]	1.22 [0.98–1.51]	**0.68** [0.51–0.91]
Work hours per week[b]				
< 25	**1.54** [1.20–1.98]	**1.41** [1.14–1.76]	1.27 [1.08–1.50]	**1.55** [1.25–1.92]
25–40	Reference			
40+	1.04 [0.88–1.23]	0.96 [0.83–1.11]	1.01 [0.91–1.12]	0.94 [0.81–1.08]
Not working	**1.45** [1.08–1.95]	**1.39** [1.08–1.79]	1.14 [0.94–1.39]	**1.65** [1.28–2.11]
Household monthly income (Baht)				
≤ 10,000	1.04 [0.86–1.24]	**1.24** [1.07–1.44]	1.10 [0.98–1.24]	1.03 [0.88–1.21]
> 10,000–30,000	Reference			
> 30,000	1.01 [0.86–1.19]	0.88 [0.76–1.02]	0.90 [0.82–1.00]	0.97 [0.84–1.11]
Hours sitting per day[c]				
0–4	**1.39** [1.17–1.65]	**1.52** [1.32–1.76]	1.11 [0.98–1.24]	**1.21** [1.03–1.41]
5–8	Reference			
9+	**0.77** [0.65–0.91]	**0.83** [0.72–0.96]	0.90 [0.82–1.00]	0.82 [0.71–0.94]
Hours standing per day[c]				
0–4	1.15 [0.96–1.34]	0.95 [0.83–1.09]	1.05 [0.95–1.17]	1.17 [1.01–1.36]
5–8	Reference			
9+	**1.40** [1.07–1.84]	0.91 [0.71–1.16]	**1.33** [1.12–1.58]	**1.49** [1.18–1.89]
Physical activity (moderate or rigorous)[c]				
< 3 sessions/week	Reference			
3–6 sessions/week	0.89 [0.76–1.04]	0.91 [0.80–1.04]	**0.79** [0.72–0.87]	**0.83** [0.72–0.95]
7+ sessions/week	1.06 [0.86–1.32]	**1.32** [1.11–1.57]	0.93 [0.81–1.07]	1.05 [0.87–1.27]
Body mass index (Asian cut offs)[c]				
Underweight (<18.5)	1.06 [0.79–1.43]	1.09 [0.84–1.41]	0.89 [0.72–1.10]	**0.71** [0.51–0.97]

Table 3 Association between 2009 and 2013 longitudinal low back pain dynamics and 2013 functional limitations adjusting for potential covariates, Thai cohort study (Continued)

Normal (18.5 to <23)	Reference			
Overweight (23 to <25)	**1.25** [1.04–1.51]	**1.21** [1.03–1.42]	**1.33** [1.18–1.49]	**1.60** [1.35–1.89]
Obese I (25 to <30)	**1.42** [1.19–1.70]	**1.33** [1.13–1.55]	**1.73** [1.54–1.93]	**2.39** [2.06–2.79]
Obese II (> = 30)	**1.85** [1.43–2.40]	**1.68** [1.33–2.12]	**2.47** [2.11–2.88]	**3.03** [2.44–3.71]

[a]Bold figures were statistically significant at $p < 0.05$
[b]Covariates available in 2013
[c]Average values of covariate confounders in 2009 and 2013

greater than for those with 'reverting' LBP. The lowest ADL limitation rate was among those who had never reported LBP and we classified that as the reference rate. Such a longitudinal study of low back pain is important because it enables comparisons across time and between countries and permits causal analyses. Evidence on back pain and its effects is limited in low and middle-income countries. Similar to findings in Western economically advanced countries, our results reveal that low back pain was common and associated with clinically important limitations in activities of daily living among middle-aged and older Thai adults.

Our findings highlight the high prevalence of low back pain across all age groups in our Thai population, as reported for studies in other groups [1, 5]. Low household income was associated with both functional limitations and low back pain in our study, and this has also been reported elsewhere [2, 18]. The relationships between physical activity and presence of low back pain have also been reported previously [19–21]. We also noted an association between reduced physical activity and increased likelihood of low back pain. As well, we found an association between reduced physical activity and increasing functional limitations for ADL among Thai adults. Being obese has been reported to be associated with functional limitations [22, 23], and this was also found in our study.

We note some grounds for caution in interpreting our findings. First, our study data are drawn from a self-administered questionnaire and are subject to imperfect recall and varying individual thresholds for reporting LBP [24]. Second, while we followed the recommended international guideline for definition of low back pain for use in epidemiologic studies [13], also used by the Global Burden of Disease 2010 study [1, 5], there were slight differences in the pain diagram, with a greater area indicated in 2013. This may have resulted in higher prevalence estimates in 2013 compared with 2009. Also, our cohort was not a random population sample; even though our prevalence results may not be generalisable, the relative effects (odds ratios) should be valid. Our cohort members were open university students, all of whom had completed high school education or had equivalent experience making them better educated than

average for the Thai population. On the other hand, cohort members were average working Thais in terms of their modest incomes and their geographic locations embedded in communities throughout Thailand. Lastly, we also examined the potential impact of non-response in 2013 of drop-outs ($n = 17,784$); in 2009 these were only slightly higher than the response group (2% for low back pain in 2009 and 0.5% for serious low back pain).

Another consideration is that the questions about functional limitations in activities of daily living were not linked with the question on LBP status. The ADL questions also had no direct link to LBP questions, hence our interest in hypothetical associations was not revealed. However, we cannot conclude for every individual reporting both LBP and limited ADL that there was a link. But for the population it is reasonable to see the results as showing an adverse effect of LBP on ADL given the statistical evidence that the relationship is unlikely to be due to chance and further given the clinically reasonable connection between LBP and ADL. In fact, it should be noted that our study is longitudinal and measures exposure variables at the beginning of the observation period. This design feature is an advantage with all prospective cohort studies and improves the analyses of potentially causal relationships.

Suitable lifestyle and behavioural interventions to prevent and mitigate LBP remain elusive but the high frequency of the conditions and their associated impacts warrant population health attention. Relevant LBP risk factors such as physical inactivity and obesity are complex and follow up of a prospective cohort over 10–20 years could provide insight into causal processes and mechanisms for LBP effects on population. This is particularly important for boosting knowledge in Asia for which information is limited.

LBP causes an enormous global burden, and this is generally increasing in developing countries such as Thailand. Initiatives aimed at the prevention and management of LBP, as with all musculoskeletal conditions, must be well-integrated with other non-communicable disease programs, rather than being stand alone [25]. This will avoid duplication of efforts and will help to promote a more-streamlined, cost-effective approach to overall health system strengthening.

Abbreviations
ADL: Activities of Daily Living; AOR: Adjusted Odds Ratio; CI: Confidence Interval; LBP: Low Back Pain

Acknowledgements
We would like to thank our cohort members for their participation in the study and editorial support from Peter Sbirakos on the earlier version of the manuscript.

Funding
The Thai Cohort Study was supported by the International Collaborative Research Grants Scheme with joint grants from the Wellcome Trust UK (GR071587MA) and the Australian National Health and Medical Research Council (268055), and as a global health grant from the NHMRC (585426). RB is supported by an NHMRC Senior Principal Research Fellowship.

Authors' contributions
VY conceptualised the study, with input and guidance from DH, RB, CB, and AS. VY analysed data and wrote up the findings. DH, RB, CB, and AS provided critical comments through various iterations of the draft manuscripts. SS and AS led the Thai Cohort Study. All authors read and approved the final manuscript.

Competing interests
The authors declare that they have no competing interests.

Consent to publication
Not applicable.

Author details
[1]Centre for Research on Ageing, Health and Wellbeing and Department of Global Health, Research School of Population Health, The Australian National University, Canberra, Australia. [2]Research, Evidence and Information Programme, Public Health Division, Secretariat of the Pacific Community, Noumea, New Caledonia. [3]Department of Epidemiology & Preventive Medicine, School of Public Health and Preventive Medicine, Monash University, Melbourne, Australia. [4]Monash Department of Clinical Epidemiology, Cabrini Institute, Melbourne, Australia. [5]QIMR Berghofer Medical Research Institute, Brisbane, Australia. [6]School of Human Ecology, Sukhothai Thammathirat Open University, Nonthaburi, Thailand. [7]National Centre for Epidemiology and Population Health, Research School of Population Health, The Australian National University, Canberra, Australia.

References
1. Hoy D, Brooks P, Blyth F, Buchbinder R. The Epidemiology of low back pain. Best Pract Res Clin Rheumatol. 2010;24(6):769–81.
2. Stewart Williams J, Ng N, Peltzer K, Yawson A, Biritwum R, Maximova T, Wu F, Arokiasamy P, Kowal P, Chatterji S. Risk Factors and Disability Associated with Low Back Pain in Older Adults in Low- and Middle-Income Countries. Results from the WHO Study on Global AGEing and Adult Health (SAGE). PLoS One. 2015;10(6):e0127880.
3. Dunn KM, Hestbaek L, Cassidy JD. Low back pain across the life course. Best Pract Res Clin Rheumatol. 2013;27(5):591–600.
4. Froud R, Patterson S, Eldridge S, Seale C, Pincus T, Rajendran D, Fossum C, Underwood M. A systematic review and meta-synthesis of the impact of low back pain on people's lives. BMC Musculoskelet Disord. 2014;15:50.
5. Hoy D, March L, Brooks P, Blyth F, Woolf A, Bain C, Williams G, Smith E, Vos T, Barendregt J, et al. The global burden of low back pain: estimates from the Global Burden of Disease 2010 study. Ann Rheum Dis. 2014;73(6):968–74.
6. Global Burden of Disease Study C. Global, regional, and national incidence, prevalence, and years lived with disability for 301 acute and chronic diseases and injuries in 188 countries, 1990–2013: a systematic analysis for the Global Burden of Disease Study 2013. Lancet. 2015;386(9995):743–800.
7. Volinn E. The epidemiology of low back pain in the rest of the world. A review of surveys in low- and middle-income countries. Spine (Phila Pa 1976). 1997;22(15):1747–54.
8. Hoy D, Toole MJ, Morgan D, Morgan C. Low back pain in rural Tibet. Lancet. 2003;361(9353):225–6.
9. Jin K, Sorock GS, Courtney TK. Prevalence of low back pain in three occupational groups in Shanghai, People's Republic of China. J Safety Res. 2004;35(1):23–8.
10. Janwantanakul P, Sitthipornvorakul E, Paksaichol A. Risk factors for the onset of nonspecific low back pain in office workers: a systematic review of prospective cohort studies. J Manipulative Physiol Ther. 2012;35(7):568–77.
11. Sleigh A, Seubsman S. Studying the Thai Health-Risk Transition. In: Butler C, Dixon J, Capon A, editors. Health of people, places and planet : reflections based on Tony McMichael's four decades of contribution to epidemiological understanding. Canberra: ANU Press; 2015. p. 155–76.
12. Sleigh AC, Seubsman SA, Bain C. Cohort profile: The Thai Cohort of 87,134 Open University students. Int J Epidemiol. 2008;37(2):266–72.
13. Dionne CE, Dunn KM, Croft PR, Nachemson AL, Buchbinder R, Walker BF, Wyatt M, Cassidy JD, Rossignol M, Leboeuf-Yde C, et al. A consensus approach toward the standardization of back pain definitions for use in prevalence studies. Spine (Phila Pa 1976). 2008;33(1):95–103.
14. Katz S. Assessing self-maintenance: activities of daily living, mobility, and instrumental activities of daily living. J Am Geriatr Soc. 1983;31(12):721–7.
15. Lim LL, Seubsman SA, Sleigh A. Validity of self-reported weight, height, and body mass index among university students in Thailand: Implications for population studies of obesity in developing countries. Popul Health Metr. 2009;7:15.
16. Yiengprugsawan V, Banwell C, Zhao J, Seubsman SA, Sleigh AC. Relationship between body mass index reference and all-cause mortality: evidence from a large cohort of Thai adults. J Obes. 2014;2014:708606.
17. Yiengprugsawan V, Horta BL, Motta JV, Gigante D, Seubsman SA, Sleigh A. Body size dynamics in young adults: 8-year follow up of cohorts in Brazil and Thailand. Nutr Diabetes. 2016;6(7):e219.
18. Carr JL, Moffett JA. The impact of social deprivation on chronic back pain outcomes. Chronic Illn. 2005;1(2):121–9.
19. Ryan CG, Grant PM, Dall PM, Gray H, Newton M, Granat MH. Individuals with chronic low back pain have a lower level, and an altered pattern, of physical activity compared with matched controls: an observational study. Aust J Physiother. 2009;55(1):53–8.
20. Henchoz Y, Kai-Lik So A. Exercise and nonspecific low back pain: a literature review. Joint Bone Spine. 2008;75(5):533–9.
21. Heneweer H, Staes F, Aufdemkampe G, van Rijn M, Vanhees L. Physical activity and low back pain: a systematic review of recent literature. Eur Spine J. 2011;20(6):826–45.
22. Hu HY, Chen L, Wu CY, Chou YJ, Chen RC, Huang N. Associations among low back pain, income, and body mass index in Taiwan. Spine J. 2013; 13(11):1521–6.
23. Shiri R, Karppinen J, Leino-Arjas P, Solovieva S, Viikari-Juntura E. The association between obesity and low back pain: a meta-analysis. Am J Epidemiol. 2010; 171(2):135–54.
24. Johansson SR. Measuring the cultural inflation of morbidity during the decline in mortality. Health Transit Rev. 1992;2(1):78–89.
25. Hoy D, Geere JA, Davatchi F, Meggitt B, Barrero LH. A time for action: Opportunities for preventing the growing burden and disability from musculoskeletal conditions in low- and middle-income countries. Best Pract Res Clin Rheumatol. 2014;28(3):377–93.

14

Association between sarcopenia and low back pain in local residents prospective cohort study from the GAINA study

Shinji Tanishima[1]* [ID], Hiroshi Hagino[2,3], Hiromi Matsumoto[3], Chika Tanimura[2] and Hideki Nagashima[1]

Abstract

Background: Low back pain (LBP) is one of the most common ailments that people experience in their lifetime. On the other hands, Sarcopenia also leads to several physical symptoms and contributes to reducing the quality of life of elderly people.The purpose of this study is to investigate the association between sarcopenia and low back pain among the general population.

Methods: The subjects included 216 adults (79 men and 137 women; mean age, 73.5 years) undergoing a general medical examination in Hino, Japan. Skeletal muscle index (SMI), The percentage of young adults' mean (%YAM) of the calcaneal bone mass using with quantitative ultrasound (QUS) method and walking speed were measured, and subjects who met the criteria of the Asian Working Group for Sarcopenia were assigned to the sarcopenia group. Subjects with decreased muscle mass only were assigned to the pre-sarcopenia group, and all other subjects were assigned to the normal group. Then, we compared the correlations with low back pain physical finding. The Oswestry Disability Index (ODI) and the low back pain visual analogue scale (VAS) were used as indices of low back pain. Statistical analysis was performed among three groups with respect their characteristic, demographics, data of sarcopenia determining factor, VAS and ODI. We also analysed prevalence of LBP and sarcopenia. We investigated the correlations between ODI and the sarcopenia-determining factors of walking speed, muscle mass and grip strength.

Results: Sarcopenia was noted in 12 subjects (5.5%). The pre-sarcopenia group included 38 subjects (17.6%), and the normal group included 166 subjects (76.9%). The mean ODI score was significantly higher in the sarcopenia group (25. 2% ± 12.3%; $P < 0.05$) than in the pre-sarcopenia group (11.2% ± 10.0%) and the normal group (11.9% ± 12.3%). %YAM and BMI were significantly lower in the sarcopenia group than in other groups ($P < 0.05$). A negative correlation existed between walking speed and ODI ($r = -0.32$, $P < 0.001$).

Conclusions: The results of this study suggested that decreased physical ability due to quality of life in residents with LBP may be related to sarcopenia.

Keywords: Sarcopenia, Low back pain, Muscle strength, Osteoporosis

Background

Low back pain (LBP) is one of the most common ailments that people experience in their lifetime. The lifetime prevalence of LBP is approximately 84% [1]. LBP is caused by many factors. Wan et al. reported that muscle atrophy may lead to chronic LBP at multiple levels of the lumbar spine [2]. Several studies have reported that atrophy of the back muscles is a factor that causes LBP [2–4]; however, no consensus has been reached on an association between sarcopenia and LBP. Sarcopenia is defined as the pathophysiology caused by decreased muscle strength accompanying ageing [5]. Sarcopenia results in several disorders, such as hypertension, obesity, osteoporosis and diabetes mellitus [6, 7]. Sarcopenia also leads to several physical symptoms and contributes to reducing the quality of life of elderly people [8, 9].

The relationship between sarcopenia and LBP is unclear, and has been explored by only few studies. The

* Correspondence: shinji@sanmedia.or.jp
[1]Department of Orthopedic Surgery,Faculty of Medicine, Tottori University, 36-1 Nishi-cho, Yonago, Tottori 683-8504, Japan
Full list of author information is available at the end of the article

current study aimed to clarify the association between sarcopenia and LBP.

Methods

Subjects

This study was based on the results obtained from a prospective cohort of subjects enrolled in the Good Ageing and Intervention Against Nursing Care and Activity Decline (GAINA) study. The GAINA study, which began in 2014, is a population-based study of cohorts from Hino, Tottori Prefecture, Japan. The population comprised 3352 subjects in September 2016, with an ageing rate of approximately 45%. The subjects were recruited from individuals who underwent an annual town-sponsored medical check-up. A self-administered questionnaire was sent to 1450 subjects aged >40 years who were eligible to receive the medical check-up. We sent the consent form for The GAINA study together with medical check-up form to all subjects before an annual town-sponsored medical check-up. We enrolled the subjects who agreed The GAINA study. The baseline assessment was performed between May and June 2014 on 273 individuals undergoing the medical check-up. The inclusion criteria for subjects in the study were 1) living independently, 2) the ability to walk to where the survey was performed and 3) agreement to provide self-reported data. Fifty-seven subjects were excluded for lack of data because of omission of recording of medical check-up form. A total of 216 subjects (79 men and 137 women) participated in the baseline assessment. All subjects provided written informed consent, and the study was approved by the local ethics committee of the Faculty of Medicine, Tottori University (No. 2354).

Baseline measurements

Baseline characteristics, such as age, sex, height, body weight, body mass index (BMI), smoking habit and alcohol habit were recorded. We regarded the subjects who answered "yes" against this question "Do you feel low back pain in your daily life lately?" were LBP subjects. The position of low back was defined by each subject. Subjects were asked to make a vertical mark through a 100-mm horizontal VAS Scale.

We also used the Oswestry Disability Index (ODI) to assess functional outcomes associated with LBP. The results of the self-administered questionnaire were then checked for accuracy by researchers who personally interviewed each subject.

Assessment of sarcopenia

The participants were classified as having sarcopenia based on muscle mass, muscle strength and physical performance. The classification was based on the recommendations of the Asian Working Group for Sarcopenia [10]. The Recommendations of the Asian Working Group for

Sarcopenia defined Sarcopenia as the Subjects were classified as having sarcopenia if they were aged >60 years and had a low handgrip strength (<26 kg in men and <18 kg in women) and/or a lower walking speed (<0.8 m/s) with a low muscle mass (<7.0 kg/m^2 in men and 5.7 kg/m^2 in women).

In this study, some subjects had low muscle mass under 60 years, so we defined subjects were classified as having sarcopenia if they were aged >40 years and had a low handgrip strength (<26 kg in men and <18 kg in women) and/or a lower gait speed (<0.8 m/s) with a low muscle mass (<7.0 kg/m^2 in men and 5.7 kg/m^2 in women). Subjects were classified as having pre-sarcopenia if they were aged >40 years and had a low handgrip strength (<26 kg in men and <18 kg in women) and/or a lower walking speed (<0.8 m/s) without a low muscle mass (<7.0 kg/m^2 in men and 5.7 kg/m^2 in women). Subjects without low muscle mass or strength or low physical performance were classified as normal (Fig. 1).

Body function and structure measurements

Handgrip strength was measured using a TKK 5401 dynamometer (Takei Co, Niigata City, Japan). The subjects were asked to squeeze the dynamometer twice with each hand. The highest scores for the left and right hands were summed. Muscle mass was measured by bioelectrical impedance analysis (BIA) with a MC-780A Body Composition Analyzer (Tanita Co., Tokyo, Japan). The BIA method requires the subjects onto a platform and remain in the standing position for approximately 30 s. Skeletal mass index was calculated by dividing the limb muscle mass (kg) by the square of the height (m). We used quantitative ultrasound (QUS) to assess the calcaneal bone mass [11, 12]. The speed of sound through the calcaneus was evaluated using a CM-200 sonometer (Furuno Co., Nishinomiya City, Japan). The subject was seated and was asked to place the right heel on the QUS device. Coupling gel was applied to the heel to facilitate the transmission of ultrasound to the skeletal site being examined. The sum of the percentage of young adult mean was calculated. Gait parameters were obtained using the Opto Gait (Microgate Co., Bolzano, Italy) designed for optical-sensitive gait analysis. We prepared a 10-m walking line. Walking section and measurement section were set respectively. The subjects completed a single trial at free speed with the instruction to 'walk at your normal speed '. Walking speed was calculated with specific software (OPTO Gait analysis software, version 1.6.4.0, Microgate S.r.L, Italy).

Statistical analysis

All data were expressed as mean ± standard deviation. The subjects were divided into normal, pre-sarcopenia and sarcopenia groups. Differences characteristic, demographics, data of sarcopenia determining factor, VAS and

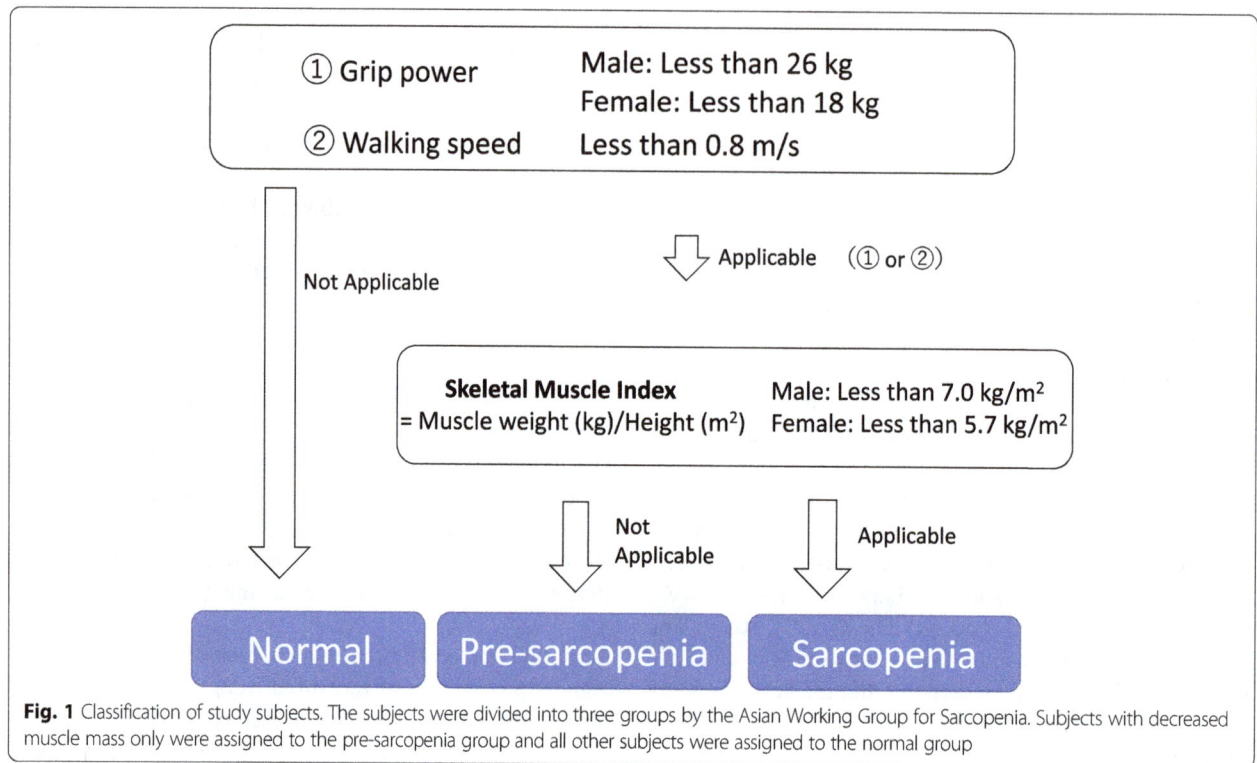

Fig. 1 Classification of study subjects. The subjects were divided into three groups by the Asian Working Group for Sarcopenia. Subjects with decreased muscle mass only were assigned to the pre-sarcopenia group and all other subjects were assigned to the normal group

ODI of the subjects among three groups were examined using Steel-Dwass test. The differences of prevalence of LBP among three groups analysed with Chi-square for independence test, m × n contingency table.

The differences of prevalence of LBP between men and women analysed with the Pearson's chi-square test or Fisher's exact test. We performed Fisher's exact test when expected cell size is <5. To investigate the correlations between ODI and the sarcopenia-determining factors, we used a partial correlation analysis with controlling the age and BMI available.

Data were analysed with StatMate for windows, version 4.01 (ATMS Corporation, Tokyo, Japan).

Results
Prevalence of sarcopenia
The prevalence of sarcopenia was approximately 5.5% (12 subjects; 5 men and 7 women). %YAM and BMI were significantly lower in the sarcopenia group than in the Normal groups. BMI in the Pre-sarcopenia group were significantly lower in the other groups (Table 1). The prevalence of sarcopenia in men and women were 8.4% in men and 4.3% in women. There was not significantly different in gender (Chi-square test; $P = 0.32$, data not shown).

Prevalence of LBP
One hundred-forty out of 216 subjects complained LBP. The overall prevalence of complaints of LBP was 64.8%

(140/216 subjects). More than 60% of the subjects in each group complained of LBP. The prevalence of LBP was not significantly different among the three groups (Table 2). The prevalence LBP in men and women were 72.2% (52/79 subjects) and 65.0% (88/137 subjects). There was not significantly different in gender (Chi-square test; $P = 0.89$, data not shown).

Table 1 Characteristic and demographics of the subjects

	Normal	Pre-sarcopenia	Sarcopenia
	($n = 166$)	($n = 38$)	($n = 12$)
Age (years)	73.0 ± 7.8	72.2 ± 8.5	84.9 ± 5.0 **
Gender (M:F)	63:103	11:27	5:7
%YAM (%)	78.9 ± 13.7	78.3 ± 15.9	63.8 ± 8.7 **
BMI (Kg/m²)	22.8 ± 2.3	18.9 ± 2.0**	20.6 ± 2.4*
Smoking habit (%)	25.6	26.3	8.3
Alcohol habit (%)	30.1	42.1	25.0

(Mean ± SD)
Steel-Dwass *$P < 0.05$,**$P < 0.01$
%YAM: the percentage of young adult mean
BMI: Body mass index
M:male
F: female
Sarcopenia was noted in 12 of 216 subjects (5.5%). %YAM and BMI were significantly lower in the sarcopenia group than in the Normal groups. BMI in the Pre-sarcopenia group were significantly lower in the other groups. %YAM and BMI were significantly lower in the sarcopenia group than in the other groups (Steel-Dwass test, *: $P < 0.05$, **:$P < 0.01$). There were no significant differences among the three groups about smoking habit and alcohol habit (Chi-square for independence test, m × n contingency table)

Table 2 Prevalence of low back pain

	LBP(−)	LBP(+)	Prevalence of LBP (%)
Normal (n = 166)	61	105	60.1 (105/166)
Pre-sarcopenia (n = 38)	13	25	65.8 (25/38)
Sarcopenia (n = 12)	2	10	83.3 (10/12)
Total (n = 216)	76	140	64.8 (140/216)

There were no significant differences among the three groups

Sarcopenia and LBP

The mean VAS score was the highest in the sarcopenia group, although there were no significant differences among the groups. The mean ODI score in sarcopenia group was 24.3%. This score was significantly higher in the Sarcopenia group than in the other groups. The mean walking speed in the sarcopenia group was significantly lower than in the other groups. Grip power in the Pre-sarcopenia and Sarcopenia group were significantly lower than in the normal group. SMI in the Pre-sarcopenia and Sarcopenia group were significantly lower than in the normal group ($6.9kg/m^2$ in Pre-sarcopenia and $6.5kg/m^2$ in Sarcopenia vs $6.9kg/m^2$ in Normal, $P < 0.05$) (Table 3).

Association between sarcopenia and ODI

We investigated the correlations between ODI and the sarcopenia-determining factors of walking speed, muscle mass and grip strength. The only correlation was a negative correlation with walking speed (correlation confident −0.32, $P < 0.001$) (Table 4).

Discussion

We investigated the association between sarcopenia and LBP in local residents, focussing on elderly people. Sarcopenia was defined as 'age-related loss of muscle mass and function' by Rosenberg [5]. Musculoskeletal disorders are greatly influenced by sarcopenia. Baumgartner et al. reported that the prevalence of sarcopenia was more than 50% in people aged >80 years in Mexico and that more people with sarcopenia had physical disabilities [13]. Janssen et al. reported that fifth decades people begin to

start decreasing their muscle volume [14] and people with low skeletal muscle mass index existed in third to sixth decades with same prevalence of over six decades in their study for 4504 American adults [15]. We included residents who are around fifth decades in this study for this reason.

The prevalence of sarcopenia was only 12% in this study, this was lower than other study. The inclusion criteria for subjects in the study were 1) living independently, 2) the ability to walk to where the survey was performed.

This criterion might affect that low prevalence of sarcopenia in this study.

LBP is one of the most common symptoms treated in daily medical practice. Park et al. investigated the prevalence of sarcopenia and lumbar spinal stenosis in Korea [16]. The prevalence of sarcopenia was higher in people with lumbar spinal stenosis than in normal people. They suggested that LBP with lumbar spinal stenosis led to low physical activity, causing sarcopenia. Although the present study showed that the prevalence of LBP was not significantly different among the three groups, the ODI scores were significantly higher in the sarcopenia group than in the other groups. The mean VAS score in the sarcopenia group was the highest among the three groups, although there were no significant differences among the groups.

The overall prevalence rate of LBP was 64.8%. Suka et al. performed a big survey for 3048 men and 1885 women in Japan to investigate the prevalence rate of LBP. They reported the prevalence rate of LBP was 26.5%. This prevalence was lower than our study [17]. In this study, most subjects over seventies and work as a former in this study, this situation might have relationship with high prevalence rate of LBP.

We consider that sarcopenia is not the cause of LBP. However, we focused on LBP in this study. LBP is induced by many factors, such as osteoporosis and muscle disorders [18]. The sarcopenia group in this study had low %YAM and BMI. The average %YAM in the sarcopenia group was 63.8% ± 8.7%. Verschueren et al. reported that sarcopenia was associated with low BMD in

Table 3 Sarcopenia and low back pain

	Normal (n = 166)	Pre-sarcopenia (n = 38)	Sarcopenia (n = 12)
VAS (mm)	20.5 ± 25.4	21.3 ± 25.8	23.5 ± 22.0
ODI (%)	11.9 ± 12.3	11.2 ± 10.0	25.2 ± 12.3 **
Walking speed (m/s)	1.2 ± 0.3	1.3 ± 0.3	0.9 ± 0.4**
Grip power (kg)	29.8 ± 8.3	26.3 ± 6.4*	20.7 ± 6.0**
SMI (Kg/m²)	7.0 ± 0.9	5.8±0.7**	6.1±0.6**

(Mean ± SD)
Steel-Dwass
*$P < 0.05$ **$P < 0.01$
Oswestry Disability Index scores were significantly higher in the sarcopenia group than in the other groups ($P < 0.05$). The mean visual analogue scale score in the sarcopenia group was the highest among the three groups, although there were no significant differences among the groups. The mean walking speed in the sarcopenia group was significantly lower than in the other groups. Grip power in the Pre-sarcopenia and Sarcopenia group were significantly lower than in the normal group. SMI in the Pre-sarcopenia and Sarcopenia group were significantly lower than in the normal group

Table 4 Association between sarcopenia and Oswestry Disability Index (ODI)

	Correlation coefficient	P Value
Walking speed	−0.32	<0.001
Grip power	−0.26	0.05
Skeletal muscle index	−0.26	0.70

(Partial correlation analysis: control the age and BMI variable)
BMI:Body mass index
The only relationship was a negative correlation between walking speed and ODI. (Partial correlation analysis: control the age and BMI variable)

middle-aged and elderly European men [19]. In Japan, under 70% YAM is one of the criteria for osteoporosis [20]. Based on this criterion, most subjects with sarcopenia in our study may have had osteoporosis. Generally, the prevalence of osteoporosis is higher in elderly women than in men [21, 22]. The fact that more than 50% of the subjects in this study were women may affect these results. It is a well-known fact that osteoclasts are highly active in osteoporosis. The relationship between bone cancer pain and osteoclast activity is well known [23, 24]. There are no reports showing a relationship between osteoclast activity and osteoporotic bone pain.

In the periosteum, the A-delta and C-sensory nerve fibres are arranged in a fishnet-like pattern, which appears to be designed to act as a "neural net" to detect mechanical injury or distortion of the underlying cortical bone [25]. Park et al. mentioned that the following mechanisms contribute to generating and maintaining pain in osteoporosis: 1) the increasing density of the bone sensory nerve fibres in the elderly; 2) the expression of nociceptors by sensory nerve fibres sensitised by lower pH (as observed during osteoclastic activity) and 3) pathological modifications of bone sensory nerve fibres. The periosteum receives more sensory innervation than any other part of the skeleton [26]. We did not investigate the mechanism of LBP induced by osteoporosis in this study. As most subjects were elderly women, the presence of osteoporosis could not be neglected. We consider that the subjects who complained of LBP had low bone mineral density (BMD)-induced bone pain, especially elderly women.

We also investigated correlations between ODI and the sarcopenia-determining factors of walking speed, muscle mass and grip strength. ODI was associated with walking speed. Muscle power and volume did not affect LBP. Previous studies reported that exercising the lumbar muscles improved chronic LBP [27, 28].

We did not assess the volume and strength of the lumbar muscles and the effect of lumbar exercise of local residents. The relationship between the strength of these muscles and LBP is unclear. Among the sarcopenia-determining factors, only walking speed correlated with ODI.

Low walking speed associated ODI. We consider that low walking speed equates to low physical ability. Low physical activity might have association with low muscle volume and %YAM. We consider that low physical ability may associate with sarcopenia. In this study, although we could not be determined whether low physical activity is a cause or a result of sarcopenia and osteoporosis, measures against low physical ability, such as exercise and osteoporosis therapy, may help prevent sarcopenia.

This study had several limitations. First, being a cross-sectional study, it did not reveal the causal relationships between sarcopenia and LBP. We did not investigate the causes of LBP without sarcopenia, such as disc herniation, lumbar spinal stenosis and spinal deformity. Second, the study may have had a subject selection bias because the subjects voluntarily participated in the medical check-up. We performed this study in a small town in mountains and most of subject who were recruited were over 70's. Our inclusion criteria were living independently and the ability to walk to where the survey was performed. As a result, subjects who could attend the check-up may have had higher levels of activities of daily living. These factors affect the result of our research as a selection bias. Especially, this bias may have relationship with the low prevalence of sarcopenia in this study. Third, sample size was too small.

Conclusion

Low back pain was associated with osteoporosis and cause low physical activity. As a result, these situations caused sarcopenia. We consider that exercise against low physical activity and osteoporosis therapy may affect sarcopenia.

Abbreviations
%YAM: The percentage of young adult mean; BIA: Bioelectrical impedance analysis; BMD: Bone mineral density; GAINA: Good Ageing and Intervention Against Nursing Care and Activity Decline; LBP: Low back pain; ODI: Oswestry Disability Index; QUS: Quantitative ultrasound; SMI: Skeletal muscle index; VAS: Visual analogue scale

Acknowledgements
The authors sincerely acknowledge all staff members of the GAINA study involved in this study. The authors also acknowledge Shinichi Taniguchi, Eri Kobayashi, Kyohei Nakata, Takeshi Sota, Taro Omori, Takashi Wada, Tetsuji Morita, Naoyuki Nakaso, Tomoko Akita, Nao Nakata, Takuya Sugimura and Naoko Ikuta for their support and Ryoko Ikehara for her secretarial assistance.

Funding
This study was supported by a Ministry of Education, Culture, Sports, Science and Technology Grant (Chi-no kyoten seibi jigyou) and a Japanese Society for Musculoskeletal Medicine Grant.

Authors' contributions
ST designed the study and participated in this study, and did the acquisition, analysis, and interpretation of data of the work and drafting of the manuscript. HH, CT and HM help designed the study and participated in this study, and did the acquisition, analysis, and interpretation of data of the work. HN contributed

to the designs and drafted the manuscript. All authors read and approved the final version of the manuscript.

Consent for publication
Not applicable.

Competing interests
HN received research funding from Nippon Zoki Pharmaceutical Co.,ltd(Osaka, Japan), TEIJIN PHARMA LIMITED (Tokyo, Japan) and Taisho Toyama Pharmaceutical Co., Ltd.(Tokyo, Japan).
HM received grant from Ministry of Education,Culture,Sports,Scince and Technology Grant and Japanese Society for Musculoskeletal Medicine Grant. Other authors have non-financial competing interests.

Author details
[1]Department of Orthopedic Surgery,Faculty of Medicine, Tottori University, 36-1 Nishi-cho, Yonago, Tottori 683-8504, Japan. [2]School of Health Science, Tottori University Faculty of Medicine, 86 Nishi-cho, Yonago, Tottori 683-8503, Japan. [3]Rehabilitation Division, Tottori University Hospital, 36-1 Nishi-cho, Yonago, Tottori 683-8504, Japan.

References

1. Airaksinen O, Brox JI, Cedraschi C, Hildebrandt J, Klaber-Moffett J, Kovacs F, Mannion AF, Reis S, Staal JB, Ursin H, et al. Chapter 4. European guidelines for the management of chronic nonspecific low back pain. European spine journal : official publication of the European Spine Society, the European Spinal Deformity Society, and the European Section of the Cervical Spine Research Society. 2006;15(Suppl 2):S192–300.
2. Wan Q, Lin C, Li X, Zeng W, Ma C. MRI assessment of paraspinal muscles in patients with acute and chronic unilateral low back pain. Br J Radiol. 2015; 88(1053):20140546.
3. Goubert D, Oosterwijck JV, Meeus M, Danneels L. Structural changes of lumbar muscles in non-specific low back pain: a systematic review. Pain Physician. 2016;19(7):E985–E1000.
4. Teichtahl AJ, Urquhart DM, Wang Y, Wluka AE, Wijethilake P, O'Sullivan R, Cicuttini FM. Fat infiltration of paraspinal muscles is associated with low back pain, disability, and structural abnormalities in community-based adults. Spine J. 2015;15(7):1593–601.
5. Rosenberg IH. Sarcopenia: origins and clinical relevance. J Nutr. 1997;127(5 Suppl):990S–1S.
6. Aagaard T, Roed C, Dahl B, Obel N. Long-term prognosis and causes of death after spondylodiscitis: a Danish nationwide cohort study. Infectious diseases. 2016;48(3):201–8.
7. Kalyani RR, Tra Y, Yeh HC, Egan JM, Ferrucci L, Brancati FL. Quadriceps strength, quadriceps power, and gait speed in older U.S. adults with diabetes mellitus: results from the National Health and nutrition examination survey, 1999-2002. J Am Geriatr Soc. 2013;61(5):769–75.
8. Hida T, Shimokata H, Sakai Y, Ito S, Matsui Y, Takemura M, Kasai T, Ishiguro N, Harada A. Sarcopenia and sarcopenic leg as potential risk factors for acute osteoporotic vertebral fracture among older women. European spine journal : official publication of the European Spine Society, the European Spinal Deformity Society, and the European Section of the Cervical Spine Research Society. 2016;25(11):3424–31.
9. Kim SH, Kim TH, Hwang HJ. The relationship of physical activity (PA) and walking with sarcopenia in Korean males aged 60 years and older using the fourth Korean National Health and nutrition examination survey (KNHANES IV-2, 3), 2008-2009. Arch Gerontol Geriatr. 2013;56(3):472–7.
10. Chen LK, Liu LK, Woo J, Assantachai P, Auyeung TW, Bahyah KS, Chou MY, Chen LY, Hsu PS, Krairit O, et al. Sarcopenia in Asia: consensus report of the Asian working Group for Sarcopenia. J Am Med Dir Assoc. 2014; 15(2):95–101.
11. Camozzi V, De Terlizzi F, Zangari M, Luisetto G. Quantitative bone ultrasound at phalanges and calcaneus in osteoporotic postmenopausal women: influence of age and measurement site. Ultrasound Med Biol. 2007;33(7):1039–45.
12. Pisani P, Renna MD, Conversano F, Casciaro E, Muratore M, Quarta E, Paola MD, Casciaro S. Screening and early diagnosis of osteoporosis through X-ray and ultrasound based techniques. World J Radiol. 2013;5(11):398–410.
13. Baumgartner RN, Koehler KM, Gallagher D, Romero L, Heymsfield SB, Ross RR, Garry PJ, Lindeman RD. Epidemiology of sarcopenia among the elderly in New Mexico. Am J Epidemiol. 1998;147(8):755–63.
14. Janssen I, Heymsfield SB, Wang ZM, Ross R. Skeletal muscle mass and distribution in 468 men and women aged 18-88 yr. J Appl Physiol. 2000; 89(1):81–8.
15. Janssen I, Heymsfield SB, Ross R. Low relative skeletal muscle mass (sarcopenia) in older persons is associated with functional impairment and physical disability. J Am Geriatr Soc. 2002;50(5):889–96.
16. Park S, Kim HJ, Ko BG, Chung JW, Kim SH, Park SH, Lee MH, Yeom JS. The prevalence and impact of sarcopenia on degenerative lumbar spinal stenosis. The bone & joint journal. 2016;98-B(8):1093–8.
17. Suka M, Yoshida K. The national burden of musculoskeletal pain in Japan: projections to the year 2055. Clin J Pain. 2009;25(4):313–9.
18. Chou R, Qaseem A, Snow V, Casey D, Cross JT Jr, Shekelle P, Owens DK. Clinical efficacy assessment Subcommittee of the American College of P, American College of P, American pain society low back pain guidelines P: diagnosis and treatment of low back pain: a joint clinical practice guideline from the American College of Physicians and the American pain society. Ann Intern Med. 2007;147(7):478–91.
19. Verschueren S, Gielen E, O'Neill TW, Pye SR, Adams JE, Ward KA, FC W, Szulc P, Laurent M, Claessens F, et al. Sarcopenia and its relationship with bone mineral density in middle-aged and elderly European men. Osteoporos Int. 2013;24(1):87–98.
20. Soen S, Fukunaga M, Sugimoto T, Sone T, Fujiwara S, Endo N, Gorai I, Shiraki M, Hagino H, Hosoi T, et al. Diagnostic criteria for primary osteoporosis: year 2012 revision. J Bone Miner Metab. 2013;31(3):247–57.
21. Yoshimura N, Muraki S, Oka H, Kawaguchi H, Nakamura K, Akune T. Cohort profile: research on osteoarthritis/osteoporosis against disability study. Int J Epidemiol. 2010;39(4):988–95.
22. Yoshimura N, Muraki S, Oka H, Mabuchi A, En-Yo Y, Yoshida M, Saika A, Yoshida H, Suzuki T, Yamamoto S, et al. Prevalence of knee osteoarthritis, lumbar spondylosis, and osteoporosis in Japanese men and women: the research on osteoarthritis/osteoporosis against disability study. J Bone Miner Metab. 2009;27(5):620–8.
23. Campbell MK, James A, Hudson MA, Carr C, Jackson E, Oakes V, Demissie S, Farrell D, Tessaro I. Improving multiple behaviors for colorectal cancer prevention among african american church members. Health Psychol. 2004;23(5):492–502.
24. Clohisy DR, Perkins SL, Ramnaraine ML. Review of cellular mechanisms of tumor osteolysis. Clin Orthop Relat Res. 2000;373:104–14.
25. Martin CD, Jimenez-Andrade JM, Ghilardi JR, Mantyh PW. Organization of a unique net-like meshwork of CGRP+ sensory fibers in the mouse periosteum: implications for the generation and maintenance of bone fracture pain. Neurosci Lett. 2007;427(3):148–52.
26. Mattia C, Coluzzi F, Celidonio L, Vellucci R. Bone pain mechanism in osteoporosis: a narrative review. Clinical cases in mineral and bone metabolism : the official journal of the Italian Society of Osteoporosis, Mineral Metabolism, and Skeletal Diseases. 2016;13(2):97–100.
27. Deutsch FE. Isolated lumbar strengthening in the rehabilitation of chronic low back pain. J Manip Physiol Ther. 1996;19(2):124–33.
28. Jeong UC, Sim JH, Kim CY, Hwang-Bo G, Nam CW. The effects of gluteus muscle strengthening exercise and lumbar stabilization exercise on lumbar muscle strength and balance in chronic low back pain patients. J Phys Ther Sci. 2015;27(12):3813–6.

15

Associations between disc space narrowing, anterior osteophytes and disability in chronic mechanical low back pain

Romain Shanil Perera[1*], Poruwalage Harsha Dissanayake[2], Upul Senarath[3], Lalith Sirimevan Wijayaratne[4], Aranjan Lional Karunanayake[5] and Vajira Harshadeva Weerabaddana Dissanayake[6]

Abstract

Background: Radiographic features of lumbar disc degeneration (LDD) are common findings in patients with chronic mechanical low back pain; however, its role in disability and intensity of pain is debatable. This study aims to investigate the associations of the x-ray features of LDD and lumbar spondylolisthesis with severity of disability and intensity of pain.

Methods: A cross-sectional study was conducted on 439 patients with chronic mechanical low back pain who attended the rheumatology clinic, National Hospital of Sri Lanka, Colombo, from May 2012 to May 2014. Severity of disability was measured using Modified Oswestry Disability Index and intensity of pain was assessed using numeric rating scale (0–100). X-ray features of LDD (disc space narrowing, anterior osteophytes and overall LDD) and spondylolisthesis were assessed in lateral recumbent lumbar x-rays (L1/L2 to L5/S1) and graded by a consultant radiologist blinded to clinical data. Generalised linear model with linear response was used to assess the associations of x-ray features of LDD with severity of disability and intensity of pain adjusting for age, gender, body mass index and pain radiating into legs.

Results: Mean age was 48.99 ± 11.21 and 323 (73.58%) were females. 87 (19.82%) were obese. Mean severity of disability was 30.95 ± 13.67 and mean intensity of pain was 45.50 ± 20.37. 69 (15.72%), 26 (5.92%) and 85 (19.36%) patients had grade 2 disc space narrowing, anterior osteophytes and overall LDD, respectively. 51 (11.62%) patients had lumbar spondylolisthesis. Grade of disc space narrowing and overall LDD were not associated with severity of disability or intensity of pain. The presence of lumbar spondylolisthesis was associated with severity of disability. Female gender and pain radiating into legs were associated with severity of disability and intensity of pain. Advancing age was associated with x-ray features of LDD and lumbar spondylolisthesis.

Conclusions: Lumbar spondylolisthesis is associated with severity of disability in patients with chronic mechanical low back pain. Associations of x-ray features of LDD with severity of disability and intensity of pain are inconclusive. Female gender and pain radiating into legs are significant confounders.

Keywords: Disability, Disc space narrowing, Anterior osteophytes, Low back pain, Lumbar disc degeneration

* Correspondence: romaingl@med.cmb.ac.lk
[1]Department of Allied Health Sciences, Faculty of Medicine, University of
Colombo, 25, Kynsey Road, Colombo 8, Sri Lanka
Full list of author information is available at the end of the article

Background

Disability due to chronic low back pain is one of the leading health care problems in most regions of the world including South Asia [1]. It affects all aspects of life including physical, mental, and social well-being [2]. Disabling chronic low back pain is reported to be a major issue in occupational health in Sri Lanka [3, 4]. Most chronic low back pains are related to mechanical causes including injuries of the musculoskeletal structures of the spine and pathologies associated with lumbar disc degeneration (LDD) [5, 6]. LDD is a common finding in the aging spine and symptoms of chronic mechanical low back pain are not always correlated with the radiological features of LDD. Patients with chronic low back pain receive routine spinal imaging (lumbar x-ray, computed tomography, or magnetic resonance imaging [MRI]) and MRI of lumbar spine has become the popular choice for routine imaging as it gives a direct visualisation of the disc without exposure to the radiation. However MRI is not a cost effective method in routine spinal imaging in developing countries and clinicians in developing countries like Sri Lanka regularly use x-ray lumbar spine as a feasible option for assessing features related to LDD [7].

There are mixed evidence for the association of LDD with chronic mechanical low back pain and disability. Although, routine x-ray of lumbar spine does not affect the outcome of the treatment of uncomplicated acute and subacute low back pain [8], x-ray features related to LDD may benefit the clinical diagnosis and management of chronic low back pain and disability when combined with other factors such as proper history taking, severity of symptoms, surgical risks and costs [8]. Disc space narrowing and anterior osteophytes are the main x-ray features of LDD [9] and are proven to be highly correlated with the morphological stages of LDD [10]. Disc space narrowing is associated with lumbar spinal stenosis, disc herniation and spondylolisthesis which are also related to the pain and disability [11]. Disc space narrowing is associated with the presence of chronic low back pain [9, 12] and intensity of pain [13]. This association becomes stronger with increasing severity of disc space narrowing [12, 13]. Mostly these associations are reported in population based studies and their study samples were limited to middle aged and elderly individuals [9, 12, 13]. There are a limited number of studies which have investigated the association of disc space narrowing with disability [9]. Although anterior osteophyte is the most frequently observed degenerative feature of the aging lumbar spine, it has variably correlated results on its association with intensity of pain [9, 13]. With regard to disability, we could not find enough evidence to prove its association with anterior osteophytes [9, 14]. Both disc space narrowing and anterior

osteophytes have been used to determine the grade of overall LDD [15] and high variability exists among the associations between the overall LDD and intensity of pain/disability [14, 16, 17].

Severity of disability/intensity of pain and x-ray features of LDD are further influenced by the effects of age, gender, body mass index (BMI) and the presence of pain radiating into legs. Advancing age increases the susceptibility for severe disability [18]. In most studies females have reported increased intensity of pain and severe disability [19, 20]. In addition obese patients have a higher risk for recurrent disabling low back pain [21]. Furthermore pain radiating into legs is associated with symptomatic disc herniation contributing to severe pain and disability [22]. Age, gender, BMI and the presence of pain radiating into legs may be helpful in predicting the severity of x-ray features of LDD. Advancing age increases the susceptibility for severe degeneration [23, 24]. In addition, there is evidence that males have more degenerative changes compared to females [9], but there are other studies that have given contradicting results [25]. Certain studies have reported that higher BMI has an add-on effect on LDD [26, 27]. However the evidence for associations of gender, BMI and the presence of pain radiating into legs with grade of x-ray features of LDD are inconsistent and need further investigation.

Routine x-ray of lumbar spine is carried out during the management of chronic low back pain in developing countries. Details about age, gender, BMI and the presence of pain radiating into legs are helpful in deciding to prescribe x-ray of lumbar spine as these variables might be useful in predicting the grade of x-ray features of the spine, clinical outcomes and deciding treatment options. Disc space narrowing has significant association with chronic low back pain while anterior osteophytes and LDD have variably correlated results. Most of these studies were population based studies and conducted in middle aged and elderly individuals. There is lack of studies which have assessed the associations of x-ray features of LDD with severity of disability and intensity of pain in patients with chronic mechanical low back pain in clinical settings. There is a wide variation in intensity of pain and disability among patients with chronic mechanical low back pain and patients with severe symptoms require comprehensive care. If there is an association between the grade of x-ray features of LDD, spondylolisthesis and severity of disability and intensity of pain, it would greatly benefit the clinical management with regard to both resource allocation and type of treatment to administer. We hypothesised that the patients with x-ray features of advanced LDD/spondylolisthesis have increased severity of disability and intensity of pain. The objective of our study was to assess the associations of the x-ray features of lumbar disc degeneration and lumbar spondylolisthesis with severity of disability and intensity of pain in patients with chronic mechanical low back pain adjusting for age, gender, BMI and pain radiating into legs. In addition we assessed the associations of x-ray features of LDD with age, gender, BMI and pain radiating into legs.

Methods

Study design, setting and participants

A descriptive cross-sectional study was conducted on consecutive patients with chronic mechanical low back pain who attended the rheumatology clinic, National Hospital of Sri Lanka, Colombo, from May 2012 to May 2014. Both male and female patients of Sri Lankan origin with chronic mechanical low back pain aged 20 to 69 years were recruited to the study. Both patients with and without x-ray evidence of LDD and spondylolisthesis were included. Low back pain was defined as pain, muscle tension, or stiffness localized below the costal margin and above the inferior gluteal folds, with or without pain radiating into the leg [19]. Back pain during day time worsening in the latter part of the day due to movements was considered to be due to a mechanical cause [28]. Chronicity was defined as pain on most days of the week for at least three months [2]. Patients with back pain due to inflammatory causes (seronegative spondyloarthropathies, diffuse idiopathic skeletal hyperostosis, rheumatoid arthritis), visceral origin (urinary tract infections, inflammatory pelvic disease), systemic infections affecting spine (spinal tuberculosis), metabolic bone diseases (osteoporosis and osteomalacia), fractures in the vertebral column, past surgeries in the spine, and spinal tumours were excluded. Pregnant females and patients who refuse to participate in the study were also excluded. The study was carried out in accordance with the Declaration of Helsinki and with the approval of the Ethics Review Committee of the Faculty of Medicine, University of Colombo. Patients who fulfilled the inclusion and exclusion criteria were recruited to the study after obtaining written informed consent.

Clinical evaluation

Demographic (age and gender) and clinical data (intensity of pain, severity of disability, presence of pain radiating into legs, and BMI) were recorded using a pretested interviewer administered questionnaire and clinical examination. The intensity of pain was measured using a 101 (0 to 100) point numeric rating scale. Patients were asked to score the average intensity of pain experienced during the past 7 days out of 100 [29–31]. Disability was assessed using the Modified Oswestry Disability Index (MODI). MODI is a low back pain specific disability questionnaire with ten items which assess pain and its impact on the activities of daily living including personal care, lifting, walking, sitting, standing, sleeping, travelling, social work, home and work duties. Each item has six responses where higher values represent greater disability. Sum of responses was calculated and presented as a percentage [32, 33]. Pain radiating into legs was positive if the pain radiated below the knee of either one or both legs. Height (cm) and weight (kg) of the patients were recorded with light clothing and without shoes to the nearest 0.1 cm and 0.1 kg, respectively, and BMI was calculated (kg/m^2) [34]. International cut off values were used for categorisation of BMI [35].

Radiographic evaluation

Static lateral lumbar x-rays were obtained from all patients. Patients were in lateral recumbent position on the table flexing the knees and hips just enough to achieve comfortable position and a small sandbag was kept between the knees. Midaxillary plane was aligned to the middle of the table and the central x-ray beam was directed perpendicular to the body of the L3 vertebra [36]. Collected lateral lumbar x-rays were evaluated by a consultant radiologist blinded to the clinical details of the patients. The intervertebral disc spaces (L1/L2 to L5/S1) in lateral lumbar x-rays were assessed for the disc space narrowing, anterior osteophytes and lumbar spondylolisthesis. Reduction of the height of the disc space compared to the adjacent normal disc space was defined as the disc space narrowing and presence of bony outgrowths of the vertebral body arising from the borders of superior and inferior surfaces extending anteriorly was defined as anterior osteophyte. Disc space narrowing was graded as follows: grade 0 = none; grade 1 = definite (mild) narrowing; grade 2 = moderate to severe narrowing. Anterior osteophyte was graded as follows: grade 0 = none; grade 1 = small osteophyte and grade 2 = moderate to large osteophyte. Based on these features, overall grading was given for the LDD: grade 0 = normal (grade 0 disc space narrowing and grade 0 anterior osteophyte); grade 1 = grade 1 disc space narrowing and/or grade 1 anterior osteophyte; grade 2 = grade 2 disc space narrowing and/or grade 2 anterior osteophyte (Fig. 1) [37]. End plate sclerosis was not taken into account due to its low interobserver reliability [9, 15]. A particular grade of disc space narrowing/anterior osteophyte/LDD was identified for each of the lumbar levels, and the highest available grade out of the five lumbar levels was used as the final grade for that particular spine. Lumbar spondylolisthesis was defined as presence of displacement of one vertebral body relative to the next most inferior vertebral body and assessed in lateral recumbent lumbar x-ray [11]. However the ability to assess the spondylolisthesis in lateral recumbent lumbar x-ray is limited. Interobserver reproducibility was assessed using a second medical officer who

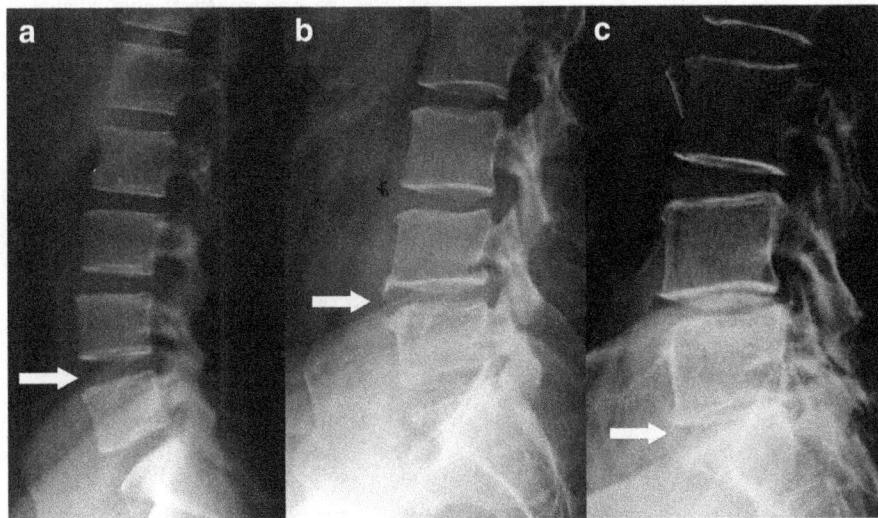

Fig. 1 Assesment of the x-ray features of lumbar disc degeneration - lateral x-ray of lumbar spine. Arrows - **a** – no disc space narrowing/anterior osteophyte (grade 0 lumbar disc degeneration), **b** – mild disc space narrowing and small anterior osteophyte, (grade 1 lumbar disc degeneration) **c** – moderate disc space narrowing and small anterior osteophyte (grade 2 lumbar disc degeneration)

was trained on radiographic evaluation according to the Lane atlas. On random evaluation of 25% of the radiographs were reported by the second medical officer who was blinded to the first reader's interpretations.

Statistical analysis

Descriptive statistics were calculated to summarise the sample characteristics. Both univariable and multivariable analyses were carried out. For the univariable analysis, severity of disability and intensity of pain were defined as continuous outcome/dependent variables and independent samples t-test was used when there were two categories and Analysis of Variance (ANOVA) was used when there were more than two categories.

Multivariable analysis was performed using different regression models considering the nature of the outcome/dependent variables. Multivariable generalised linear model with linear response was used when the severity of disability and intensity of pain were used as the continuous outcome variables. X-ray features of LDD (disc space narrowing, anterior osteophytes and overall LDD) and presence of lumbar spondylolisthesis were defined as main independent variables/predictor variables and were treated as categorical variables. Separate linear regression models were created for each feature. In each multivariable generalised linear model with linear response, the magnitude of the association was presented as β coefficients with 95% confidence intervals (CI). Multivariable ordinal logistic regression was used when the severity of x-ray features of LDD (disc space narrowing, anterior osteophytes and overall LDD) were used as the ordinal outcome variables (0, 1 and 2). Multivariable logistic regression analysis was used when the

presence of lumbar spondylolisthesis (yes/no) was used as a binary outcome variable. Magnitude of the associations was presented as adjusted odds ratios (aOR) with 95% CI in logistic regression models. Age, gender, BMI and presence of pain radiating into legs were defined as confounder variables in all regression models. Age and BMI were treated as continuous variables and gender (male/female) and presence of pain radiating into legs (yes/no) were treated as categorical variables.

Assumptions of ANOVA, independent samples t-test and regression models were verified. P value < 0.05 was used as the level of significance. Statistical analysis was carried out using SPSS version 17.

Results
Characteristics of the participants

Table 1 summarises the characteristics of the study participants. Among 689 patients with chronic mechanical low back pain, 439 patients were recruited according to eligibility criteria. Thirteen patients had missing data for the variable BMI. Mean age ± SD was 48.99 ± 11.21 and 323 (73.58%) were females. BMI ± SD was 26.39 ± 4.65 and 87 (19.82%) were obese. Mean severity of disability was 30.95 ± 13.67 and mean intensity of pain was 45.50 ± 20.37. In addition, 110 (25.10%) patients had pain radiating into legs. With regard to interobserver reproducibility, intra-class correlation coefficient (ICC) of two readers for disc space narrowing was 0.88 (0.82-0.91) and ICC for anterior osteophytes was 0.81 (0.75 – 0.85). Among patients, 176 (40.09%) had disc space narrowing and 201 (45.78%) had anterior osteophytes with 69 (15.72%) and 26 (5.92%) having grade 2 disc space narrowing and grade 2 anterior osteophytes, respectively.

Table 1 Summary of sample characteristics

Variable	All $N = 439$ n ((n/N) %)
Age	
20–29 years	26 (5.92)
30–39 years	72 (16.40)
40–49 years	118 (26.88)
50–59 years	141 (32.12)
60–69 years	82 (18.68)
Gender	
Female	323 (73.58)
Male	116 (26.42)
Radiation of pain into legs	
Yes	110 (25.10)
No	329 (74.90)
Body mass index	
Normal (18–24.9 kg/m^2)	178 (40.55)
Overweight (25–29.9 kg/m^2)	160 (36.45)
Obese (≥30 kg/m^2)	87 (19.82)
X-ray features	
Disc space narrowing	
Grade 0	263 (59.91)
Grade 1	107 (24.37)
Grade 2	69 (15.72)
Anterior osteophytes	
Grade 0	238 (54.21)
Grade 1	175 (39.86)
Grade 2	26 (5.92)
Lumbar disc degeneration	
Grade 0	164 (37.36)
Grade 1	190 (43.28)
Grade 2	85 (19.36)
Lumbar spondylolisthesis	
Yes	51 (11.62)
No	388 (88.38)

LDD was present in 275 (62.64%) and 85 (19.36%) had grade 2 LDD. Lumbar spondylolisthesis was present in 51 (11.62%) patients.

Associations of x-ray features of lumbar disc degeneration, spondylolisthesis with severity of disability

There were no significant differences in severity of disability with the severity of disc space narrowing, anterior osteophytes and LDD according to ANOVA and generalised linear models with linear response (Table 2 and 3). Patients with the presence of lumbar spondylolisthesis had significantly severe disability in contrast to the patients without lumbar spondylolisthesis in both univariable and multivariable analysis (Table 2 and 3). Female gender and presence of pain radiating into legs were significantly associated with the severity of disability in all the multivariable generalised linear models (Table 3).

Associations of x-ray features of lumbar disc degeneration, spondylolisthesis with intensity of pain

Disc space narrowing and LDD were not associated with intensity of pain in either univariable or multivariable regression analyses (Table 2 and 3). However patients with grade 1 anterior osteophytes had significantly higher intensity of pain compared to the patients with grade 0 anterior osteophytes. The presence of lumbar spondylolisthesis was not associated with the intensity of pain. Female gender and pain radiating into legs were associated with the intensity of pain in all multivariable generalised linear models (Table 3). In addition increasing age was associated with two linear regression models involving anterior osteophytes and LDD (Table 3).

Associations of age, gender, BMI and presence of pain radiating into legs with x-ray features of lumbar disc degeneration and spondylolisthesis

The presence of grade 2 disc space narrowing was reported from 20 – 29 years age group, but presence of grade 2 anterior osteophytes was reported from 40 – 49 years age group. Furthermore the presence of lumbar spondylolisthesis was reported from 30 – 39 years age group. Advancing age was strongly associated with the severity of disc space narrowing, anterior osteophytes, LDD (Table 4) and presence of lumbar spondylolisthesis (aOR 1.15; 95% CI: 1.1 – 1.21) after adjusting for gender, BMI and pain radiating into legs. Male gender was associated with the severity of anterior osteophytes, but was not associated with disc space narrowing, overall LDD and lumbar spondylolisthesis. Furthermore, BMI was significantly associated with grades of anterior osteophytes and LDD.

Discussion

In this study we assessed the associations of x-ray features of LDD and lumbar spondylolisthesis with severity of disability and intensity of pain in patients with chronic mechanical low back pain adjusting for age, gender, BMI and pain radiating into legs. In addition we assessed the associations of x-ray features of LDD with age, gender, BMI and presence of pain radiating into legs. We found that, the associations of x-ray features of LDD with severity of disability or intensity of pain (except anterior osteophytes) were inconclusive. The presence of lumbar spondylolisthesis was associated with increased severity of disability. However the Female gender and presence of pain radiating into legs were

Table 2 Means of severity of disability/intensity of pain according to the severity of x-ray features of lumbar disc degeneration and lumbar spondylolisthesis – univariable analysis

Variable	Mean disability ± SD	p value	Mean intensity of pain ± SD	p value
Disc space narrowing		0.115		0.504
Grade 0	30.48 ± 12.92		44.63 ± 19.58	
Grade 1	30.10 ± 13.84		47.31 ± 21.69	
Grade 2	34.07 ± 15.81		46.01 ± 21.33	
Anterior osteophytes		0.076		0.200
Grade 0	30.05 ± 13.61		44.10 ± 20.20	
Grade 1	32.65 ± 14.15		47.64 ± 20.73	
Grade 2	27.79 ± 9.17		43.87 ± 18.93	
Lumbar disc degeneration		0.207		0.534
Grade 0	29.75 ± 12.85		44.13 ± 19.05	
Grade 1	31.07 ± 13.79		46.11 ± 21.32	
Grade 2	32.98 ± 14.79		46.79 ± 20.77	
Lumbar spondylolisthesis		0.001*		0.289
Yes	36.65 ± 13.58		48.34 ± 19.97	
No	30.20 ± 13.52		45.13 ± 20.42	

* - p value < 0
SD standard deviation

associated with increased severity of disability and intensity of pain. Furthermore, x-ray features of LDD and lumbar spondylolisthesis were strongly associated with advancing age.

Lumbar intervertebral discs are fibrocartilage pads between adjacent lumbar vertebral bodies which distribute compressive loading evenly on to the vertebral bodies. Intervertebral discs contribute to spinal stability along with the apophyseal joints and supported by surrounding muscles and ligaments [38]. With LDD the normal architecture of the disc is disrupted leading to abnormal biomechanical force distribution which may cause severe and disabling low back pain. With degeneration, the height of the disc can be reduced due to inward or outward herniation of the disc material and is visible as disc space narrowing in x-ray lumbar spine. This results in abnormal load distribution to the surrounding structures and lead to segmental instability and spondylolisthesis. Formation of osteophytes is a compensatory mechanism to distribute increasing axial forces of spine on a larger articulating surface to prevent spinal instability [11]. Although x-ray features of LDD are not correlated with the outcome of the treatment, they can give important details for managing chronic mechanical low back pain especially in the presence of severe symptoms [39].

Disc space narrowing is used as a surrogate variable for LDD and many studies found positive association with the presence of chronic low back pain in population based studies [9, 15, 24]. However, studies done in clinical settings did not find significant association between disc space narrowing and intensity of pain [17].

Similarly in our study disc space narrowing was not associated with intensity of pain. There are limited cross sectional clinical studies which have assessed the association of LDD with disability. A study on 172 consecutive patients with chronic low back pain in United Kingdom did not find significant association between LDD (based on x-ray findings) and disability [15]. Authors of the previous study did not assess the association of features of LDD separately as disc space narrowing and anterior osteophytes, but rather assessed the overall LDD. According to our univariable and multivariable analyses disc space narrowing was not associated with disability, but gender and presence of pain radiating into legs had significant association with disability.

Comparatively, the association between anterior osteophytes and chronic low back pain is largely considered as not significant, unless there is a higher grade of anterior osteophytes [9, 24]. As mentioned previously we could not find cross sectional clinical studies which have assessed the associations between anterior osteophytes and disability. Higher grades of anterior osteophytes are frequently seen in elderly individuals (above 65 years). Our sample was restricted to patients below 70 years and there were only 26 patients with grade 2 anterior osteophytes. In our results, grade of anterior osteophytes was not associated with the severity of disability. However the patients with grade 1 anterior osteophytes had higher intensity of pain in contrast to patients with grade 0 anterior osteophytes. The overall association between the grades of anterior osteophytes and intensity of pain was inconsistent as there was no

Table 3 Associations of x-ray features of lumbar disc degeneration and spondylolisthesis with severity of disability and intensity of pain – multivariable generalised linear models with linear response

Variables	Severity of disability		Intensity of pain	
	β coefficient (95% confidence itervals)	p value	β coefficient (95% confidence intervals)	p value
Regression model 1				
Intercept	22.945 (14.589 – 31.301)	<0.001*	47.375 (34.766 – 59.984)	<0.001*
Severity of disc space narrowing				
Grade 0	0.000		0.000	
Grade 1	-0.311 (-3.301 – 2.679)	0.839	3.896 (-0.616 – 8.408)	0.091
Grade 2	2.751 (-0.934 – 6.437)	0.143	2.007 (-3.555 – 7.569)	0.479
Age (years)	-0.014 (-0.133 – 0.106)	0.824	-0.173 (-0.352 – 0.007)	0.060
Gender				
Male	0.000		0.000	
Female	7.369 (4.446 – 10.293)	<0.001*	4.899 (0.488 – 9.311)	0.030*
Body mass index (kg/m^2)	0.042 (-0.236 – 0.320)	0.765	-0.049 (-0.468 – 0.370)	0.819
Pain radiating into legs				
No	0.000		0.000	
Yes	6.989 (4.174 – 9.803)	<0.001*	12.262 (8.015 – 16.508)	<0.001*
Regression model 2				
Intercept	22.049 (13.736 – 30.362)	<0.001*	49.630 (37.099 – 62.161)	<0.001*
Severity of anterior osteophyte				
Grade 0	0.000		0.000	
Grade 1	2.136 (-0.565 – 4.838)	0.121	4.836 (0.764 – 8.908)	0.020*
Grade 2	-2.309 (-7.727 – 3.108)	0.403	2.931 (-5.235 – 11.097)	0.482
Age	0.001 (-0.118 – 0.120)	0.989	-0.200 (-0.379 – -0.021)	0.029*
Gender				
Male	0.000		0.000	
Female	7.374 (4.448 – 10.301)	<0.001*	5.507 (1.096 – 9.918)	0.014*
Body mass index (kg/m^2)	0.037 (-0.241 – 0.315)	0.794	-0.130 (-0.550 – 0.289)	0.543
Pain radiating into legs				
No	0.000		0.000	
Yes	6.889 (4.076 – 9.702)	<0.001*	12.045 (7.805 – 16.285)	<0.001*
Regression model 3				
Intercept	22.710 (14.255 – 31.164)	<0.001*	49.254 (36.523 – 61.985)	<0.001*
Severity of lumbar disc degeneration				
Grade 0	0.000		0.000	
Grade 1	0.976 (-1.885 – 3.838)	0.252	3.642 (-0.688 – 7.951)	0.098
Grade 2	2.243 (-1.599 – 6.086)	0.504	4.559 (-1.227 – 10.345)	0.122
Age	-0.020 (-0.144 – 0.105)	0.758	-0.207 (-0.394 – -0.020)	0.030*
Gender				
Male	0.000		0.000	
Female	7.320 (4.391 – 10.249)	<0.001*	5.240 (0.829 – 9.651)	0.020*
Body mass index (kg/m^2)	0.045 (-0.234 – 0.324)	0.753	-0.111 (-0.531 – 0.310)	0.606
Pain radiating into legs				
No	0.000		0.000	
Yes	7.009 (4.191 – 9.828)	<0.001*	12.167 (7.923 – 16.412)	<0.001*

Table 3 Associations of x-ray features of lumbar disc degeneration and spondylolisthesis with severity of disability and intensity of pain – multivariable generalised linear models with linear response (Continued)

Regression model 4				
Intercept	23.304 (15.086 – 31.523)	<0.001*	48.248 (35.749 – 60.748)	<0.001*
Presence of lumbar spondylolisthesis				
No	0.000		0.000	
Yes	5.670 (1.684 – 9.656)	0.005*	3.549 (-2.514 – 9.612)	0.251
Age	-0.040 (-0.156 – 0.076)	0.501	-0.168 (-0.345 – 0.009)	0.063
Gender				
Male	0.000		0.000	
Female	7.011 (4.114 – 9.908)	<0.001*	4.824 (0.418 – 9.231)	0.032*
Body mass index (kg/m^2)	0.078 (-0.197 – 0.353)	0.578	-0.055 (-0.473 – 0.363)	0.795
Pain radiating into legs				
No	0.000		0.000	
Yes	6.820 (4.019 – 9.621)	<0.001*	12.128 (7.868 – 16.388)	<0.001*

Main predictor (independent) variables were analysed as follows:
Regression model 1: severity of disc space narrowing (grade 0, 1 and 2)
Regression model 2: severity of anterior osteophytes (grade 0, 1 and 2)
Regression model 3: severity of lumbar disc degeneration (grade 0, 1 and 2)
Regression model 4: presence of lumbar spondylolisthesis (yes/no)
* - p value < 0.05

significant association between intensity of pain and grade 2 anterior osteophytes in contrast to grade 0 anterior osteophytes.

In most studies, overall LDD poorly correlated with clinical symptoms including severity of disability and intensity of pain [14, 40]. In our results we could not find a significant association between LDD and severity of disability or LDD and intensity of pain, which agree with the findings of the previous evidence [15]. Most radiographic scoring systems including the Lane atlas have used disc space narrowing or anterior osteophytes or both features to determine the overall LDD. Accordingly, either higher grades of disc space narrowing or higher grades of anterior osteophytes could determine higher grades of LDD. Although grade 1 anterior osteophytes was associated with intensity of pain (in contrast to patients with grade 0 anterior osteophytes), we could not find a significant association between overall LDD and intensity of pain. The strength of the association might have become further attenuated when both features (disc

Table 4 Associations of age, gender and BMI with x-ray features of lumbar disc degeneration – multivariable ordinal logistic regression model

Variable	Disc space narrowing			Anterior osteophytes			Disc degeneration		
	Parameter estimates (β)	aOR (95% CI)	p value	Parameter estimates (β)	aOR (95% CI)	p value	Parameter estimates (β)	aOR (95% CI)	p value
Age	0.074	1.077 (1.056 – 1.100)	<0.001*	0.075	1.078 (1.056 –1.100)	<0.001*	0.090	1.094 (1.072 –1.115)	<0.001*
BMI	0.023	1.023 (0.980 –1.069)	0.301	0.058	1.059 (1.013 –1.108)	0.012*	0.060	1.062 (1.018 –1.108)	0.005*
Gender									
Male	-0.245	1.277 (0.792 – 2.059)	0.316	0.517	1.676 (1.042 –2.696)	0.033*	0.371	1.450 (0.928 –2.265)	0.103
Female	0.000			0.000			0.000		
Pain radiating into legs									
No	-0.161	0.851 (0.542 – 1.335)	0.483	-0.118	0.888 (0.566 –1.394)	0.606	-0.168	0.845 (0.551 –1.296)	0.441
Yes	0.000	1.175 (0.749 –1.844)		0.000			0.000		

* - p value <0.05
aOR adjusted odds ratios, CI confidence interval

space narrowing and anterior osteophytes) were considered in overall LDD.

Degenerative lumbar spondylolisthesis is related to LDD and degenerative changes of the apophyseal joints [11]. In our results presence of lumbar spondylolisthesis was associated with the increasing grade of disc space narrowing and overall LDD, and was more frequent at the L4–L5 level. The presence of lumbar spondylolisthesis was associated with increased severity of disability in our study, but it was not associated with the intensity of pain. Narrowing of the disc space is associated with advanced LDD, annular tears and disc herniation, but these features do not always correlate well with the intensity of pain. Furthermore it can adversely affect the biomechanical stability of the lumbar spine which will increase the strain on apophyseal joints and surrounding structures where the combined effects can reduce the flexibility and stability of the spine leading to severe disability [11].

X-ray features of LDD are age related [9, 24] and our study results are compatible with the previous evidence. Interestingly, disc space narrowing was seen from an early age (20 –39 years), but anterior osteophytes was seen from the middle age group (40 –49 years) onwards. Although previous studies have found significantly higher degenerative features in males [9], we found positive association only with anterior osteophytes. Furthermore, increasing BMI was associated with increasing grade of anterior osteophytes and LDD which was compatible with previous findings [26, 27].

There is evidence that females are more susceptible to higher intensity of pain and disability and our results were compatible with the existing evidence. Finding reasons for this is beyond the objectives of our study, however, certain studies have suggested that females have higher sensitization to pain, higher chance of reporting of pain and differences in response to analgesics [41–43]. The presence of pain radiating into legs was strongly associated with severity of disability and intensity of pain. Pain radiating into legs is associated with symptomatic disc herniation, annular tears and nerve impingement which can cause severe disability and pain [22]. These two variables have strong confounding effect on the associations between x-ray features of LDD/lumbar spondylolisthesis and severity of disability/intensity of pain.

As there are less certain radiographic recommendations for uncomplicated chronic mechanical low back pain [44], regular radiographic assessment (x-ray lumbar spine) are taken into account during the decision making on different treatment options. In management of chronic mechanical low back pain weight training is a viable option in patients with mild LDD, but presence of moderate to severe features of LDD make this option

unjustifiable. Furthermore, patients with lumbar spondylolisthesis may require specific flexion strengthening exercises during the management to reduce the pain and disability [45]. The presence of lumbar spondylolisthesis, female gender and pain radiating into legs increased the severity of disability in our patients and these features might provide helpful information when assessing the severity of disability and management decision on type of treatment to administer.

There are a few limitations in the study. Our study is cross-sectional and was conducted in a specific group of patients with chronic mechanical low back pain at a single centre. We have not assessed the other associated factors with disability and pain such as depression, anxiety and fear avoidance. In addition we have not assessed the dynamic stability of the lumbar spine which could have contributed to the severity of disability and intensity of pain. X-ray lumbar spine cannot visualise the intervertebral disc directly. There may be increased risk of type 1 error due to multiple comparisons and it may affect the significance of the findings.

Conclusions

This study shows that the predictive ability of x-ray features of LDD for severity of disability and intensity of pain is weak among the patients with chronic mechanical low back pain. However the presence of lumbar spondylolisthesis is associated with severe disability. Female gender and the presence of pain radiating into legs are associated with increased severity of disability and intensity of pain, hence acting as strong confounders. Advancing age is associated with x-ray features of advanced LDD including spondylolisthesis. The presence of lumbar spondylolisthesis, gender and pain radiating into legs are good predictive factors of severe disability and higher intensity of pain which may facilitate the decision making process in management of chronic mechanical low back pain.

Abbreviations
aOR: Adjusted odds ratios; BMI: Body mass index; CI: Confidence intervals; ICC: Intra-class correlation coefficient; LDD: Lumbar intervertebral disc degeneration; MODI: Modified oswestry disability index; SD: Standard deviation

Acknowledgements
A special thanks to staff of the Rheumatology Clinic, NHSL and all the patients participated in the study.

Funding
This work was funded by the University Grants Commission, Sri Lanka (UGC/ICD/2/RG2011/02/08) and the University of Colombo, Sri Lanka (AP/3/2012/PG/03).

Authors' contributions

RSP participated in the conception and design, acquisition of data, performed the statistical analysis and interpretation, and drafted the manuscript. PHD participated in the conception and design and helped to revise the manuscript. US performed the statistical analysis and interpretation and helped to draft and revise the manuscript. LSW participated in the conception and design, acquisition of data and helped to revise the manuscript. ALK participated in the conception and design, helped to perform the statistical analysis and interpretation and revised the manuscript. VHWD participated in the conception and design, helped to perform the statistical analysis and interpretation and revised the manuscript. All authors reviewed and approved the final version of the manuscript.

Competing interests

The authors declare that they have no competing interest.

Consent for publication

Not applicable.

Author details

[1]Department of Allied Health Sciences, Faculty of Medicine, University of Colombo, 25, Kynsey Road, Colombo 8, Sri Lanka. [2]Department of Anatomy, Faculty of Medical Sciences, University of Sri Jayewardenepura, Gangodawila, Nugegoda, Sri Lanka. [3]Department of Community Medicine, Faculty of Medicine, University of Colombo, 25, Kynsey Road, Colombo 8, Sri Lanka. [4]National Hospital of Sri Lanka, Colombo 10, Sri Lanka. [5]Department of Anatomy, Faculty of Medicine, University of Kelaniya, Annasihena Road, Ragama, Sri Lanka. [6]Department of Anatomy, Faculty of Medicine, University of Colombo, 25, Kynsey Road, Colombo 8, Sri Lanka.

References

1. Vos T, Flaxman AD, Naghavi M, Lozano R, Michaud C, Ezzati M, et al. Years lived with disability (YLDs) for 1160 sequelae of 289 diseases and injuries 1990-2010: a systematic analysis for the global burden of disease study 2010. Lancet. 2012;380(9859):2163–96. doi:10.1016/s0140-6736(12)61729-2.

2. North RB, Shipley J, Wang H, Mekhail N. A review of economic factors related to the delivery of health care for chronic low back pain. Neuromodulation. 2014;17 Suppl 2:69–76. doi:10.1111/ner.12057.

3. Warnakulasuriya SS, Peiris-John RJ, Coggon D, Ntani G, Sathiakumar N, Wickremasinghe AR. Musculoskeletal pain in four occupational populations in Sri Lanka. Occup Med (Lond). 2012;62(4):269–72. doi:10.1093/occmed/kqs057.

4. Lombardo SR, Vijitha De Silva P, Lipscomb HJ, Ostbye T. Musculoskeletal symptoms among female garment factory workers in Sri Lanka. Int J Occup Environ Health. 2012;18(3):210–9. doi:10.1179/1077352512z.00000000029.

5. Boos N, Weissbach S, Rohrbach H, Weiler C, Spratt KF, Nerlich AG. Classification of age-related changes in lumbar intervertebral discs: 2002 Volvo award in basic science. Spine. 2002;27(23):2631–44. doi:10.1097/01.brs.0000035304.27153.5b.

6. Deyo RA, Weinstein JN. Low back pain. N Engl J Med. 2001;344(5):363–70. doi:10.1056/NEJM200102013440508.

7. Muhogora WE, Ahmed NA, Almosabihi A, Alsuwaidi JS, Beganovic A, Ciraj-Bjelac O, et al. Patient doses in radiographic examinations in 12 countries in Asia, Africa, and eastern Europe: initial results from IAEA projects. AJR Am J Roentgenol. 2008;190(6):1453–61. doi:10.2214/ajr.07.3039.

8. Chou R, Qaseem A, Snow V, Casey D, Cross Jr JT, Shekelle P, et al. Diagnosis and treatment of low back pain: a joint clinical practice guideline from the American college of physicians and the American pain society. Ann Intern Med. 2007;147(7):478–91.

9. de Schepper EI, Damen J, van Meurs JB, Ginai AZ, Popham M, Hofman A, et al. The association between lumbar disc degeneration and low back pain: the influence of age, gender, and individual radiographic features. Spine. 2010;35(5):531–6. doi:10.1097/BRS.0b013e3181aa5b33.

10. Benneker LM, Heini PF, Anderson SE, Alini M, Ito K. Correlation of radiographic and MRI parameters to morphological and biochemical assessment of intervertebral disc degeneration. Eur Spine J. 2005;14(1):27–35. doi:10.1007/s00586-004-0759-4.

11. Modic MT, Ross JS. Lumbar degenerative disk disease. Radiology. 2007;245(1):43–61. doi:10.1148/radiol.2451051706.

12. Pye SR, Reid DM, Smith R, Adams JE, Nelson K, Silman AJ, et al. Radiographic features of lumbar disc degeneration and self-reported back pain. J Rheumatol. 2004;31(4):753–8.

13. Cho NH, Jung YO, Lim SH, Chung CK, Kim HA. The prevalence and risk factors of low back pain in rural community residents of Korea. Spine. 2012;37(24):2001–10. doi:10.1097/BRS.0b013e31825d1fa8.

14. Peterson CK, Bolton JE, Wood AR. A cross-sectional study correlating lumbar spine degeneration with disability and pain. Spine. 2000;25(2):218–23.

15. Kettler A, Wilke HJ. Review of existing grading systems for cervical or lumbar disc and facet joint degeneration. Eur Spine J. 2006;15(6):705–18. doi:10.1007/s00586-005-0954-y.

16. Muraki S, Akune T, Oka H, Ishimoto Y, Nagata K, Yoshida M, et al. Incidence and risk factors for radiographic lumbar spondylosis and lower back pain in Japanese men and women: the ROAD study. Osteoarthritis Cartilage. 2012;20(7):712–8. doi:10.1016/j.joca.2012.03.009.

17. Hicks GE, Morone N, Weiner DK. Degenerative lumbar disc and facet disease in older adults: prevalence and clinical correlates. Spine. 2009;34(12):1301–6. doi:10.1097/BRS.0b013e3181a18263.

18. Scheele J, Enthoven WT, Bierma-Zeinstra SM, Peul WC, van Tulder MW, Bohnen AM, et al. Characteristics of older patients with back pain in general practice: BACE cohort study. Eur J Pain. 2014;18(2):279–87. doi:10.1002/j.1532-2149.2013.00363.x.

19. Manek NJ, MacGregor AJ. Epidemiology of back disorders: prevalence, risk factors, and prognosis. Curr Opin Rheumatol. 2005;17(2):134–40.

20. Gerdle B, Bjork J, Henriksson C, Bengtsson A. Prevalence of current and chronic pain and their influences upon work and healthcare-seeking: a population study. J Rheumatol. 2004;31(7):1399–406.

21. Vincent HK, Omli MR, Day T, Hodges M, Vincent KR, George SZ. Fear of movement, quality of life, and self-reported disability in obese patients with chronic lumbar pain. Pain Med. 2011;12(1):154–64. doi:10.1111/j.1526-4637.2010.01011.x.

22. Lin CW, Verwoerd AJ, Maher CG, Verhagen AP, Pinto RZ, Luijsterburg PA, et al. How is radiating leg pain defined in randomized controlled trials of conservative treatments in primary care? a systematic review. Eur J Pain. 2014;18(4):455–64. doi:10.1002/j.1532-2149.2013.00384.x.

23. Kalichman L, Guermazi A, Li L, Hunter DJ. Association between age, sex, BMI and CT-evaluated spinal degeneration features. J Back Musculoskelet Rehabil. 2009;22(4):189–95. doi:10.3233/bmr-2009-0232.

24. Goode AP, Marshall SW, Renner JB, Carey TS, Kraus VB, Irwin DE, et al. Lumbar spine radiographic features and demographic, clinical, and radiographic knee, hip, and hand osteoarthritis. Arthritis Care Res (Hoboken). 2012;64(10):1536–44. doi:10.1002/acr.21720.

25. Siemionow K, An H, Masuda K, Andersson G, Cs-Szabo G. The effects of age, sex, ethnicity, and spinal level on the rate of intervertebral disc degeneration: a review of 1712 intervertebral discs. Spine. 2011;36(17):1333–9. doi:10.1097/BRS.0b013e3181f2a177.

26. Samartzis D, Karppinen J, Chan D, Luk KD, Cheung KM. The association of lumbar intervertebral disc degeneration on magnetic resonance imaging with body mass index in overweight and obese adults: a population-based study. Arthritis Rheum. 2012;64(5):1488–96. doi:10.1002/art.33462.

27. Hassett G, Hart DJ, Manek NJ, Doyle DV, Spector TD. Risk factors for progression of lumbar spine disc degeneration: the Chingford study. Arthritis Rheum. 2003;48(11):3112–7. doi:10.1002/art.11321.

28. Walker BF, Williamson OD. Mechanical or inflammatory low back pain. What are the potential signs and symptoms? Man Ther. 2009;14(3):314–20. doi:10.1016/j.math.2008.04.003.

29. Williamson A, Hoggart B. Pain: a review of three commonly used pain rating scales. J Clin Nurs. 2005;14(7):798–804. doi:10.1111/j.1365-2702.2005.01121.x.

30. Bijur PE, Latimer CT, Gallagher EJ. Validation of a verbally administered numerical rating scale of acute pain for use in the emergency department. Acad Emerg Med. 2003;10(4):390–2.

31. Jensen MP, Karoly P, Braver S. The measurement of clinical pain intensity: a comparison of six methods. Pain. 1986;27(1):117–26.

32. Fritz JM, Irrgang JJ. A comparison of a modified oswestry Low back pain disability questionnaire and the Quebec back pain disability scale. Phys Ther. 2001;81(2):776–88.

33. Fairbank JC, Pynsent PB. The oswestry disability index. Spine. 2000;25(22):2940–52. discussion 52.

34. Arambepola C, Ekanayake R, Fernando D. Gender differentials of abdominal obesity among the adults in the district of Colombo, Sri Lanka. Prev Med. 2007;44(2):129–34. doi:10.1016/j.ypmed.2006.11.004.

35. Katulanda P, Jayawardena MA, Sheriff MH, Constantine GR, Matthews DR. Prevalence of overweight and obesity in Sri Lankan adults. Obes Rev. 2010; 11(11):751–6. doi:10.1111/j.1467-789x.2010.00746.x.

36. Whitley AS, Sloane C, Hoadley G, Moore AD. Clark's Positioning in Radiography 12Ed. Boca Raton: CRC Press; 2005.

37. Lane NE, Nevitt MC, Genant HK, Hochberg MC. Reliability of new indices of radiographic osteoarthritis of the hand and hip and lumbar disc degeneration. J Rheumatol. 1993;20(11):1911–8.

38. Adams MA. Biomechanics of back pain. Acupunct Med. 2004;22(4):178–88.

39. Vining RD, Potocki E, McLean I, Seidman M, Morgenthal AP, Boysen J, et al. Prevalence of radiographic findings in individuals with chronic low back pain screened for a randomized controlled trial: secondary analysis and clinical implications. J Manipulative Physiol Ther. 2014;37(9):678–87. doi:10.1016/j.jmpt.2014.10.003.

40. Muraki S, Oka H, Akune T, Mabuchi A, En-Yo Y, Yoshida M, et al. Prevalence of radiographic lumbar spondylosis and its association with low back pain in elderly subjects of population-based cohorts: the ROAD study. Ann Rheum Dis. 2009;68(9):1401–6. doi:10.1136/ard.2007.087296.

41. Fillingim RB, Doleys DM, Edwards RR, Lowery D. Clinical characteristics of chronic back pain as a function of gender and oral opioid use. Spine. 2003;28(2):143–50. doi:10.1097/01.BRS.0000041582.00879.D3.

42. Stewart Williams J, Ng N, Peltzer K, Yawson A, Biritwum R, Maximova T, et al. Risk factors and disability associated with Low back pain in older adults in Low- and middle-income countries. Results from the WHO study on global AGEing and adult health (SAGE). PLoS One. 2015;10(6):e0127880. doi:10.1371/journal.pone.0127880.

43. Bartley EJ, Fillingim RB. Sex differences in pain: a brief review of clinical and experimental findings. Br J Anaesth. 2013;111(1):52–8. doi:10.1093/bja/aet127.

44. Chou R, Fu R, Carrino JA, Deyo RA. Imaging strategies for low-back pain: systematic review and meta-analysis. Lancet. 2009;373(9662):463–72. doi:10.1016/S0140-6736(09)60172-0.

45. Kalichman L, Hunter DJ. Diagnosis and conservative management of degenerative lumbar spondylolisthesis. Eur Spine J. 2008;17(3):327–35. doi:10.1007/s00586-007-0543-3.

16

Fat in the lumbar multifidus muscles-predictive value and change following disc prosthesis surgery and multidisciplinary rehabilitation in patients with chronic low back pain and degenerative disc

Kjersti Storheim[1,2*], Linda Berg[3,4,5,6], Christian Hellum[7], Øivind Gjertsen[8], Gesche Neckelmann[3], Ansgar Espeland[3,4], Anne Keller[9,10] and on behalf of the Norwegian Spine Study Group

Abstract

Background: Evidence is lacking on whether fat infiltration in the multifidus muscles affects outcomes after total disc replacement (TDR) surgery and if it develops after surgery. The aims of this study were 1) to investigate whether pre-treatment multifidus muscle fat infiltration predicts outcome 2 years after treatment with TDR surgery or multidisciplinary rehabilitation, and 2) to compare changes in multifidus muscle fat infiltration from pre-treatment to 2-year follow-up between the two treatment groups.

Methods: The study is secondary analysis of data from a trial with 2-year follow-up of patients with chronic low back pain (LBP) and degenerative disc randomized to TDR surgery or multidisciplinary rehabilitation. We analyzed (aim 1) patients with both magnetic resonance imaging (MRI) at pre-treatment and valid data on outcome measures at 2-year follow-up (predictor analysis), and (aim 2) patients with MRI at both pre-treatment and 2-year follow-up. Outcome measures were visual analogue scale (VAS) for LBP, Oswestry Disability Index (ODI), work status and muscle fat infiltration on MRI. Patients with pre-treatment MRI and 2-year outcome data on VAS for LBP ($n = 144$), ODI ($n = 147$), and work status ($n = 137$) were analyzed for prediction purposes. At 2-year follow-up, 126 patients had another MRI scan, and change in muscle fat infiltration was compared between the two treatment groups. Three radiologists visually quantified multifidus muscle fat in the three lower lumbar levels on MRI as <20% (grade 0), 20–50% (grade 1), or >50% (grade 2) of the muscle cross-section containing fat. Regression analysis and a mid-P exact test were carried out.

Results: Grade 0 pre-treatment multifidus muscle fat predicted better clinical results at 2-year follow-up after TDR surgery (all outcomes) but not after rehabilitation. At 2-year follow-up, increased fat infiltration was more common in the surgery group (intention-to-treat $p = 0.03$, per protocol $p = 0.08$) where it was related to worse pain and ODI.

(Continued on next page)

* Correspondence: Kjersti.storheim@medisin.uio.no
[1]Research and Communication unit for musculoskeletal disorders (FORMI), Oslo University Hospital Ullevål, Postbox 4956, Nydalen 0424, Oslo, Norway
[2]Faculty of Medicine, University of Oslo, Postbox 1078, Blindern 0316, Oslo, Norway
Full list of author information is available at the end of the article

(Continued from previous page)

Conclusions: Patients with less fat infiltration of multifidus muscles before TDR surgery had better outcomes at 2-year follow-up, but findings also indicated a negative influence of TDR surgery on back muscle morphology in some patients. The rehabilitation group maintained their muscular morphology and were unaffected by pre-treatment multifidus muscle fat.

Keywords: Multifidus muscle fat, Predictive value, Change over time, Chronic degenerative low back pain, Multidisciplinary rehabilitation, Physiotherapy, Surgery, Total disc replacement

Background

During the past 25 years, total disc replacement (TDR) surgery has become an option for selected patients with chronic low back pain (LBP) traditionally treated conservatively or with spinal fusion [1]. Randomized trials have found clinical outcome of TDR to be at least equivalent to that of fusion [2]. In the first study to compare TDR to non-surgical treatment, TDR was more effective than multidisciplinary rehabilitation at 2-year follow-up, based on patient reported outcomes like disability, pain, quality of life, and patient satisfaction [3].

A variety of muscles, including the superficial and deep layers of the paraspinal muscles, contributes to stabilization and movement of the spine [4–8]. Altered paraspinal muscle morphology – such as fat infiltration in the lumbar multifidus muscles [9] – may be related to back pain [9–15] and low physical activity [15]. Physical exercises can improve and maintain muscular fitness [16] and resistance exercise can prevent fat infiltration in skeletal muscle [17]. However, it is not clear whether such muscle alterations affect outcomes after TDR surgery. In the only previous study of this issue, less paraspinal muscle fat preoperatively was related to better results 2 years after surgery [18]. It is also unclear whether TDR surgery affects the paraspinal muscles. Surgical techniques more invasive to the back muscles (like posterior lumbar fusion) can change back muscle morphology, possibly explained by muscle denervation [19–25]. TDR surgery with anterior access is hypothesized to minimize back muscle injury and thereby prevent nerve injury and subsequent altered muscle morphology. Another possible advantage of TDR surgery is maintained mobility at the operated level, which also may be favorable for the back muscles [26].

New surgical interventions should be compared with conservative treatment [27] and the present study is an analysis of the lumbar multifidus muscles of patients included in the first randomized trial of TDR surgery with such a design [3]. Our *a priori* aims were 1) to investigate whether pre-treatment multifidus muscle fat infiltration predicts outcome 2 years after treatment with TDR surgery or multidisciplinary rehabilitation, and 2) to compare changes in fat infiltration between the two treatment groups from pre-treatment to 2-year follow-up.

Methods

This is a secondary analysis of patients included in a randomized trial evaluating the effect of surgery with disc prosthesis versus rehabilitation [3]. The trial included 173 patients who were randomized and treated with TDR surgery or multidisciplinary rehabilitation between May 2004 and September 2007: 86 were randomized to surgery and 87 to rehabilitation. Patients underwent pre-treatment magnetic resonance imaging (MRI) of the lumbar spine 0–12 months prior to inclusion and a follow-up MRI with clinical investigation 2 years after treatment. The Regional Committees for Medical Research Ethics in east Norway approved the study (43-04013) and all participants gave written informed consent. The trial was conducted in accordance with the Helsinki Declaration and the ICH-GCP guidelines and registered at www.clinicaltrial.gov under the identifier NCT 00394732.

Eligibility criteria and study sample

As detailed elsewhere [3], inclusion criteria for the main trial were age 25–55 years, LBP as the main symptom for at least 1 year, structured physiotherapy or chiropractic treatment for at least 6 months without sufficient effect, Oswestry Disability Index (ODI) ≥30%, and degenerative disc at L4/L5 and/or L5/S1 defined by the following MRI findings: A) ≥40% reduction of disc height [28] and/or B) at least two of these three findings: Modic changes type I and/or II [29], posterior high intensity zone (HIZ) in the disc [30], and dark/black nucleus pulposus on T2-weighted images (i.e. grade 2 or 3 signal intensity changes) [31]. Exclusion criteria were any of the four MRI findings in A) or B) at any higher lumbar level (L1-L4), spondylolysis, spondylolisthesis, arthritis (e.g., ankylosing spondylitis), osteoporosis, prior fracture L1-S1, prior spinal fusion, deformity, osteoporosis, symptomatic disc herniation/spinal stenosis, generalized chronic pain, ongoing psychiatric or somatic disease that excluded either one or both treatment alternatives, drug abuse, or inability to understand Norwegian.

In the present study, we analyzed: 1) patients with both a pre-treatment MRI and valid visual analogue scale (VAS) score for LBP, ODI score and data of work status at 2-year follow-up (predictor analysis), and: 2) patients with MRI at both pre-treatment and 2-year follow-up (to compare change in fat infiltration over time between treatment groups). See CONSORT flow diagram for details of patients included in these secondary analyses (Fig. 1). In the predictor analysis, patients crossing over from rehabilitation to TDR surgery during the 2-year follow-up period were analyzed in the surgical group, and patients randomized to surgery who refused surgery and underwent rehabilitation were analyzed in the rehabilitation group according to as-treated principles. Patients not

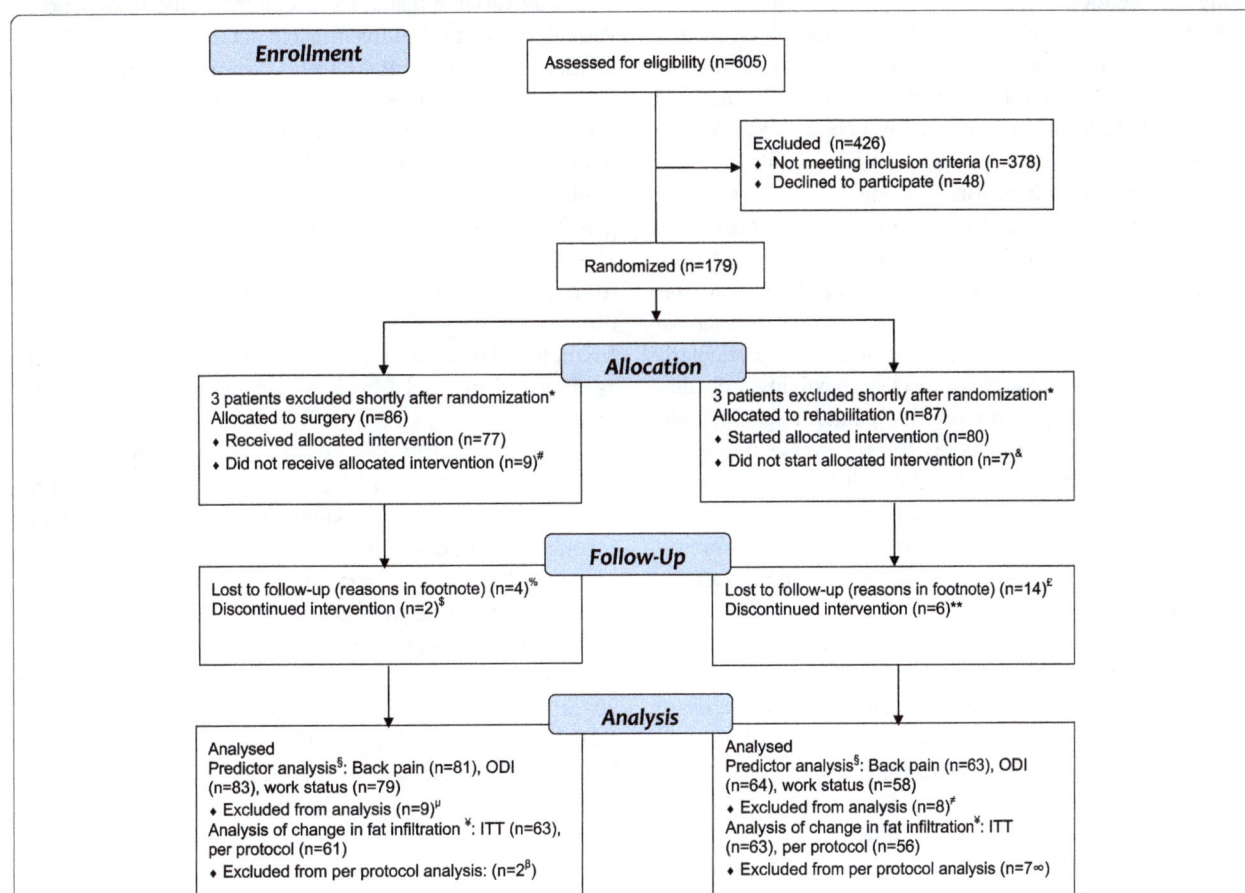

Fig. 1 CONSORT flow diagram. * Heart attack some days after randomization ($n = 1$), obvious exclusion criterion discovered some days after randomization (earlier large abdominal operation ($n = 1$)), degenerative change insufficient to satisfy inclusion criteria ($n = 2$) or present in more than two lower lumbar discs ($n = 2$)). # Changed their mind and declined surgery after randomization (3 had social reasons for not receiving treatment, 1 had work related economic reasons, and 5 wanted guaranteed success). & Changed their mind after randomization and did not attend the rehabilitation program (2 had work-related economic reasons, 1 was treated elsewhere with surgery for lumbar disc herniation, 1 had social reasons, and 2 needed to travel long distances/could not stay away from home). % Dropped out after total disc replacement (TDR) surgery (1 had serious complications with a vascular injury and leg amputation, 2 did not want to attend the follow-up and 1 could not be contacted after surgery). £ 6 patients dropped out during the rehabilitation program (1 did not find the program good enough, 1 had lumbar disc herniation during treatment and underwent microdiscectomi, 1 did not manage to go through the training program, 1 developed diabetes during or just before treatment, 1 had psychosocial reasons, and 1 had hypertension and the family doctor did not recommend training), 8 dropped out after completing the treatment (1 took part in another study, 1 patient did not complete the questionnaire, 1 patient moved, 1 patient died of cancer, 3 did not want to attend the follow-up, and there was 1 for whom the reason was unknown). $ Two patients underwent surgery with instrumented fusion before 2-year follow-up. ** One patient crossed over to surgery between 6 months and 1 year and five patients between 1 year and 2 years. Five patients underwent TDR surgery and one patient fusion. § Subjects relevant for analysis were patients with both a pre-treatment MRI and valid score for back pain, Oswestry Disability Index (ODI) score and data on work status at 2-year follow-up. Patients randomized to rehabilitation who crossed over and underwent TDR surgery before 2-year follow-up within ($n = 5$) or outside ($n = 5$) the study setting are analyzed in the surgery group, patients who refused TDR surgery and underwent rehabilitation were analyzed in the rehabilitation group ($n = 2$), according to as-treated principles. μ Refused surgery ($n = 7$), re-operated upon with a fusion ($n = 2$). ‡ Did not start the rehabilitation program ($n = 7$), received a primary fusion ($n = 1$). ¥ Randomized design (RCT) includes patients with MRI at both pre-treatment and 2-year follow-up. β Re-operated upon with a fusion. ∞ Crossed over to surgery ($n = 5$ to TDR and $n = 1$ to fusion), did not complete the rehabilitation program ($n = 1$)

undergoing allocated interventions and patients operated upon with a fusion were excluded from the predictor analysis. When comparing change in fat infiltration over time between treatment groups, all available patients were examined according to the intention-to-treat (ITT) analysis, but in a secondary per protocol analysis we excluded patients deviating from the study protocol (Fig. 1).

Study interventions

Interventions have been described in detail elsewhere [3]. *The rehabilitation intervention* was based on the treatment model described by Brox et al and consisted of supervised physical exercise with a cognitive approach [32]. Patients were treated in groups by a multidisciplinary team of physiotherapists and specialists in physical medicine and rehabilitation (plus other professions if required) at the hospitals' outpatient clinics for about 60 h over 3–5 weeks / 12–15 days. The multidisciplinary rehabilitation program included general exercise for increasing overall fitness (cardiovascular, strength (particularly thighs, back- and abdominal muscles), flexibility, coordination, body awareness and relaxation), and for specific individual needs (strength (including the transverse abdominal muscles and multifidus muscles, flexibility, endurance, etc.). Examples of general exercise are group exercise accompanied by music ("Aerobics"), circuit training, swimming / water games, biking, Nordic walking, treadmill walking, cross country skiing and games (i.e. ball games). Patients had two or three workout sessions per treatment day, at least one "heavy" and one "light" and one group based and one individual session. Intensity was gradually increased during the rehabilitation period. Physiotherapists supervised most exercise, but patients were also encouraged to exercise by themselves at home and after ended rehabilitation period. Overall goal for the training was to increase patients' belief and confidence in being able to perform daily activities of life and to increase functional capacity although the back may hurt. *The surgical intervention* was replacement of the degenerative intervertebral lumbar disc with an artificial lumbar disc (ProDisc II, Synthes Spine). There were no major postoperative restrictions and patients were not referred for postoperative physiotherapy, but at 6-week follow-up they could be referred for physiotherapy if required (emphasizing general mobilization and exercise). All patients were treated within 3 months after randomization.

Measurement of outcomes and possible predictors

The only variable tested for predictive value (independent variable) was multifidus muscle fat on MRI. MRI performed at the different trial sites typically included sagittal T1- and T2-weighted images and axial images of the three lower lumbar levels (T2-, T1-, and/or proton density-weighted); image characteristics are given in Table 1. Typically, slice thickness was 3 – 5 mm, interslice gap 0 – 1.4 mm, field of view 28 – 35 cm for sagittal and 17 – 30 cm for axial images, and matrix 512×512 (varied from 160×256 to 1024×1024). The images were obtained directly in Digital Imaging and Communications in Medicine (DICOM) format or, for seven examinations, as digitized printed film hard copies stored in DICOM format.

Fat in the multifidus muscles was visually graded at levels L3/L4, L4/L5 and L5/S1 using the axial T2-weighted image (T1 if T2 was lacking) closest to an axial plane through the mid-sagittal posterior and anterior caudal corners of the upper vertebrae. The grading was based on the criteria used by Kjaer et al [9], but adjusted as recommended by Solgaard-Sørensen et al [33]: 0 = 0 or < 20% of total cross-section (left plus right side) contains fat, 1 = 20–50% of cross-section contains fat, 2= >50% of cross-section contains fat (Fig. 2). One radiologist, experienced in musculoskeletal MRI (reader A), and two neuroradiologists (readers B and C) from three different institutions evaluated the images independently, retrospectively, and blinded to clinical data. Each reader had more than 10 years' experience in MRI of the lumbar spine. Readers A and B evaluated the images using the eFilm Lite software version 2.1.2 (Merge Healthcare, Hartland,

Table 1 Magnetic resonance imaging characteristics

Characteristics	Predictor analysis (137 patients, 137 examinations)	Analysis of change in fat infiltration (126 patients, 252 examinations)
1.5 T	121 / 137 examinations (88%)	235 / 252 examinations (93%)
Sagittal T1-weighted images	128 / 137: FSE (TR / TE, 350 – 911 ms / 7.4 – 20 ms) 8 / 137: FLAIR images (TR / TE, 1984 – 2130 ms / 20 – 22.1 ms)	244 / 252 FSE (TR / TE, 360 – 911 ms / 7 – 22 ms) 7 / 252 FLAIR images (TR / TE, 1984 – 2130 ms / 20 – 22 ms)
Sagittal T2-weighted images	136 / 137 FSE (TR / TE, 2511 – 4760 ms / 70 – 140 ms)	251[a] / 252 FSE (TR / TE, 2000 – 5070 ms / 70 – 140 ms) and/or DRIVE images (FSE with 90° Flip-Back Pulse: TR / TE 700 ms / 135 – 140 ms): 236 FSE only (126 pre-treatment and 110 2-year) 12 DRIVE only (all 2-year), and 3 both FSE and DRIVE (all 2-year)
Axial images at L3/L4, L4/L5 and L5/S1	134 / 137 (105 T2-weighted, 27 T1-weighted, and 19 proton density-weighted images)	247 / 252 (213 T2-weighted, 31 T1-weighted, and 19 proton density-weighted images)

TR repetition time, *TE* echo time, *FLAIR* fluid-attenuated inversion-recovery, *FSE* fast spin echo
[a]one examination lacked sagittal T2-weighted FSE images at 2 years but included sagittal STIR (short tau inversion-recovery) images

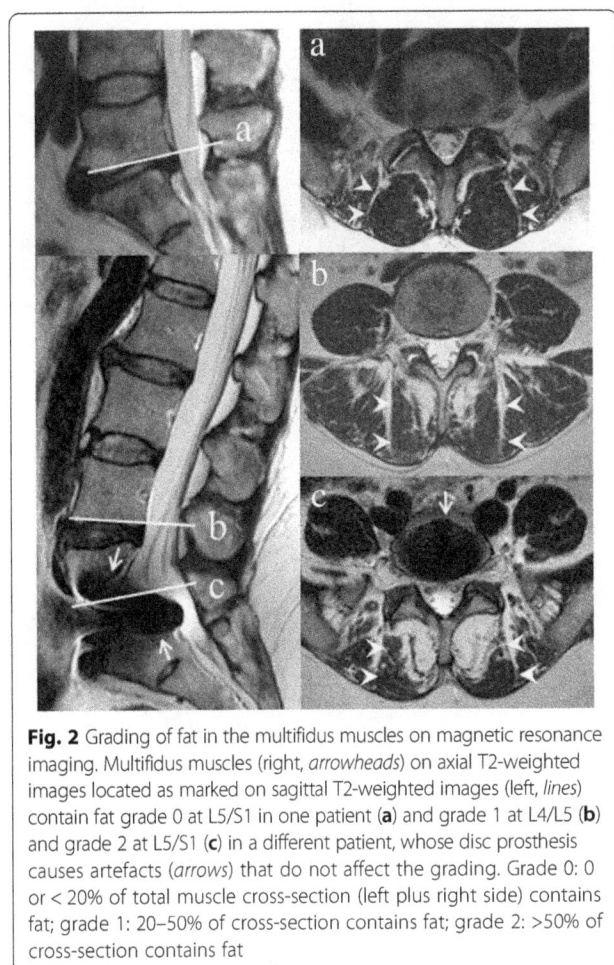

Fig. 2 Grading of fat in the multifidus muscles on magnetic resonance imaging. Multifidus muscles (right, *arrowheads*) on axial T2-weighted images located as marked on sagittal T2-weighted images (left, *lines*) contain fat grade 0 at L5/S1 in one patient (**a**) and grade 1 at L4/L5 (**b**) and grade 2 at L5/S1 (**c**) in a different patient, whose disc prosthesis causes artefacts (*arrows*) that do not affect the grading. Grade 0: 0 or < 20% of total muscle cross-section (left plus right side) contains fat; grade 1: 20–50% of cross-section contains fat; grade 2: >50% of cross-section contains fat

Wisconsin), while reader C used the Agfa Impax 4.5 (Agfa HealthCare, Mortsel, Belgium). The images were anonymized and presented in random order.

Readers B and C independently graded pre-treatment fat in the lumbar multifidus muscles [9, 33] (kappa 0.42–0.51 for interobserver agreement on grade 0 versus grade 1 or 2 at L3/L4, L4/L5, and L5/S1 in the original sample of 170 MRIs). When a grading was agreed upon it was considered to be conclusive; otherwise the majority or median grading by readers A, B, and C determined the conclusive grading. The conclusive grade was 0 at all levels in 45.3% of the patients and 2 at one level in one patient; hence, patients were dichotomized as having grade 0 muscle fat at all evaluated levels versus grade 1 or 2 muscle fat at any level.

Change in fat in the multifidus muscles was rated by comparing the 2-year follow-up and the pre-treatment images. Any progress or regress of at least one grading category was reported. Readers A and B independently evaluated the images (the prevalence- and bias-adjusted kappa, used due to low prevalence of change, was 0.57 – 0.97 and indicated moderate to very good interobserver agreement on progress or not at L3/L4, L4/L5, and L5/S1

in the 126 patients studied). When reader A and B disagreed, reader C independently rated the actual level(s), and the majority or median rating was used.

Outcome measures (dependent variables) in the predictor analysis were pain, back specific function and work status at 2-year follow-up. Pain (LBP during the preceding week) was measured by a horizontal VAS, ranging from 0 to 100 mm with respective end anchors "no pain" and "worst pain imaginable" [34]. Back specific function was evaluated by the Norwegian ODI version 2.0 [35, 36]. The ODI ranges from 0 to 100, with a lower score indicating less severe disability. Work status at 2-year follow-up was obtained from the patients and from the National Insurance of employees and categorized into working/not working (working part or full time, being a student or homemaker = working).

Possible effect moderators: to test if the predictive value of fat in the multifidus muscles is influenced by effect moderators, the following other variables were controlled for (based on literature search): age, gender, leisure time physical activity [37], body mass index (BMI), and smoking. These data were collected at baseline.

Statistical analysis

All data were analyzed using SPSS (version 18, SPSS Inc., Chicago, IL, USA). Dependent and independent variables and possible effect moderators were selected *a priori* before statistical analysis commenced. Patients were analyzed according to as-treated-principles in the predictor analysis and according to randomization (ITT) when comparing change in fat infiltration over time between treatment groups. A Chi-Square Test (Continuity Correction) was used to compare groups at baseline (proportion of patients with grade 0 *versus* grade 1 or 2 pre-treatment fat in the lumbar multifidus muscles) and to compare work status at baseline and at 2-year follow-up between patients with grade 0 *versus* grade 1 or 2 muscle fat in each treatment group. An independent-samples t-test (two-tailed) was used to compare pain and ODI at baseline and at 2 year follow-up between patients with grade 0 *versus* grade 1 or 2 fat in each treatment group.

Multiple regression analysis (linear) was carried out with pain and ODI as dependent variables, and logistic regression analysis was conducted with work status as dependent variable. The models were adjusted for age (years), gender, BMI, current smoking (yes/no), and leisure time physical activity [37] (grade 0–3), and assessed for normality, homoscedasticity, and collinearity by residuals and variance inflation factor (VIF). In addition, we adjusted for baseline pain in analysis of pain at 2 years as a dependent variable, and baseline ODI in analysis of ODI at 2 years as a dependent variable.

The Mid-P exact test was used to compare change in fat infiltration over time between treatment groups [38].

Table 2 Patient characteristics at baseline

	Predictor analysis ($n = 147$)	Analysis of change in fat infiltration ($n = 126$)
Age (mean (SD))	41.0 (7.2)	41.6 (7.1)
Gender (women (n %))	77 (52.4)	65 (51.6)
BMI (mean (SD))	25.3 (3.2)	25.4 (3.2)
Current smoker (n % yes)	66 (44.9)	58 (46.0)
Previous back surgery (n % yes)[a]	44 (29.9)	37 (29.4)
Work status [b] (n % working)	31 (21.1)	25 (19.8)
Duration of back pain, years (mean (SD))	6.3 (5.9)	6.5 (6.1)
Daily consumption of opioids (n % yes)	34 (23.1)	30 (23.8)
ODI score, 0-100[c] (mean (SD))	42.3 (9.0)	41.8 (8.4)
EQ-5D index, -0.59–1[d] (mean (SD))	0.28 (0.30)	0.28 (0.30)
HSCL-25, 1-4[c] (mean (SD))	1.80 (0.51)	1.81 (0.50)
FABQ-physical, 0-24[c] (mean (SD))	13.2 (5.6)	13.3 (5.4)
FABQ-work, 0-42[c] (mean (SD))	26.5 (10.6)	26.0 (10.4)
Back Pain, 0-100[c] (mean (SD))	70.0 (14.9)	69.4 (15.0)
Leg Pain, 0-100[c] (mean (SD))	44.5 (26.8)	47.0 (25.7)

BMI body mass index (weight in kilograms divided by height in meters squared), *ODI* Oswestry Disability Index, EQ-5D = EuroQol-5 Dimensions, *HSCL-25* Hopkins Symptom Checklist, *FABQ* Fear Avoidance Beliefs Questionnaire

[a]There were no differences in fat infiltration between patients with/without previous back surgery

[b]Working versus not working; including part-time work as working

[c]Lower scores indicate less severe symptoms

[d]Higher scores indicate better quality of life

Changes were collapsed into reduced fat infiltration or no change *versus* increased fat infiltration (≥ 1 grade at 1 or more levels). A per protocol analysis excluding patients deviating from the study protocol was also conducted.

All *P* values are 2-sided and the significance level was 5%. No formal power calculation was conducted since the present study is a secondary analysis of patients included in a randomized controlled trial and therefore has a fixed sample size.

Results

Out of 173 patients included in the original trial (of 605 patients screened for eligibility) [3], in these secondary predictor analyzes 144, 147, and 137 patients had pre-treatment MRI and valid 2-year data on back pain, ODI, and work status, respectively (Fig. 1). For comparing change in fat infiltration over time between treatment

groups, 126 patients had MRI at both pre-treatment and 2-year follow-up and were included in the ITT analysis, and 117 were included in the per protocol analysis. Patients included in the predictor analyzes and in the between groups analysis of change in fat infiltration over time were similar at baseline (Table 2); mean age about 45 years with chronic LBP for well over 6 years, BMI just above the limit for normal weight, and ODI-score of about 42 points on average. Only 20% were gainfully employed.

Results for grading of pre-treatment fat in the multifidus muscles are shown in Tables 3 and 4. Almost half of the patients, 67 (45.6%) included in the predictor analysis and 59 (46.8%) of patients analyzed for change in fat infiltration over time, had fat grade 0 in the multifidus muscles at any evaluated level, about 5% had $\geq 20\%$ fat in all three levels (Table 4). In only one patient at one level did >50% of the muscle cross-section (left plus

Table 3 Visual grading of fat in the multifidus muscles in the two analysis- / treatment groups by level at pre-treatment

	Predictor analysis ($n = 147$)						Analysis of change in fat infiltration ($n = 126$)					
	Rehab ($n = 64$)			Surgery ($n = 83$)			Rehab ($n = 63$)			Surgery ($n = 63$)		
Grade[a]	0	1	2	0	1	2	0	1	2	0	1	2
L3/L4 (n / %)	60 (93.8)	4 (6.3)	0 (0)	77 (92.8)	6 (7.2)	0 (0)	60 (95.2)	3 (4.8)	0 (0)	58 (92.1)	5 (7.9)	0 (0)
L4/L5 (n / %)	48 (75.0)	16 (25.0)	0 (0)	61 (73.5)	22 (26.5)	0 (0)	47 (74.6)	16 (25.4)	0 (0)	49 (77.8)	14 (22.2)	0 (0)
L5/S1 (n / %)	33 (51.6)	31 (48.4)	0 (0)	36 (43.4)	46 (55.4)	1 (1.2)	32 (50.8)	31 (49.2)	0 (0)	29 (46.0)	33 (52.4)	1 (1.6)

[a]Grading according to the criteria Kjaer et al [9] and Solgaard et al [31]: Grade 0: 0 or <20% of total cross-section (left plus right side) contains fat, Grade 1: 20%–50% of cross-section (left plus right side) contains fat, Grade 2: >50% of cross-section (left plus right side) contains fat

Table 4 Number of levels registered with fat (grade 1 or 2) in the multifidus muscles at pre-treatment in the two analysis- / treatment groups

	Predictor analysis (n = 147)		Analysis of change in fat infiltration (n = 126)	
	Rehab (n = 64)	Surgery (n = 83)	Rehab (n = 63)	Surgery (n = 63)
0 levels with fat (n / %)	31 (48.4)	36 (43.4)	30 (47.6)	29 (46.0)
1 level with fat (Grade[a] 1 or 2; n / %)	18 (28.1)	24 (28.9)	18 (28.6)	19 (30.2)
2 levels with fat (Grade[a] 1 or 2; n / %)	12 (18.8)	18 (21.7)	13 (20.6)	11 (17.5)
3 levels with fat (Grade[a] 1 or 2; n / %)	3 (4.7)	5 (6.0)	2 (3.2)	4 (6.3)

[a]Grading according to the criteria by Kjaer et al [9] and Solgaard et al [31]: Grade 0: 0 or < 20% of total cross-section (left plus right side) contains fat, Grade 1: 20%–50% of cross-section (left plus right side) contains fat, Grade 2: >50% of cross-section (left plus right side) contains fat

right side) contain fat (Table 3). Fat was more common at the lower levels. Patients analyzed in the rehabilitation group and in the surgical group did not differ in presence of (yes/no), or number of levels of, pre-treatment multifidus muscle fat (valid for both predictor analysis and between groups analysis of change in fat over time).

In explorative comparison of baseline and 2-year clinical outcome (pain, ODI, work status) between patients with grade 0 versus grade 1–2 pre-treatment multifidus muscle fat in the two treatment groups, patients in the surgical group with fat grade 0 had better 2 year values for ODI and work status (but not pain). No such findings were seen in the rehabilitation group (Table 5). Unadjusted regression analysis revealed that patients with grade 0 pre-treatment multifidus muscle fat in the surgery group had significantly better ODI and work status after 2 years. Further strengthening this finding, grade 0 pre-treatment muscle fat was significantly related to lower pain scores in the surgery group at 2-year follow-up after adjusting for age, gender, BMI, smoking, and leisure time physical activity (and baseline pain/ODI in analysis of 2-year pain/ODI as dependent variable). The regression analysis showed no significant results for patients treated with rehabilitation (Tables 6 and 7).

Analysis of normality, homoscedasticity, collinearity, and VIFs did not reveal any violation of these factors to the assumptions of the models.

More patients had increased multifidus muscle fat in the surgical group at 2-year follow-up than in the rehabilitation group (11.1%, 7 of 63 patients vs. 1.6%, 1 of 63 patients, $p = 0.03$, Mid-P exact test, 2x2 table for increase versus reduction or no change; raw data shown in Table 8). The difference remained but was not significant ($p = 0.08$) in the per protocol analysis. Explorative analysis revealed that clinical outcomes in the surgery group at 2-year follow-up were worse for patients with increased multifidus muscle fat versus those without (Table 9). The differences remained significant for pain ($p < 0.01$) and ODI ($p = 0.03$) in the per protocol analysis. Another explorative analysis showed that the difference in pain and ODI was present already 6 weeks postoperatively (data not shown, $p = 0.06$ (pain) and $p < 0.01$ (ODI), independent-sample t-test).

Discussion

This study on multifidus muscle fat had three main findings. First, less fat on pre-treatment MRI predicted better 2-year clinical outcomes after TDR surgery (i.e.

Table 5 Exploring pain, ODI, and work status in patients with grade 0 versus grade 1–2 multifidus muscle fat in patients included in the predictor analysis[a]

	Rehabilitation			Surgery		
	Grade 0 fat at pre-treatment (n = 31)	Fat grad 1-2 at pre-treatment (n = 33)	p-value	Grade 0 fat at pre-treatment (n = 36)	Fat grade 1-2 at pre-treatment (n = 47)	p-value
Pain baseline (mean (SD))	75.1 (11.7)	70.8 (14.2)	0.19*	70.5 (15.6)	65.5 (15.8)	0.16*
Pain 2 year (mean (SD))	50.4 (28.9)	42.8 (26.5)	0.29*	25.9 (28.2)	33.3 (27.1)	0.24*
ODI baseline (mean (SD))	42.8 (8.6)	41.8 (8.0)	0.65*	40.0 (8.0)	44.1 (10.6)	0.05*
ODI 2 year (mean (SD))	28.9 (15.1)	25.5 (12.3)	0.33*	15.0 (17.1)	22.4 (14.6)	0.04*
Work status baseline (n / % working)	4 (12.9)	7 (21.2)	0.51#	12 (33.3)	8 (17.4)	0.12#
Work status 2 year (n / % working)	15 (48.4)	11 (33.3)	0.11#	24 (72.7)	22 (46.8)	0.04#

ODI Oswestry Disability Index
*Independent-samples t-test
#Chi-Square Test (Continuity Correction)
[a]n = 144 for pain, n = 147 for ODI, n = 137 for work status

Table 6 Multiple regression analysis (unadjusted and adjusted) of effect of grade 1–2 pre-treatment multifidus muscle fat on pain and ODI at 2 years in each treatment group

		Pain			ODI		
		B	95% CI for β	p-value	B	95% CI for β	p-value
Rehab (n = 63 (pain)/64 (ODI))	Unadjusted	-7.56	-21.56–6.45	0.29	-3.36	-10.23–3.51	0.33
	Adjusted[a]	-5.93	-25.18–13.31	0.54	-1.49	-10.46–7.48	0.74
Surgery (n = 81 (pain)/83 (ODI))	Unadjusted	7.40	-4.93–19.73	0.24	7.35	0.40–14.29	0.04
	Adjusted[a]	15.36	0.92–29.79	0.04	10.39	2.50–18.28	0.01

ODI Oswestry Disability Index

[a]The model is adjusted for age, gender, body mass index, smoking, and leisure time physical activity. In addition, the model for 2-year pain is adjusted for baseline pain, and the model for 2-year ODI is adjusted for baseline ODI

more fat predicted worse outcomes). Second, more patients had increased fat at 2-year follow-up in the surgery group than in the rehabilitation group. Third, increased fat at 2-year follow-up was related to a less favorable clinical outcome in the surgical group.

Discussion of findings

Less pre-treatment multifidus muscle fat was also related to a better clinical result (lower ODI, i.e. better function) at 2-year follow-up after TDR surgery in the only former study on this issue [18]. This indicates that less multifidus muscle fat is favorable prior to TDR surgery. Exercise can prevent fat infiltration of other muscles [17] and might perhaps help to prevent multifidus muscle fat as well. Exercise science states that muscular strength reduces the risk of developing functional limitations [39]. A recent report lists no and low physical activity as risk factors for disability [40]. Further, low physical activity is found to be associated with fat in the multifidus muscles in a dose-dependent manner [15]. Presence of pre-treatment fat may indicate physical inactivity not caught by our categorical leisure time physical activity variable controlled for in the analysis. Less favorable clinical outcome in patients with grade 1 or 2 pre-treatment fat in the surgical group might also be caused by pain-induced alterations of paraspinal morphology not solved by surgery. It is hypothesized that pain-induced muscular alterations is caused by long-loop inhibition of the multifidus together with a combination of reflex inhibition and substitution patterns

of the trunk muscles [10]. Localized multifidus morphology changes corresponding to painful levels has been described previously [10–12]. Similar hypotheses are postulated for other muscle groups [41–43].

Lack of structured post-operative rehabilitation and possible post-operative inactivity may partly explain why increased multifidus muscle fat at 2-year follow up was more common in the surgery group than in the rehabilitation group. The surgery group did not receive post-operative rehabilitation by routine and may have tended to remain inactive, whereas the rehabilitation group received comprehensive general and specific functional and muscular restoration and was encouraged to continue exercising and being active after the rehabilitation program ended [3, 32]. This may also explain maintenance of muscle morphology in all but one patient in the rehabilitation group. Exercises have proved useful for maintaining and improving muscle condition in patients with LBP [11, 20, 44–46]. Additionally, the surgery itself may have induced muscular alterations. Biomarkers have indicated general muscle atrophy following surgery [47] and atrophy of back muscles has been reported after lumbar interbody fusion surgery [22, 24, 25]. Another explanation may be neuromuscular deficits as reported following other surgical techniques that cause minimal muscle damage [41, 42]. Our finding of increased multifidus muscle fat in the surgery group at 2-year follow-up should be assessed in further studies, also because all increases in fat infiltration were of only one grade (from grade 0 to grade 1, or grade 1 to grade 2; footnote Table 8). The finding was weakened in the per protocol analysis, perhaps due to few cases (*n* = 7) with increased fat.

Our explorative analyses indicated that increased multifidus muscle fat in the surgical group at follow-up was related to a worse clinical outcome. Interestingly, the difference in pain and ODI reported at 2-year follow-up between patients with and without increased fat in the surgery group is considerable (33.8 mm for pain and 25.8 points for ODI respectively, Table 9) and well above suggested limits for clinically important outcomes for differences in pain (20 mm) and ODI (10 points) [48].

Table 7 Logistic regression model (unadjusted and adjusted) predicting likelihood of working at 2 years in each treatment group

		p-value	B	OR	95% CI for OR	
					Lower	Upper
Rehab (n = 58)	Unadjusted	0.08	0.957	2.603	0.896	7.563
	Adjusted[a]	0.25	0.779	2.179	0.575	8.261
Surgery (n = 79)	Unadjusted	0.03	1.068	2.909	1.114	7.598
	Adjusted[a]	0.03	1.357	3.886	1.107	13.638

OR odds ratio, *CI* confidence interval

[a]The model is adjusted for age, gender, body mass index, smoking, and leisure time physical activity

Table 8 Change in multifidus muscle fat in the two treatment groups from pre-treatment to 2-year follow-up

	Rehabilitation (n = 63)	Surgery (n = 63)
Improvement in 1 level	1[a]	0
No change	61	56
Deterioration in 1 level	1[b]	5[c]
Deterioration in 2 levels	0	2[d]

[a]Change from grad 1 to grade 0
[b]Change from grade 0 to grade 1
[c]All changes were from grade 0 to grade 1
[d]One patient changed from grade 0 to grade 1 in two levels, one patient changed from grade 0 to grade 1 in one level and from grade 1 to grade 2 in one level

The worse pain being present already 6 weeks postoperatively may have contributed to increased muscular alterations [10, 12, 25, 41–43]. Again, since only 7 patients in the surgery group had increased fat, these results should be interpreted with caution and ought to be re-examined in further studies. Still it is possible that severe pain and reduced mobility among these few patients led to increased fat infiltration.

Strengths and limitations

MRI is a valid method for evaluating muscle fat infiltration [49]. In our study, three experienced radiologists blinded to clinical data performed independent evaluations so that none of them had undue influence on the results [50]. The interobserver agreement was only moderate but the use of multiple readers likely increased the consistency of the conclusive ratings compared to studies with a single reader [51]. The direct comparison of post- and pre-treatment images, as in routine clinical practice, is the preferred method for evaluating changes in MRI findings over time [52–54]. It may reduce erroneous rating of changes due to ambiguous findings or minor differences in MRI technique, and can provide a more reliable rating (moderate to very good interobserver agreement) than separate evaluations of post- and pre-treatment images [52]. We used MRI rather than computed tomography, since MRI is without radiation exposure and can provide better soft tissue resolution and contrast and slightly more reliable muscle evaluations [55]. Muscle fat was graded visually also in former studies [9, 18]. However, single-voxel proton MR spectroscopy

detects smaller fat amounts not visible on conventional MRI; this method identified more fat in the multifidus muscles in chronic LBP patients than in asymptomatic volunteers, despite no difference was seen on conventional MRI [49]. Hence, results might have differed had we used alternative or more sophisticated fat evaluation methods.

The study had a well-defined sample of patients with chronic non-specific LBP and localized MRI findings, and it included the three most important outcome variables for evaluating LBP patients [56, 57]. The follow-up rate was fair: 79–85% (137-147/173) had 2-year data for the predictor analysis and 73% (126/173) had data for comparing change in fat infiltration over time between treatment groups. Our study design allowed, for the first time within the field, comparisons of MRI findings between patients treated with and without surgery. According to the literature, the length of follow-up is sufficient to evaluate change in muscle morphology over time [16]. Our regression models included only one candidate predictor, five other variables, and ≥137 patients (the adjusted models lacked data on some variables). The models were therefore well within the recommended limit of at least ten observations for each exposure variable studied [58]. The decision to analyze patients according to as-treated-principles in the predictor analysis was based on our *a priori* decided research questions. We could have analyzed patients in a single merged cohort and controlled for treatment group in the regression models, but this procedure may be more relevant with multiple clinical questions. We could also have controlled for other potential effect moderators, as we know that diabetes mellitus and cardiovascular disease can affect muscle fat [59, 60], but only 20% of patients had comorbidities. We could not compare muscle fat to muscle function, which was not tested. The significance level of 0.05 in multiple explorative analyses implied a risk of wrong conclusions. Finally, smaller differences and changes in muscle fat (and perhaps more convincing associations) might have been detected if more categories (or a continuous measure) of fat had been used and/or MRI to assess fat had been performed more than once during the follow-up period.

Table 9 Clinical outcome at 2-year follow-up in the surgery group for patients with increased multifidus muscle fat *versus* those without

	No change in multifidus muscle fat	Increased multifidus fat in 1 or 2 levels	p-value
Pain at 2 year (mean (SD)) (n = 54/7)	29.2 (26.2)	63.0 (33.5)	<0.01*
ODI at 2 year (mean (SD)) (n = 56/7)	16.8 (14.2)	42.6 (20.3)	<0.001*
Work status at 2 year (n/ % working) (n = 55/6)	36 (65.5)	1 (16.7)	0.03#

ODI, Oswestry Disability Index
*Independent-sample t-test
#Mid-P exact test

Potential implications

Better outcome for patients with less multifidus muscle fat before treatment may be a result of a better starting point and a clinical implication could be that patients scheduled for TDR surgery should optimize their back muscle condition before surgery. Since we found worse outcome in patients with increased muscle fat at 2-year follow-up after TDR surgery, postoperative rehabilitation may also be relevant. This may be supported by a study of patients receiving back fusion [61] and may be especially relevant for those with substantial postoperative back pain. However, our findings should be re-examined in further studies.

Conclusions

In this secondary analysis of data from a randomized trial comparing clinical efficacy of multidisciplinary rehabilitation versus TDR surgery, patients with less fat infiltration of multifidus muscles before TDR surgery had better outcomes at 2-year follow-up. Our findings also indicated a negative influence of TDR surgery on back muscle morphology in some patients. The rehabilitation group maintained their muscular morphology and were unaffected by pre-treatment multifidus muscle fat.

Abbreviations

BMI: Body mass index; DICOM: Digital Imaging and Communications in Medicine; HIZ: High intensity zone; ITT: Intention-to-treat; LBP: Low back pain; MRI: Magnetic resonance imaging; ODI: Oswestry Disability Index; TDR: Total disc replacement; VAS: Visual analogue scale

Acknowledgements

Many thanks to the patients who participated in the study and to all our colleagues in The Norwegian Spine Study Group.
The Norwegian Spine study Group:
University Hospital North Norway, Tromsø: Odd-Inge Solem department of orthopaedic surgery), Jens Munch-Ellingsen (department of neurosurgery), and Franz Hintringer, Anita Dimmen Johansen, Guro Kjos (department of physical medicine and rehabilitation).
Trondheim University Hospital, Trondheim: Øystein P Nygaard, Lars Gunnar Johnsen, Ivar Rossvoll, Hege Andresen, Helge Rønningen, Kjell Arne Kvistad (national centre for spinal disorders, department of neurosurgery), Magne Rø, Bjørn Skogstad, Janne Birgitte Børke, Erik Nordtvedt, Gunnar Leivseth (multidiscipline spinal unit, department of physical medicine and rehabilitation).
Haukeland University Hospital, Bergen: Sjur Braaten, Turid Rognsvåg, Gunn Odil Hirth Moberg (Kysthospitalet in Hagevik, department of orthopaedic surgery), Jan Sture Skouen, Lars Geir Larsen, Vibeche Iversen, Ellen H Haldorsen, Elin Karin Johnsen, Kristin Hannestad (Outpatient Spine Clinic, department of physical medicine and rehabilitation).
Stavanger University Hospital, Stavanger: Endre Refsdal (department of orthopaedic surgery).
Oslo University Hospital, Oslo: Oliver Grundnes, Jens Ivar Brox, Vegard Slettemoen, Kenneth Nilsen, Kjersti Sunde, Helenè E Skaara (department of orthopaedics), Berit Johannessen, Anna Maria Eriksdotter (department of physical medicine and rehabilitation).
We also want to thank Eira Kathleen Ebbs for help with the language.

Funding

This work received financial support from the Norwegian Fund for Post-Graduate Training in Physiotherapy, the South Eastern Norway Regional Health Authority, the Western Norway Regional Health Authority, Haakon and Sigrun Ødegaard's Fund at the Norwegian Society of Radiology.

Authors' contributions

KS, LB, CH, ØG, GN, AE and AK have contributed to the conception and design of the study, interpretation of data, revision of the manuscript and approval of the final draft. KS was the major contributor in writing the manuscript. LB, ØG, GN and AE interpreted all MRI scans. KS performed the statistical analysis. All authors read and approved the final manuscript.

Competing interests

The authors declare that they have no competing interests.

Consent for publication

All participants gave written informed consent. The consent stated that clinical data collected would be used for the publication of research reports. All presented data are anonymized and risk of identification is low.

Author details

[1]Research and Communication unit for musculoskeletal disorders (FORMI), Oslo University Hospital Ullevål, Postbox 4956, Nydalen 0424, Oslo, Norway. [2]Faculty of Medicine, University of Oslo, Postbox 1078, Blindern 0316, Oslo, Norway. [3]Department of Radiology, Haukeland University Hospital, Postbox 1400, 5021 Bergen, Norway. [4]Section for Radiology, Department of Clinical Medicine, University of Bergen, Postbox 7804, N-5020 Bergen, Norway. [5]Department of Radiology, Nordland Hospital, Postbox 1480, 8092 Bodø, Norway. [6]Institute of Clinical Medicine, UiT, The Arctic University of Norway, Postbox 6050, Langnes 9037, Tromsø, Norway. [7]Department of Orthopaedics, Oslo University Hospital Ullevål, Postbox 4956, Nydalen 0424, Oslo, Norway. [8]Department of Radiology and Nuclearmedicine, Oslo University Hospital Rikshospitalet, Postbox 4950, Nydalen 0424, Oslo, Norway. [9]Department of Physical Medicine and Rehabilitation, Oslo University Hospital Ullevål, Postbox 4956, Nydalen 0424, Oslo, Norway. [10]Center for Rheumatology and Spine Diseases, National Hospital, 2600 Glostrup, Denmark.

References

1. van den Eerenbeemt KD, et al. Total disc replacement surgery for symptomatic degenerative lumbar disc disease: a systematic review of the literature. Eur Spine J. 2010;19(8):1262–80.
2. Yajun W, et al. A meta-analysis of artificial total disc replacement versus fusion for lumbar degenerative disc disease. Eur Spine J. 2010;19(8):1250–61.
3. Hellum C, et al. Surgery with disc prosthesis versus rehabilitation in patients with low back pain and degenerative disc: two year follow-up of randomised study. BMJ. 2011;342:d2786.
4. Panjabi MM. The stabilizing system of the spine. Part I. Function, dysfunction, adaptation, and enhancement. J SpinalDisord. 1992;5(4):383–9.
5. Panjabi M, et al. Spinal stability and intersegmental muscle forces. A biomechanical model. Spine. 1989;14(2):194–200.
6. Moseley GL, Hodges PW, Gandevia SC. Deep and superficial fibers of the lumbar multifidus muscle are differentially active during voluntary arm movements. Spine. 2002;27(2):E29–36.
7. Solomonow M, et al. The ligamento-muscular stabilizing system of the spine. Spine (Phila Pa). 1998;23(23):2552–62.
8. Wagner H, et al. Musculoskeletal support of lumbar spine stability. Pathophysiology. 2005;12(4):257–65.
9. Kjaer P, et al. Are MRI-defined fat infiltrations in the multifidus muscles associated with low back pain? BMC Med. 2007;5:2.
10. Danneels LA, et al. CT imaging of trunk mucles in chronic low back pain patients and healthy control subjects. Eur Spine J. 2000;9(4):266–72.
11. Hides JA, et al. Evidence of lumbar multifidus muscle wasting ipsilateral to symptoms in patients with acute/subacute low back pain. Spine. 1994;19(2):165–72.
12. Wallwork TL, et al. The effect of chronic low back pain on size and contraction of the lumbar multifidus muscle. Man Ther. 2009;2009(5):496–500.
13. Kalichman L, et al. Changes in paraspinal muscles and their association with low back pain and spinal degeneration: CT study. Eur Spine J. 2010;2010(7):1136–44.
14. Kalichman L, et al. Computed tomography-evaluated features of spinal degeneration: prevalence, intercorrelation, and association with self-reported low back pain. Spine J. 2010;2010(3):200–8.

15. Teichtahl AJ, et al. Physical inactivity is associated with narrower lumbar intervertebral discs, high fat content of paraspinal muscles and low back pain and disability. Arthritis Res Ther. 2015;17:114.

16. American College of Sports Medicine Position Stand. The recommended quantity and quality of exercise for developing and maintaining cardiorespiratory and muscular fitness, and flexibility in healthy adults. Med Sci Sports Exerc. 1998;30(6):975-91. PMID 9624661.

17. Hamrick MW, McGee-Lawrence ME, Frechette DM. Fatty Infiltration of Skeletal Muscle: Mechanisms and Comparisons with Bone Marrow Adiposity. Front Endocrinol (Lausanne). 2016;7:69.

18. Le Huec JC, et al. Influence of facet and posterior muscle degeneration on clinical results of lumbar total disc replacement: two-year follow-up. J Spinal Disord Tech. 2005;18(3):219-23.

19. Sihvonen T, et al. Local denervation atrophy of paraspinal muscles in postoperative failed back syndrome. Spine. 1993;18(5):575-81.

20. Keller A, et al. Trunk muscle strength, cross-sectional area, and density in patients with chronic low back pain randomized to lumbar fusion or cognitive intervention and exercises. Spine (Phila Pa 1976). 2004;29(1):3-8.

21. Stevens KJ, et al. Comparison of minimally invasive and conventional open posterolateral lumbar fusion using magnetic resonance imaging and retraction pressure studies. J Spinal Disord Tech. 2006;19(2):77-86.

22. Motosuneya T, et al. Postoperative change of the cross-sectional area of back musculature after 5 surgical procedures as assessed by magnetic resonance imaging. J Spinal Disord Tech. 2006;19(5):318-22.

23. Fan S, et al. Multifidus muscle changes and clinical effects of one-level posterior lumbar interbody fusion: minimally invasive procedure versus conventional open approach. Eur Spine J. 2010. 19(2):316-24.

24. Putzier M. et al., Minimally invasive TLIF leads to increased muscle sparing of the multifidus muscle but not the longissimus muscle compared with conventional PLIF-a prospective randomized clinical trial. Spine J. 2016;16(7):811-9.

25. Waschke A, et al. Denervation and atrophy of paraspinal muscles after open lumbar interbody fusion is associated with clinical outcome–electromyographic and CT-volumetric investigation of 30 patients. Acta Neurochir (Wien). 2014;156(2):235-44.

26. Jacobs WC et al., Total Disc Replacement for Chronic Discogenic Low-Back Pain: A Cochrane Review. Spine (Phila Pa 1976). 2012;38(1):24-36.

27. Brox JI. The contribution of RCTs to quality management and their feasibility in practice. Eur Spine J. 2009;18 Suppl 3:279-93.

28. Masharawi Y, et al. The reproducibility of quantitative measurements in lumbar magnetic resonance imaging of children from the general population. Spine (Phila Pa). 2008;33(19):2094-100.

29. Modic MT et al., Degenerative disk disease: assessment of changes in vertebral body marrow with MR imaging. Radiology. 1988; 166(1:Pt 1):193-9.

30. Aprill C, Bogduk N. High-intensity zone: a diagnostic sign of painful lumbar disc on magnetic resonance imaging. Br J Radiol. 1992;65(773):361-9.

31. Luoma K, et al. Low back pain in relation to lumbar disc degeneration. Spine (Phila Pa). 2000;25(4):487-92.

32. Brox JI, et al. Randomized Clinical Trial of Lumbar Instrumented Fusion and Cognitive Intervention and Exercises in Patients with Chronic Low Back Pain and Disc Degeneration. Spine. 2003;28(17):1913-21.

33. Solgaard SJ, et al. Low-field magnetic resonance imaging of the lumbar spine: reliability of qualitative evaluation of disc and muscle parameters. Acta Radiol. 2006;47(9):947-53.

34. Revill SI, et al. The reliability of a linear analogue for evaluating pain. Anaesthesia. 1976;31(9):1191-8.

35. Fairbank JC, Pynsent PB. The oswestry disability index. Spine. 2000;25(22):2940-53.

36. Grotle M, Brox JI, Vollestad NK. Cross-cultural adaptation of the Norwegian versions of the Roland-Morris Disability Questionnaire and the Oswestry Disability Index. J Rehabil Med. 2003;35(5):241-7.

37. Leren P, et al. The Oslo study. Cardiovascular disease in middle-aged and young Oslo men. Acta Med Scand Suppl. 1975;588:1-38.

38. Lydersen S, Fagerland MW, Laake P. Recommended tests for association in 2 x 2 tables. Stat Med. 2009;28(7):1159-75.

39. Garber CE, et al. American College of Sports Medicine position stand. Quantity and quality of exercise for developing and maintaining cardiorespiratory, musculoskeletal, and neuromotor fitness in apparently healthy adults: guidance for prescribing exercise. MedSciSports Exerc. 2011;43(7):1334-59.

40. Lim SS, et al. A comparative risk assessment of burden of disease and injury attributable to 67 risk factors and risk factor clusters in 21 regions, 1990-2010: a systematic analysis for the Global Burden of Disease Study 2010. Lancet. 2012;380(9859):2224-60.

41. Ingersoll CD, et al. Neuromuscular consequences of anterior cruciate ligament injury. Clin Sports Med. 2008;27(3):383-404.

42. Konishi Y, Fukubayashi T, Takeshita D. Mechanism of quadriceps femoris muscle weakness in patients with anterior cruciate ligament reconstruction. Scand J Med Sci Sports. 2002;12(6):371-5.

43. Forth KE, Layne CS. Background muscle activity enhances the neuromuscular response to mechanical foot stimulation. Am J Phys Med Rehabil. 2007;86(1):50-6.

44. Storheim K, et al. The effect of comprehensive group training on cross-sectional area, density, and strength of paraspinal muscles in patients sick-listed for subacute low back pain. J Spinal Disord Tech. 2003;16(3):271-9.

45. Kaser L, et al. Active therapy for chronic low back pain: part 2. effects on paraspinal muscle cross-sectional area, fiber type size, and distribution. Spine. 2001;26(8):909-19.

46. Danneels LA, et al. Effects of three different training modalities on the cross sectional aera of the lumbar multifidus in patients with chronic low back pain. Br J Sports Med. 2001;35:186-91.

47. Mendias CL, et al. Changes in circulating biomarkers of muscle atrophy, inflammation, and cartilage turnover in patients undergoing anterior cruciate ligament reconstruction and rehabilitation. Am J Sports Med. 2013;41(8):1819-26.

48. Ostelo RW, de Vet HC. Clinically important outcomes in low back pain. Best Pract Res Clin Rheumatol. 2005;19(4):593-607.

49. Mengiardi B, et al. Fat content of lumbar paraspinal muscles in patients with chronic low back pain and in asymptomatic volunteers: quantification with MR spectroscopy. Radiology. 2006;2006(3):786-92.

50. Bankier AA, et al. Consensus interpretation in imaging research: is there a better way? Radiology. 2010;257(1):14-7.

51. Espeland A, Vetti N, Krakenes J. Are two readers more reliable than one? A study of upper neck ligament scoring on magnetic resonance images. BMCMedImaging. 2013;13:4.

52. Berg L, et al. Reliability of change in lumbar MRI findings over time in patients with and without disc prosthesis-comparing two different image evaluation methods. Skeletal Radiol. 2012;41(12):1547-57.

53. Wu HT, Morrison WB, Schweitzer ME. Edematous Schmorl's nodes on thoracolumbar MR imaging: characteristic patterns and changes over time. Skeletal Radiol. 2006;35(4):212-9.

54. Mitra D, Cassar-Pullicino VN, McCall IW. Longitudinal study of high intensity zones on MR of lumbar intervertebral discs. Clin Radiol. 2004;59(11):1002-8.

55. Hu ZJ, et al. An assessment of the intra- and inter-reliability of the lumbar paraspinal muscle parameters using CT scan and magnetic resonance imaging. Spine (Phila Pa). 2011;36(13):E868-74.

56. Bombardier C. Outcome assessments in the evaluation of treatment of spinal disorders: summary and general recommendations. Spine. 2000;25(24):3100-3.

57. Deyo RA, et al. Outcome measures for low back pain research. A proposal for standardized use. Spine. 1998;23(18):2003-13.

58. Moons KG, et al. Prognosis and prognostic research: what, why, and how? BMJ. 2009;338:b375.

59. Therkelsen KE, et al. Intramuscular fat and associations with metabolic risk factors in the Framingham Heart Study. Arterioscler Thromb Vasc Biol. 2013;33(4):863-70.

60. Almurdhi MM, et al. Reduced Lower-Limb Muscle Strength and Volume in Patients With Type 2 Diabetes in Relation to Neuropathy, Intramuscular Fat, and Vitamin D Levels. Diabetes Care. 2016;39(3):441-7.

61. Nielsen PR, et al. Prehabilitation and early rehabilitation after spinal surgery: randomized clinical trial. Clin Rehabil. 2010;24(2):137-48.

17

Individuals' explanations for their persistent or recurrent low back pain

Jenny Setchell[1]* [iD], Nathalia Costa[1], Manuela Ferreira[2], Joanna Makovey[2], Mandy Nielsen[1] and Paul W. Hodges[1]

Abstract

Background: Most people experience low back pain (LBP), and it is often ongoing or recurrent. Contemporary research knowledge indicates individual's pain beliefs have a strong effect on their pain experience and management. This study's primary aim was to determine the discourses (patterns of thinking) underlying people's beliefs about what causes their LBP to persist. The secondary aim was to investigate what they believed was the source of this thinking.

Methods: We used a primarily qualitative survey design: 130 participants answered questions about what caused their LBP to persist, and where they learned about these causes. We analysed responses about what caused their LBP using discourse analysis (primary aim), and mixed methods involving content analysis and descriptive statistics to analyse responses indicating where participants learnt these beliefs (secondary aim).

Results: We found that individuals discussed persistent LBP as 1) due to the body being like a 'broken machine', 2) permanent/immutable, 3) complex, and 4) very negative. Most participants indicated that they learnt these beliefs from health professionals (116, 89%).

Conclusions: We concluded that despite continuing attempts to shift pain beliefs to more complex biopsychosocial factors, most people with LBP adhere to the traditional biomedical perspective of anatomical/biomechanical causes. Relatedly, they often see their condition as very negative. Contrary to current "best practice" guidelines for LBP management, a potential consequence of such beliefs is an avoidance of physical activities, which is likely to result in increased morbidity. That health professionals may be the most pervasive source of this thinking is a cause for concern. A small number of people attributed non-physical, unknown or complex causes to their persistent LBP – indicating that other options are possible.

Keywords: Pain trajectories, Discourse analysis, Lumbar, Patient perspectives, Psychosocial

Background

Low back pain (LBP) is the leading musculoskeletal problems contributing significantly to personal and community health burden [1]. Around 40% of people globally experience LBP. For many it is persistent, recurrent and bothersome [2–4]. Reducing the impact of ongoing LBP is a major research priority – with research of trajectories over time an underexplored aspect [5]. Over the last two decades, there has been a comprehensive shift in the understanding of why LBP becomes persistent or recurrent [6, 7]. A large body of research has taken understandings of persistent pain from the predominantly biomedical model that argues LBP is reducible to anatomical or biomechanical factors, to a biopsychosocial model where persistent pain is considered to be largely modified/maintained by a complex combination of biological, psychological and social factors [8–11] that interact. For example, moderation of the biological processes of sensitisation by psychosocial features [10, 12–14], or the development of ongoing musculoskeletal conditions due to avoidance of activity resulting from a fear of exacerbating pain/damage (e.g. the Fear-Avoidance Model outlined by Lethem, Slade, Troup and Bentley [15]).

The clear linking of psychosocial factors with persistent pain highlights that how people think about their pain is an important predictor of severity and chronicity

* Correspondence: j.setchell@uq.edu.au
[1]School of Health and Rehabilitation Sciences, St Lucia, QLD 4072, Australia
Full list of author information is available at the end of the article

[16, 17]. Amongst other factors, pain beliefs contribute to prognosis [18]. For example, in a study on 1591 patients attending general practices, poor clinical outcomes 6 months after initial consultation were more likely in individuals who expected their LBP to last a long time, perceived serious consequences, and believed they had little control over their pain [19]. Further, excessively negative orientation towards pain correlates with greater pain [20, 21]. People's beliefs about how physical activity and work affect their LBP account for variance in pain and disability [22–24]. Recent best practice guidelines reflect that understanding and addressing these pain beliefs is an important component of reducing the burden of LBP (e.g., [25]).

This psychosocial understanding of painful conditions, including LBP, is inconsistently reflected in the beliefs and practices of clinicians or people with LBP. Parsons, Harding, Breen, Foster, Tamar, Vogel and Underwood [26] reviewed 22 qualitative studies concluding that physician's beliefs about painful musculoskeletal conditions were primarily biomedical and, in a cross-sectional study of 453 musculoskeletal physiotherapists, Bishop and Foster [27] highlighted that while these clinicians often recognised the importance of psychosocial factors they contradicted evidence based best practice guidelines by frequently highlighting biomedical over psychosocial factors of LBP cases. Observational studies show clinicians and patients consider risk factors for a sudden onset of LBP to be mainly biomechanical and rarely endorse psychosocial risk factors [28, 29]. Little research has considered why these beliefs and practices persist regarding LBP despite evidence this view is outdated and inaccurate.

There is insufficient knowledge about why people (including clinicians and individuals with the condition) adopt or resist considering pain beliefs (and other psychosocial factors) as contributors to ongoing LBP. One possibility is that the biopsychosocial approach involves a paradigm shift, which challenges (amongst other things) existing biomedical structures and beliefs. Change would necessarily need to be reflected in people's underlying systems of belief. Little research has investigated these belief systems. The primary aim of this study was to investigate what patterns of thinking (discourses) underlie what people say caused their LBP to persist or recur. The secondary aim was to investigate where people with the condition considered these patterns of thinking came from.

Methods
Study design
We created an online survey to elicit individuals with LBP's understanding of the patterns of their condition including questions about pain increase, condition flare, and persistence or recurrence. We report here on the answers to questions related to individual's perceptions of why their condition is persistent or recurrent.

Participant selection
A wide range of participants were purposively sampled via a range of recruitment methods including promotion through pain consumer support organisations, advertisements in local community and health centres and through social media. Inclusion criteria were 1) personal experience of LBP, 2) English language proficiency, and 3) age 18 and over. Efforts were made to include a broad range of participants with LBP by promotion through a variety of sources. Recruitment continued until a satisfactory level of participant diversity and theoretical saturation was achieved. There was no exclusion based on chronicity, currency of LBP, or comorbidities. A total of 130 participants entered full responses to the survey. Most participants were female (74.6%), from Australia (98.5%) and reported daily pain (82.0%). See Table 1 for demographic and LBP details.

Data collection/procedure
The study gained institutional ethics approval. Data were collected through an online survey, which participants consented to enter after reading an information page. They responded to two questions designed to address the aims of this study:

Table 1 Demographic characteristics of study participants

Age (years)	
Mean ± SD	43.2 ± 12.05
Gender	
Female	74.6%
Male	25.4%
Country	
Australia	98.5%
Other	1.5%
State	
Queensland	56.9%
New South Wales	16.9%
Victoria	15.4%
Other	10.8%
LBP everyday	
Yes	82%
No	18%
Time frame of LBP variation	
Daily	55.4%
Weekly	23.1%
Monthly	7.7%
Other	13.8%
Periods of no LBP	
Yes	29.7%
No	70.3%

1) What is your understanding of why your low back pain is persisting or recurring? This question required a text-box response with no word limit.

2) Where does this understanding come from? Participant could choose one or more of five options that were provided for this question i) health care provider, ii) internet, iii) family, iv) friends, or v) other. In the final option, 'other', short text-box responses were allowed.

Methodology and theoretical underpinnings

The primary methodology in this study is discourse analysis [30]. This qualitative methodology offers an approach to investigating people's patterns of thinking, or systems of belief, that underlie their perceived reasons for LBP persisting or recurring. Discourse analysis is based on the premise that the language we use has a role in creating or constituting reality, rather than simply reflecting it – thus discourses are seen as having real world effects [31]. For example, if someone believe that their LBP is due to tissue damage they may behave in particular ways, such as avoiding certain movements or taking time off work – which will have (greater or lesser) effects on their life. We do not mean to suggest that by identifying discourses we can know what individuals will do based on what they say but rather that certain ways of thinking are likely to produce certain realities more broadly (social constructionism [32]). Thus, discourse analysis does not try to simply summarise individual experiences, or try to find out what 'really happened' (in this case what caused their LBP to persist or recur), but rather tries to understand how particular patterns of talking and thinking make certain realities (in this case a particular pain belief and its consequences) more likely [32]. In this research, we sought to understand the particular discourses evident in what participants said make their condition persist or recur. This type of analysis has been used frequently in healthcare and offers different insights compared to other forms of analysis [33]. As it has been rarely used to understand painful conditions such as LBP, it has the potential to bring a novel perspective. To consider the second question we used a simple convergent parallel mixed methods design [34], employing a descriptive count analysis (content analysis where data were qualitative, and descriptive statistics were data were quantitative). This analysis produced a descriptive overview of where participants said they learnt about their condition, which we understood from a relativist perspective [32] to be likely (but not certain) to indicate what had occurred in reality.

Data analysis

Discourse analysis was conducted following procedures outlined by Willig [31]. The six-member analysis team included experienced qualitative and quantitative researchers from a range of disciplines (physiotherapy, medical, psychology, and social work). The analysis was inductive, which means that the research team did not impose a pre-existing theory on the analysis; rather it was the data that drove the development of the discourses [32], although some a priori assumptions are inevitable in any research [32]. The first author, a physiotherapist with social science training and experience in this type of analysis (JS) initially reviewed the entire data set. On a second reading, she formulated four provisional discourses. JS and another author (NC) then independently read the entire dataset and determined which discourses were represented in each participant response. These researchers then discussed to agreement any discrepancies in naming/defining the discourses and coding of the data according to discourse. The other authors then reviewed the entire dataset, and the coding and analysis of findings, with any incongruences discussed to agreement.

We used descriptive statistics to analyse the data from the second question where data were quantitative (sections 1–4), and content analysis where data were qualitative (section 5). The content analysis was initially carried out by JS and then reviewed by the entire team – results were combined using convergent analysis into final groupings so they could be related. We used the Consolidated Criteria for Reporting Qualitative Research (COREQ: [35]) to guide rigour in study design and reporting. Relevant criteria were satisfied for study design and reporting. To improve trustworthiness, data were independently analysed by two team members with other team members providing input into analysis. A researcher external to the study further confirmed trustworthiness and that the results were grounded in the data.

Results

We report results in three sections: analysis of participant responses to the first and second questions and then the cross analysis of the two.

Analysis of responses to question 1

We identified four clear patterns of thinking (discourses) in participant's responses to the question: "What is your understanding of why your low back pain is persisting or recurring?" (Table 2). We describe these discourses below using examples from the data and then highlight their relevance to our research aims in the discussion. Participants are anonymised and differentiated by numbers. Responses were typically one sentence to a paragraph in length. A small number of responses were very short (e.g., one word). All of these were easily identifiable within at least one of the discourses except for two responses "good" P110 and "my employment aggravates it" P16. These two responses were not included in the analysis as their meaning in relation to the four discourses was unclear.

Table 2 Discourses found in analysis of participant responses to the question: "What is your understanding of why your low back pain (LBP) is persistent or recurring?"

Discourse (pattern of thinking)	Explanation
1) Body as machine	The body is viewed as biomechanical (literally: the body as a machine) or anatomical. Like a machine, the body is considered to be able to break and can sometimes be repaired. LBP persists because something is physically defective.
2) LBP as permanent/ immutable	Related to the first discourse, LBP is conceptualised as a static or fixed entity that once 'broken', it cannot be 'fixed'. LBP is not dynamic or fluid but unchangeable and permanent.
3) LBP is complex	This is a counter discourse to the first two. Multiple factors can contribute to the persistence of LBP – not only biomechanical or anatomical but also possibly psychosocial or cultural factors. There is no simple explanation for ongoing LBP.
4) LBP is very negative	LBP is conceptualised as abnormal, catastrophic, or very negative experience. LBP should be avoided and/or has a large effect on life.

Discourse 1: Body as machine

"Body as a machine" was the most common discourse and was evident in almost all participant responses. Most participants viewed their body in a machine-like way – as if something mechanical was "wrong" with their body and that this caused their LBP recurrence or persistence. Described causes included: joint, muscle and nerve injury/disease; posture and "alignment" issues; muscle control, length and strength issues; and inflammatory conditions. Participants often presented a distinct picture of what they believed was wrong. For example, participant 3 wrote:

"Degeneration of the integrity of my tendons and ligaments from faulty collagen due to Ehlers-Danlos Syndrome causing instability in my spine (and other joints) resulting in herniation of spinal discs (currently 3 cervical, 1 thoracic and 2 lumbar) and degenerative disc disease at L5/S1. Also sacroiliac joint dysfunction, hip dysplasia and instability has a correlating impact to my back issues."

And participant 59 wrote:

"My motor control has suffered due to chronic low back pain initially caused by an injury and then perpetuated by degeneration in the joints. Even though there is no acute injury any more (arthritis is still there), my motor patterns are inefficient and I recruit larger muscles to stabilise my back due to pain inhibition. This means sometimes I do movements that are actually more forceful that needed and

increase joint loading at the degenerating level, which is what causes a flare up."

Like these participants, many used technical biomedical language, for example: "fusion surgery leading to sacroiliac joint problems" P8, "my L4 and L5 are rubbing together" P43, and "spondylolisthesis L5S1 with pars defect" P62. Others spoke less specifically of general physical conditions (e.g., "spinal damage caused by arthritis" P7).

Discourse 2: LBP as permanent/immutable

"I am suffering from multi-level degenerating disks. (L1-S1) There is no "mechanical fix" for my condition. And as time goes by it continues to degenerate." P105

Like the opening quote above, many responses included some indication that when LBP damage or disease occurred it would be that way forever. This discourse is related to the first, where participants viewed the body as machine-like (relatively immutable). For example, several participants referred to earlier damage that had a seemingly permanent or definitive ongoing effect: "Damage done earlier in life" P107, and "Injury from high school..." P85. These participants' attribution of an ongoing cause of their condition seemed to indicate that a prior cause for their LBP meant that it could not be changed.

Akin to the opening quote, the word 'degeneration' was commonly used by participants to indicate that damage was ongoing and worsening. For example "Now, it has become a matter of degeneration to the structure due to age and injury" P49. Other participants referred to more specific diagnoses, in this way denoting that their condition was permanent. For example, one participant said "arthritic changes in the bones" P12, and another "severe multi-level stenosis" P97. One participant (59) stated clearly that, due to their diagnosis they believed their LBP is likely to persist and worsen, "My understanding is that because of my scoliosis I may always have lower back pain – and this could increase as I get older." Overall, participants referred to damage, degeneration or LBP diagnoses as reified conditions, and almost never framed their LBP as something that is transient, reversible or temporary.

Discourse 3: LBP is complex

This discourse was much less common and contrasted with the first two discourses – it is a counter narrative to them. These participants indicated, at least in some way, that LBP can be complex; that bodies are not simply machines that are broken or not, but rather that bodies, disease states, and pain can be impermanent and complex – and variously reworked. Factors other than biomechanics and disease processes can contribute to LBP's recurrence or persistence. For example: one participant said that her LBP's persistence was "...in part my dependence on medication" P52, and another that it was "Pain patterns in brain as well as muscles that engage to 'protect' me when they don't need to." P83. Participant 50 described considerable detail complex mechanical and psychological contributors:

"I have a severe burst dispersion fracture of L1 with up to 75% of the body of L1 crushed and dissolved. I have no neurological impairment and the fracture was stabilised without surgery. In 2013 I had a 20-year MRI and consulted a private pain specialist (also ortho surgeon) and he confirmed that the root cause is mechanical. My background pain was very high for approx 1 year (mid 2012-13) during a suicidal depression period. I have several month long bouts of depression every 3-5 years but the 2012 episode was worse than others. This fed the pain which fed the depression and I started hating my pain for the first time in 22 years. Although it can be tiring and exasperating at times, I had never hated the pain or wished it gone. Interestingly, during a few months of intense psychological treatment sessions, I had a week and a half long bad pain episode but it wasn't until the 4th day that I realised that my attitude to the pain and my "automatic responses" to it had reverted back to my usual acceptance so I saw that as a step forward. The year highlighted again the direct correlation of mood to pain."

This participant highlights a complex interplay between biological, psychological and emotional contributing factors to his condition: while LBP may have an anatomical driver of a fractured vertebra, he believed his LBP was also impacted by the interplay of psychological health (depression), mood (anger) and pain beliefs (acceptance).

Participants who said they were unsure about what caused their condition also had a discourse of LBP as complex. For example, participants used statements such as: "I am not sure why this happens...." P43, "There is no understanding it, it is a combination so specific to the individual" P13, and another: "I have degeneration in the L4 and L5. No apparent reason why. Every physiotherapist, specialist, massage therapist and osteopath all have different theories why. Nothing conclusive as I have not had a significant trauma and the degeneration indicates that I have." P69. The complexity and the lack of knowledge about LBP is portrayed as a mystery, and these participants give little indication of whether this enabled or disempowered them to manage their condition. Interestingly, however, one participant indicated that not being sure of the cause of their ongoing LBP did not stop them from taking action:

"I don't really know [why my pain is ongoing or recurrent]. I do believe that there's a "learned behaviour" in my brain. I have been trying to focus on different things lately or visualise different things when my back starts to get worse, and it seems to be helping a bit. I have recently gone back to the gym and have found that I can move and perform some exercises that not only are pain free but help with my overall pain. That has shown me that movement is not the cause of my pain, but the type of movement and how I do it." P71

Two participants (P71 and P13 – both quoted above) *only* stated a complex picture of their condition without any aspect of the first two discourses ('body as machine' or 'body as permanent').

Discourse 4: LBP is very negative

Many people described their LBP very negatively, often explicitly stating this. For example, participant 3 said "Severe spinal stenosis and an awful scoliosis", and participant 31 "severe sciatica...pain never goes away". Participants frequently used negative words such as "damage", "degeneration" to denote that they believed that their body was harmed. For example, participant 33 said: "I have worn out, my L5/S1 to the point, it can't take anything else." Often participants used the word "poor" (poor posture, poor disc health, poor core strength).

The discourse of LBP being very negative was also often implicit in discourse 1 and 2 (but was not classified this way for the sake of clarity in this analysis). In itself, the idea of the body as a machine which breaks permanently is a negative conceptualization of their condition. For example, return to the quote: "My understanding is that because of my scoliosis I may always have lower back pain – and this could increase as I get older." P59. Although there are no overtly negative words used, the words 'always' and 'increase' give the statement a negative valence.

Although some participants were only mildly negative it was rare that people's reasons given for the persistence or recurrence of their LBP were neutral or normalised, and extremely rare that they indicated a positive relationship to their LBP when thinking about its persistence or recurrence. One of the few examples of a more neutral, normalised and somewhat positive response was embedded within participant 50's reply which was quoted in full above: "Although it can be tiring and exasperating at times, I had never hated the pain or wished it gone."

Analysis of responses to question 2

The second question was: "Where does this understanding come from?". Findings are summarised in Table 3. Participants could choose one or more options - with

Table 3 Number (percentage) of responses to the question "Where does this understanding come from?"

Health Care Provider n (%)	Internet n (%)	Family n (%)	Friends n (%)	Other* n (%)
116 (89)	31 (24)	12 (9)	7 (5)	16 (12) self-reflection
				9 (7) education
				4 (3) scientific lit
				3 (2) other
				1 (1) not relevant
				33 (25) Total

*In the "other" box 15 participants provided clarification or repetition of the first four options. These figures were not included separately in the analysis

most choosing only 1. Of the four possible options, the majority indicated that their understanding of their LBP came from a health professional ($n = 116$, 89%) and almost one quarter from the internet ($n = 31$, 24%), with the other options being chosen much less frequently. The option 'other' was selected by 49 people – however, some ($n = 15$) responses were simply clarifications of the other categories (so were excluded from consideration under 'other'), one response was not relevant as it was unrelated to the question. The most pertinent findings were that a small number ($n = 16$, 12%) of people discussed reflection on their own experiences (e.g., "knowing my own body" P46 and "my own reflection" P63) as informing their understanding of why their LBP was ongoing. A small number also discussed information gathering from formal health education ($n = 9$) or scientific literature ($n = 4$). This study was not intended to detect statistically significant relationships between the discourses and the reported source of their understanding of causes. However, in a simple comparison there were no indications of potential relationships between the participants' belief of where their LBP had come from and the discourses in their responses to question 1.

Discussion

The key finding of this study is that people with LBP predominantly consider their condition to persist or recur because of biomechanical or structural reasons (machines that can be broken, and if not 'fixed' will continue to be in pain/damaged). Participants discussed factors such as joint damage, nerve injury and/or muscle imbalance as the main reasons why their LBP was ongoing. While there were counter-narratives, these were much less common. This finding indicates that overwhelmingly individual's beliefs about their LBP are aligned with (Western) traditional biomedical discourses of health and the body. A secondary finding of this study was that participants overwhelmingly considered health professionals, and the internet to be sources of their understandings. This highlights the likely value of ensuring good quality information from both sources. This study can only discuss where people with LBP *say* they

learnt about the causes of their condition and thus findings may not reflect what health professionals believe or do in their healthcare practice, nor the quality of internet resources. However, as discussed, other studies have shown that health professionals, such as physicians [26] and physiotherapists [27], demonstrate primarily biomedical pain beliefs and practices, and that this is strongly associated with the beliefs of their patients [36]. This primarily Western belief system has also been shown to have potential effects across cultures [37].

Why do the LBP-related discourses found in this study matter? There is considerable evidence to suggest harm is done by this way of thinking. People might modify their behaviour in a manner that may worsen their LBP, placing emphasis on avoiding causes that are not relevant. Greater beliefs in the anatomical causes of persistent pain have been related to greater beliefs in physical disability [17] and thus avoidance of activities. There are strong associations between low perception of controllability of LBP and poor clinical outcomes [19] and this belief is likely to underpin strongly negative beliefs about pain. Encouragingly, some people have a more complex understanding of LBP, aligned with more contemporary biopsychosocial discourses, but this was rare in our data and is often largely overshadowed by biomedical discourses.

Similar findings about beliefs of individuals with LBP have been reported elsewhere. For example, Bunzli, Watkins, Smith, Schütze and O'Sullivan [38] synthesized 18 studies with 713 participants with chronic LBP, highlighting the social construction of the condition, and its psychosocial impact. The study discussed that people with chronic LBP often adhere to a biomedical model of their condition and that this results in them "putting their lives on hold" until they receive what they believe to be a viable (biomedical) diagnosis/prognosis. Consistent with our findings, the synthesis suggests that the potential harm in these beliefs is that people may undertake a misdirected search for legitimacy that prevents both acceptance of the condition as well as attention to more evidence based contributors to continuing LBP. The present findings strengthen these observations using a novel approach to uncover underlying discourses and contribute to new understandings of the trajectories of LBP. The present study also reveals that biomedical discourses are prevalent despite many efforts towards changing these beliefs (e.g., [39]), and potential positive clinical outcomes of changing them (e.g., [40]).

Interpretation of these findings poses challenges. It is important to acknowledge we must take seriously the perspectives of people living with LBP [41]. Not doing so has led to issues in the past, such as inadvertent stigmatisation [42] and inadequate attention to the often-complex psychosocial aspects of living with ongoing conditions [43, 44]. If individual perspectives are predominantly produced by an outdated (or at least, incomplete) healthcare paradigm, it is necessary to consider how this might be challenged.

Our findings offer some possible ways forward, evident in that some participants' responses included all discourses. This indicates that individuals with LBP are able to think with more than one paradigm – switching between them seemingly with little issue concerning apparent contradictions. For example:

"there is degeneration of vertebra and discs which results in pinching of nerves. A lot of soft tissue damage to core muscles front and back which makes that back more pliable. It is said that my brain is not interpreting the signals properly because of many things including PTSD, TBI, IBS..." P2.

This participant used all four discourses – but some are stronger than others. The participant speaks first about biomechanical/anatomical factors as reasons for the ongoing nature of their LBP ("degenerated vertebra and discs", "pinching of nerves", "soft tissue damage") using very definite language "there is...results in... a lot of...". This language suits the dominant form of understanding bodies and health in biomedicine: bodies are like machines that may or may not be fixed. Like a machine, when something cannot be 'fixed' it is 'permanently broken'. Notably, the participant also provides another less definite story ("it is said that..."). This choice of wording makes the subsequent statement appear not to be coming from her/his own thinking, perhaps indicating the participant has heard this information but does not really believe/understand it. In this second story, the participant discusses that LBP can persist because a number of factors can influence it (the participant mentions psychological and other physical conditions). Although the traditional view is given more emphasis, the presence of both stories suggests this person is able to adopt more than one perspective – an understanding of LBP as complex and not only biomechanical or anatomical. Such participants show an ability to integrate biopsychosocial with biomedical understandings. As other research has highlighted that sense-making processes may play a role in developing harmful LBP beliefs [45], this highlights a potentially useful way forward to assist people with LBP (and others) to helpfully reconceptualise their condition.

The findings of the discourse 'LBP as very negative' were often closely linked with the understanding of the body as 'a machine that can break' and as 'permanent'. This close relationship highlights further that underlying discourses have important effects on beliefs about LBP, which in turn affect prognosis. The conceptualisation of LBP as very negative found here and elsewhere [21] is not surprising given the underlying discourses of the body as a machine that can break, and LBP as permanent. Yet this conceptualistation contrasts with the fact that LBP is so common as to say that it is normal [2], and persistence/recurrence are also very common/normal [4]. Although not directly researched regarding LBP itself, other conditions involving injury, illness and disability have been conceptualised differently including positive possibilities such as those of 'well-being within illness' [46], hope [47], and acceptance [48]. These possibilities for more positive reconceptulisations might be a relevant to consider for future work in the LBP population. If LBP was perceived as relatively normal (although at times unpleasant) rather than something to always 'fix', potentially harmful beliefs and their negative psychosocial and clinical implications might be avoided.

There are a number of important factors to consider when interpreting the results of this study. Although survey formats have some limitations in qualitative research due to the lack of direct interaction, there are also benefits - due to the online nature of this study, participants were likely to have felt comfortable expressing their views freely. The study was Australian, consequently, care must be taken in extrapolating results to other settings – although similar Western countries are likely to find many contextual similarities. The investigatory team was comprised of researchers with a physiotherapy background (and one social worker). Physiotherapists would be expected to have views on LBP grounded in biomedical aspects and may give less attention to psychological and socio-cultural aspects [49]. Efforts were made to reduce any effect of this viewpoint by assembling a team that includes a social worker (MN), a researcher with graduate training in psychology who focuses on the socio-cultural elements of health (JS), and sourcing external review. Future research can build on the findings of this study. A similar research design could be conducted in different cultural contexts to investigate how LBP is conceptualised elsewhere.

Finding that biomedical discourses underlie most thinking about LBP has implications for how it is possible to change. These discourses challenge deep cultural understandings of what it means to have a body and to be human, including the Cartesian notion of a distinct body/mind division [50]. Changing such deeply held beliefs will not be simple – doing so challenges established institutions of healthcare and the very core of what it means to be a person with LBP, a health researcher, and a clinician [51]. This study provides a strong basis for challenging deeply held traditional beliefs and interventional studies testing these as methods for reducing the burden of LBP are indicated.

We do not want to deny possible biomedical causes of LBP or permanence of the condition. Rather, our aim is to highlight that these discourses are not necessarily true for everyone and can set people up for damaging pain beliefs such as fear avoidance. Described biomedical causes in the current study included various musculoskeletal injuries/diseases and biomechanical factors. Although some biomedical factors have support as the initial cause of LBP [13], there is currently little support for them causing ongoing or recurrent LBP which, as discussed, is likely to be more biopsychosocial and multifactorial [8–11]. There is thus a disconnection between cause of initial injury and the reason it is ongoing, which is worthy of further investigation.

Conclusions

The findings of this study support and add to other studies discussing that biomedical understandings of LBP persist and recur in those who live with musculoskeletal pain conditions. Seeking to understand underlying discourses provides a novel perspective which looks past singular causes to consider the systems of thought that make an adherence to particular patterns of beliefs possible. The findings of this study support a complex and thorough approach to shifting understandings of LBP beyond biological causes to consider psychosocial, cultural and institutional factors that constitute LBP. Finally, our finding that patients believe they learnt their potentially harmful understandings from health professionals encourages further interventions to shift thinking within healthcare.

Abbreviation
LBP: Low back pain

Acknowledgments
We thank the participants who contributed their time and experience to this study. The study was funded by the National Health and Medical Research Council of Australia (Program Grant: 1091302; Centre of Research Excellence grant: 1079078; Senior Principal Research Fellowship (PH): 1102905). MF holds a Sydney Medical Foundation Fellowship, Sydney Medical School. There are no conflicts of interest to declare.

Funding
The study was funded by the National Health and Medical Research Council of Australia (Program Grant: 1,091,302; Centre of Research Excellence grant: 1,079,078; Senior Principal Research Fellowship (PH): 1,102,905). None of the funding bodies had any involvement in any aspect of study design or implementation or reporting.

Authors contributions
All authors contributed to the design and reporting of the study. MN, MF, JM, NC and PH contributed to the design and distribution of the survey. JS, MF, PH and NC contributed to the analysis and reporting of results (which were later checked by all authors). JS, NC and PH contributed to the first draft of the manuscript. All authors contributed to subsequent and final manuscript drafts. All authors read and approved the final manuscript.

Consent for publication
Not applicable.

Competing interests
MC is a member of the editorial board of BMC Musculoskeletal Disorders. The authors declare that they have no competing interests.

Author details
[1]School of Health and Rehabilitation Sciences, St Lucia, QLD 4072, Australia. [2]Institute of Bone and Joint Research/The Kolling Institute, Sydney Medical School, The University of Sydney, St Leonards, NSW 2065, Australia.

References
1. Vos T, Flaxman AD, Naghavi M, Lozano R, Michaud C, et al. Years lived with disability (YLDs) for 1160 sequelae of 289 diseases and injuries 1990–2010: a systematic analysis for the global burden of disease study 2010. Lancet. 2013;380(9859):2163–96.
2. Hoy D, Bain C, Williams G, March L, Brooks P, Blyth F, Woolf A, Vos T, Buchbinder R. A systematic review of the global prevalence of low back pain. Arthritis Rheum. 2012;64:2028–37.
3. Young AE, Wasiak R, Phillips L, Gross DP. Workers' perspectives on low back pain recurrence: "it comes and goes and comes and goes, but it's always there". Pain. 2011;152(1):204–11.
4. Axen I, Leboeuf-Yde C. Trajectories of low back pain. Best Pract Res Clin Rheumatol. 2013;27(5):601–12.
5. Kongsted A, Kent P, Axen I, Downie A, Dunn KM. What have we learned from ten years of trajectory research in low back pain? BMC Musculoskelet Disord. 2016;17(1):220.
6. Waddell G. The back pain revolution. Edinburgh: Churchill Livingstone; 2005.
7. McMahon S, Koltzenburg M, Tracey I, Turk DC. Wall and Melzack's textbook of pain. Philadelphia: Elsevier Saunders; 2013.
8. Linton SJ. Occupational psychological factors increase the risk for back pain: a systematic review. J Occup Rehabil. 2001;11(1):53–66.
9. Linton SJ. A review of psychological risk factors in back and neck pain. Spine. 2000;25(9):1148–56.
10. Vachon-Presseau E, Roy M, Martel MO, Caron E, Marin MF, et al. The stress model of chronic pain: evidence from basal cortisol and hippocampal structure and function in humans. Brain. 2013;136(Pt 3):815–27.
11. Edwards RR, Dworkin RH, Sullivan MD, Turk DC, Wasan AD. The role of psychosocial processes in the development and maintenance of chronic pain. J Pain. 2016;17(9 Suppl):T70–92.
12. Videman T, Battie MC. Commentary: back pain epidemiology–the challenge of case definition and developing new ideas. Spine J. 2012;12(1):71–2.
13. Hoy D, Brooks P, Blyth F, Buchbinder R. The epidemiology of low back pain. Best Pract Res Clin Rheumatol. 2010;24(6):769–81.
14. Frank JW, Brooker A-S, DeMaio S, Kerr M, Maetzel A, et al. Disability resulting from occupational low back pain. Part II: what do we know about secondary prevention? A review of the scientific evidence on prevention after disability begins. Spine. 1996;21(24):2918–29.
15. Lethem J, Slade PD, Troup JD, Bentley G. Outline of a fear-avoidance model of exaggerated pain perception. Behav Res Ther. 1983;21(4):401–8.
16. Turner JA, Jensen MP, Romano JM. Do beliefs, coping, and catastrophizing independently predict functioning in patients with chronic pain? Pain. 2000; 85(2000):115–25.
17. Walsh D, Radcliffe J. Pain beliefs and perceived physical disability of patients with chronic low back pain. Pain. 2002;97:23–31.
18. Wertli MM, Rasmussen-Barr E, Weiser S, Bachmann LM, Brunner F. The role of fear avoidance beliefs as a prognostic factor for outcome in patients with nonspecific low back pain: a systematic review. Spine J. 2014;14(5):816–36. e814
19. Foster NE, Bishop A, Thomas E, Main C, Horne R, et al. Illness perceptions of low back pain patients in primary care: what are they, do they change and are they associated with outcome? Pain. 2008;136(1–2):177–87.
20. Sullivan M, Bishop S, Pivik J. The pain Catastrophizing scale: development and validations. Psychol Assess. 1995;7(4):524–32.
21. Picavet H, Vlaeyen J, Schouten J. Pain catastrophizing and kinesiophobia: predictors of chronic low back pain. Am J Epidemiol. 2002;156(11):1028–34.
22. Waddell G, Newton M, Henderson I, Somerville D, Main C. A fear-avoidance beliefs questionnaire (FABQ) and the role of fear avoidance beliefs in chronic low back pain and disability. Pain. 1993;52:157–68.
23. Fritz J, Steven G, Delitto A. The role of fear-avoidance beliefs in acute low back pain: relationships with current and future disability and work status. Pain. 2001;94
24. Vlaeyen JW, Linton SJ. Fear-avoidance and its consequences in chronic musculoskeletal pain: a state of the art. Pain. 2000;85(3):317–32.

25. Delitto A, George S, Van Dillen L, Whitman J, Sowa G, Shekelle P, et al. Low back pain: Clinicial practice guidelines linked to the international classification of functioning disability, and health from the orthopaedic section of the American Physical Therapy Association. J Orthop Sports Phys Ther. 2012;42(4):A1–A57.

26. Parsons S, Harding G, Breen A, Foster N, Tamar P, et al. The influence of patients' and primary care practitioners' beliefs and expectations about chronic musculoskeletal pain on the process of care: a systematic review of qualitative studies. Clin J Pain. 2007;23(1):91–8.

27. Bishop A, Foster NE. Do physical therapists in the United Kingdom recognize psychosocial factors in patients with acute low back pain? Spine. 2005;30(11):1316–22.

28. Stevens ML, Steffens D, Ferreira ML, Latimer J, Li Q, et al. Patients' and physiotherapists' views on triggers for low back pain. Spine. 2016;41(4):E218–24.

29. Steffens D, Maher CG, Ferreira ML, Hancock MJ, Glass T, et al. Clinicians' views on factors that trigger a sudden onset of low back pain. Eur Spine J. 2014;23(3):512–9.

30. Yates SJ, Taylor S, Wetherell M. Discourse as data: a guide for analysis. London: Sage; 2001.

31. Willig C. Discourse analysis. In: Smith J, editor. Qualitative psychology: a practical guide to research methods. Los Angeles: Sage; 2003. p. 160–5.

32. Braun V, Clarke V. Successful Qualitative Research. London, UK: Sage; 2013.

33. Wigginton B, Lee C. "but I am not one to judge her actions": thematic and discursive approaches to university students' response to women who smoke while pregnant. Qual Res Psychol. 2014;11(3):265–76.

34. Creswell JW. A concise introduction to mixed methods research. Los Angeles, CA: Sage; 2015.

35. Tong A, Sainsbury P, Craig J. Consolidated criteria for reporting qualitative research (COREQ): a 32-item checklist for interviews and focus groups. Int J Qual Health Care. 2007;19(6):349–57.

36. Darlow B, Fullen BM, Dean S, Hurley DA, Baxter GD, Dowell A. The association between health care professional attitudes and beliefs and the attitudes and beliefs, clinical management, and outcomes of patients with low back pain: a systematic review. Eur J Pain. 2012;16(1):3–17.

37. Lin IB, O'Sullivan PB, Coffin JA, Mak DB, Toussaint S, Straker LM. Disabling chronic low back pain as an iatrogenic disorder: a qualitative study in Aboriginal Australians. BMJ Open. 2013;3:e002654. doi:10.1136/bmjopen-2013-002654.

38. Bunzli S, Watkins R, Smith A, Schütze R, O'Sullivan P. Lives on hold: a qualitative synthesis exploring the experience of chronic low-back pain. Clin J Pain. 2013;29(10):907–16.

39. Butler DS, Moseley GL. Explain pain. 2nd ed. Adelaide, Australia: Noigroup Publications; 2013.

40. O'Sullivan K, Dankaerts W, O'Sullivan L, O'Sullivan PB. Cognitive functional therapy for disabling nonspecific chronic low back pain: multiple case-cohort study. Phys Ther. 2015;95(11).1478–88.

41. Greenfield BH, Jensen GM. Understanding the lived experiences of patients: application of a phenomenological approach to ethics. Phys Ther. 2010;90(8):1185–97.

42. Holloway I, Sofaer-Bennett B, Walker J. The stigmatisation of people with chronic back pain. Disabil Rehabil. 2007;29(18):1456–64.

43. Roussel NA, Neels H, Kuppens K, Leysen M, Kerckhofs E, et al. History taking by physiotherapists with low back pain patients: are illness perceptions addressed properly? Disabil Rehabil. 2016;38(13):1268–79.

44. Robinson-Papp J, George M, Simpson D. Barriers to chronic pain measurement: a qualitative study of patient perspectives. Pain Med. 2015;16(7):1256–64.

45. Bunzli S, Smith A, Schutze R, O'Sullivan P. Beliefs underlying pain-related fear and how they evolve: a qualitative investigation in people with chronic back pain and high pain-related fear. BMJ Open. 2015;5(10):e008847.

46. Carel H. Illness: the cry of the flesh. Durham, UK: Acumen; 2013.

47. Mattingly C. The hope paradox: journeys through a clinical borderland. California, USA: University of California Press; 2010.

48. McCracken L. Learning to live with the pain: acceptance of pain predicts adjustment in persons with chronic pain. Pain. 1998;74:21–7.

49. Setchell J, Nicholls DA, Gibson BE. Objecting: multiplicity and the practice of physiotherapy. Health. 2017. doi:10.1177/1363459316688519.

50. Bendelow G, Williams S. Transcending the dualisms: towards a sociology of pain. Sociol Health Illness. 1995;17(2):139–65.

51. Nicholls DA, Gibson BE. The body and physiotherapy. Physiother Theory Practice. 2010;26(8):497–509.

18

Cost-effectiveness of using a motion-sensor biofeedback treatment approach for the management of sub-acute or chronic low back pain: economic evaluation alongside a randomised trial

Terry Haines[*] [iD] and Kelly-Ann Bowles

Abstract

Background: Low back pain is a common and costly condition internationally. There is high need to identify effective and economically efficient means for managing this problem. This study aimed to explore the cost-effectiveness of a novel motion-sensor biofeedback treatment approach in addition to guidelines-based care compared to guidelines-based care alone, from a societal perspective over a 12 month time horizon.

Method: This was an incremental cost-effectiveness analysis conducted concurrently with a pilot, cluster randomized controlled trial. Health care resource use was collected using daily diaries and patient-self report at 3, 6 and 12 month follow-up assessments. Productivity was measured using industry classifications and participant self-reporting of ability to do their normal work with their present pain. Clinical effect was measured using the Patient Global Impression of Change measured at the 12 month follow-up assessment. Data were compared between groups using linear regression clustered by recruitment site. Bootstrap resampling was used to generate a visual representation of the 95% confidence interval for the incremental cost-effectiveness estimate. Two, one-way sensitivity analyses were undertaken to examine the robustness of findings to key assumptions.

Result: There were $n = 38$ participants in the intervention group who completed the 12 month assessment and $n = 45$ in the control. The intervention group had greater use of trial-related medical and therapy resources [$477 per participant (95% CI: $447, $508)], but lower use of non-trial medical and therapy resources [$-53 per participant (95% CI: $-105, $-0)], and a greater improvement in productivity [$-5123 per participant (95% CI: $-10,174, $-72)]. Overall, the intervention dominated with a saving of $478,100 and an additional 41 participants self-rating as being very or much improved compared to the control. There was >99% confidence in this finding of dominance in both the primary and sensitivity analyses.

Conclusions: The motion-sensor biofeedback treatment approach in addition to guidelines- based care appears to be both more clinically effective and economically efficient than guidelines- based care alone. This approach appears to be a viable means to manage low back pain and further research in this area should be a priority.

Keywords: Low back pain, Economic evaluation, Cost-effectiveness, Randomized trial

* Correspondence: Terrence.haines@monash.edu
Allied Health Research Unit & Physiotherapy Department, School of Primary Health Care, Monash University and Monash Health, Kingston Rd, Cheltenham 3192, Australia

Background

Low back pain presents a tremendous cost to developed nations internationally [1]. These costs can be incurred by patients directly, and by society as a whole through increased use of publicly subsidized health services and reduced paid occupational activity [2]. Loss of productivity (in both paid and unpaid occupations) has been identified as a key driver of these costs [3]. There is need to understand how this burden of disease can be minimised.

There are many interventions that have been argued as being beneficial for management of low back pain. Some approaches, such as spinal surgery, come at substantial cost to patients and/or health care providers. Other options, such as physical therapy, are less costly to deliver but the comparative cost-effectiveness of these approaches remains relatively unknown [4]. In the absence of robust evidence demonstrating the relative cost effectiveness of different treatment options, clinicians are left only with evidence examining the effectiveness of different treatments to guide their selection. There are conflicting results present in this literature and best practice guidelines now make somewhat generic recommendations regarding evaluation and management approaches for clinicians treating low back pain patients [5–7]. A review of the cost-effectiveness of these approaches has identified that interdisciplinary rehabilitation, exercise, acupuncture, spinal manipulation and cognitive-behavioural therapy may all be cost-effective for management of sub-acute or chronic low back pain [8].

Recent advances in technology have permitted development of new approaches to manage low back pain. One such approach has been the use of a motion-sensor biofeedback systems. Biofeedback has been used for the management of low back pain as far back as the 1980's with some promising short-term results [9]. These interventions however were largely restricted to laboratory settings as the equipment was not readily portable. Recent advances in the portability of this technology now allow patients to understand how their low back moves, and have their posture monitored while performing everyday activities so that clinicians can receive a detailed log of how the patient moved during the day and/or night. Using the data from the ambulatory monitoring session, the device can be personalised to notify or remind patients of optimal movements and postures based on their own condition. A recent multicentre, cluster-randomised, placebo-controlled, pilot clinical trial reported a significant and sustained improvement in pain and activity limitation that persisted several months after the initial biofeedback treatment sessions were completed using this technology [10].

Adoption of new technologies in clinical practice should be driven by evidence of both efficacy and of economic efficiency [11]. There has been much recent comment on the spiralling costs of health care being driven, in part, by the increasing costs of service provision attributable to new technologies [12]. No economic evaluation of the use of modern motion-sensor biofeedback systems for the management of low back pain has previously been presented in the literature. However, the value of adding this treatment approach to conventional, guidelines based care needs to be established. This study aimed to explore the cost-effectiveness of a novel motion-sensor biofeedback treatment approach in addition to guidelines-based care compared to guidelines-based care alone, from a societal perspective over a 12 month time horizon.

Methods

Design

Incremental cost-effectiveness study conducted concurrently with a pilot, cluster randomised trial. The cluster randomised trial included eight recruiting sites randomised to either an intervention group consisting of motion-sensor biofeedback combined with "guidelines-based care" or a "guidelines-based care" only control group. Further details of this trial can be found in the trial report paper [10]. This economic evaluation took a societal perspective over a 12 month follow-up time horizon from the date of commencing participation in the trial.

Participants and setting

This trial was conducted across eight sites (two hospitals, six outpatient primary care clinics) in Victoria, Australia. The participating clinicians were two physicians, four GPs and three physiotherapists, all with a special interest in musculoskeletal conditions. The medical practitioners had an average of 25.8 years post-graduate experience and the physiotherapists 19.0 years.

Patients approached for inclusion into this study needed to be aged between 18 and 65 years, have a primary complaint of low back pain or back-related leg pain, have an average pain intensity of three or more on a 0–10 scale, and an episode duration of at least 3 weeks. Patients were excluded from this study if they had surgery or another invasive procedure on their lumbar spine within the previous 12 months, if they were pregnant, had severe hearing impairment, had an implanted electrical medical device, had a known allergic skin reaction to tapes and plasters or any of a range of comorbid disorders including: neoplasm, infection, inflammatory or neurological disorder, fracture or other joint or medically-related disorders. The flow of participants is presented (Fig. 1).

Randomisation

This was a cluster randomised trial where clinics were the unit of randomisation. Consequently, clinicians at each clinic delivered only one type of treatment. Patient

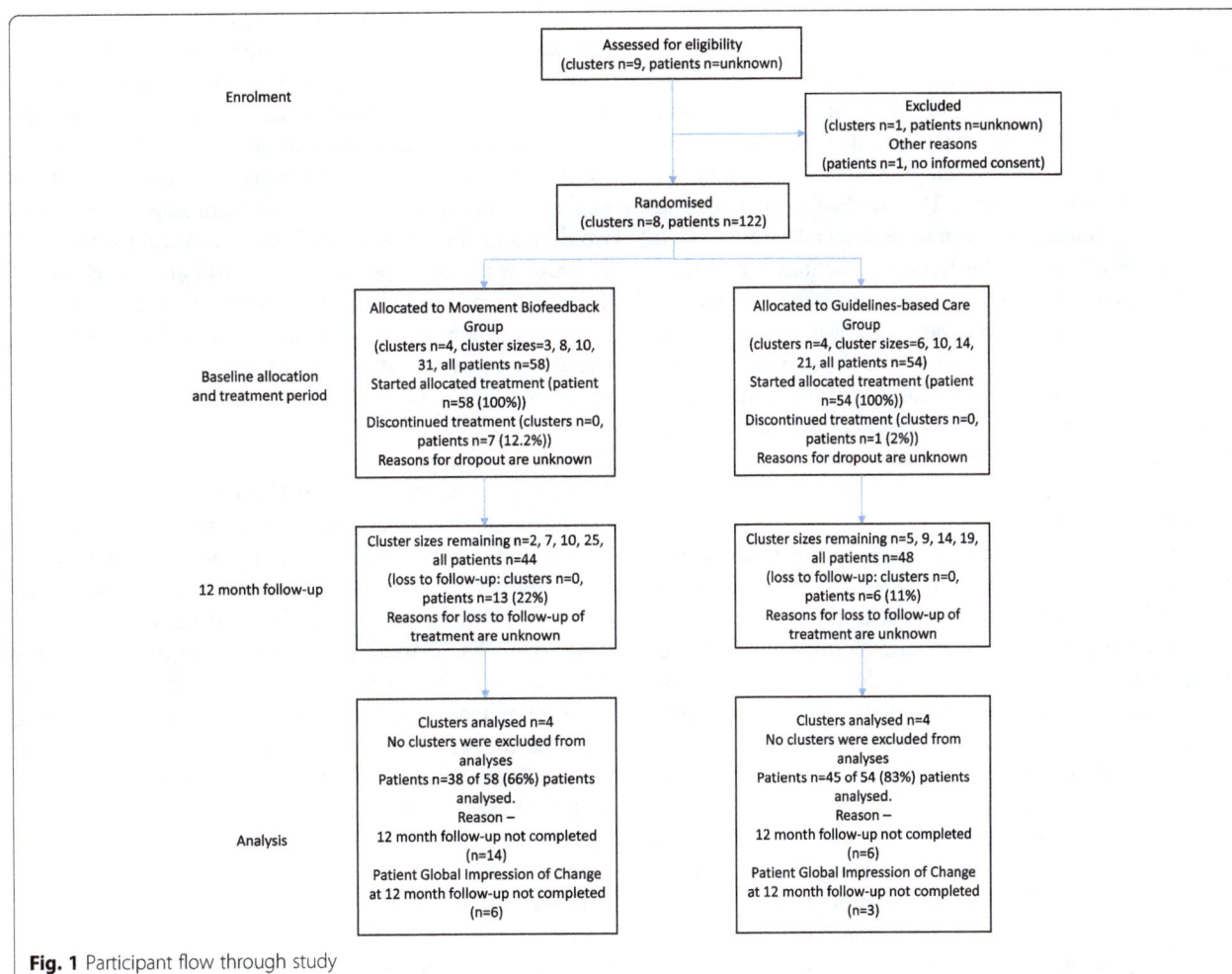

Fig. 1 Participant flow through study

recruitment occurred from each clinician's usual patient flow and clinicians were not blind to treatment allocation. Randomisation was undertaken by allocating each of the three participating physiotherapy clinics to be randomly paired with one of the participating medical clinics, and the remaining two medical clinics formed a fourth and final pair. Each pair was arbitrarily given a number from 1 to 4, and each clinic given an arbitrary code (A or B) within each pair. These four numbered and paired codes, without clinic identification (blinded), were given to a researcher (TH) who generated a random number between 0.0 and 1.0 for Clinic A in each of the four pairs using Excel (Microsoft Corp, Redmond WA, USA). If the number was >0.5, Clinic A was assigned to be a Movement Biofeedback Group clinic and its paired Clinic B to be a Guidelines-based Care Group clinic. If the number was <0.5, the assignment direction was the reverse. This procedure resulted in one physician, one GP and two physiotherapists being randomised to the intervention (movement biofeedback) group and one physician, two GPs and one physiotherapist being randomised to the control (guidelines-based care only) group.

Funding

Funding for this study was equally provided by (i) a grant from the Department of Business and Innovation (Market Validation Program), Victorian Government, Australia, and (ii) dorsaVi P/L (the Australian company who manufactures the ViMove motion-sensor system used in this study). The Department of Business and Innovation helped in the governance of the trial. DorsaVi supplied the motion-sensor equipment and coordinated the trial, assisted by a contract research organisation (Kendle P/L, Oakleigh, Victoria, Australia). All data and trial-related documentation were independently audited by Paul L Clark and Associates (Beaumaris Victoria, Australia). The authors analysed the results and wrote this paper independently of both funders, and neither funder had any influence over how these data were presented and the conclusions reached.

Description of treatments

All participants

All participants in this trial received advice on staying active and general self-management of back pain. This advice was based on the 2003 Australian National Health and Medical Research Council guidelines for the management of acute low back pain [13], and European guidelines for the management of chronic non-specific LBP [14] in the absence of similar Australian guidelines for chronic LBP. The participants could also have received whatever usual medical and physiotherapy care was deemed essential by their clinicians, and such guidelines-based [13, 14] co-interventions were noted. These treatments and advice were metered out over 6–8 sessions over a 10 week period at the commencement of the trial.

Intervention participants

The motion-sensor biofeedback system investigated in this research was the ViMove motion-sensor system (Version 5, dorsaVi.com). This system consists of: (i) two wireless motion-sensors that measure three-dimensional movement, movement velocity and acceleration, and orientation to gravity, (ii) two wireless surface electromyography (EMG) sensors that measure para-spinal muscle activation, (iii) a wireless recording device (approximately the size of a small mobile phone) that captures the sensor data, has a button that patients can push when an event occurs (such as an onset or increase in pain), an audio and vibration function that can be programmed to provide patient-specific biofeedback alerts, and (iv) a charging dock for these wireless devices. The system also has a comprehensive computer software application that clinicians use to observe movement characteristics in real-time, to download postural and movement data from the recording device captured during activities of daily living, to analyse these data with the use of graphics-rich reports, and to compare an individual's movement pattern with their previous assessments or with reference values.

Participants in the intervention group had an individualised assessment including a physical examination and biomechanical movement analysis using the ViMove system to examine potential relationships between their movement or posture and their pain. The ViMove was worn both in the clinic and during the patient's activities of daily living. The clinician then devised a patient-specific rehabilitation strategy designed to address any identified deficits in the patient's pattern of lumbo-pelvic movement and/or posture. For example, output from the ViMove device could be used to differentiate pelvic tilt movement from lumbar spine flexion movement when a participant attempted to reach towards the ground. If movement limitation was identified and found to be largely attributable to limited lumbar spine flexion rather than pelvic tilt, then the lumbar spine flexion component

could be targeted for treatment. Clinicians provided 'live training' in the clinic, where patients were instructed in how to alter their movement pattern(s) or posture using real-time on-screen biofeedback, while wearing the ViMove device. Clinicians could also program the ViMove to provide motion-sensor biofeedback alerts (audio 'beeps' and/or vibration of the wireless recording device) that would occur during 4- to 10- h periods during which participants wore the device at home. This biofeedback would prompt the patient when they 'broke a rule' that the clinician had programmed. The clinician could also prescribe specific exercises that supplemented the patient-specific movement biofeedback.

Control participants

Control participants received the care as described for "all participants" which included a combination of education and advice, exercises, imaging, manual therapy, medication and taping/bracing as previously described [10]. In addition, they wore the ViMove device 6 to 8 times over the 10-week treatment period to mitigate any potential placebo effects of wearing this equipment. Their clinicians were blocked via a software lock during the trial to any of the motion-sensor/EMG information collected. Patients in the control group were informed that the ViMove system was a measurement device.

Measurements

A range of demographic data and patient outcome questionnaires, including the Fear Avoidance Beliefs Questionnaire, the Quadruple Visual Analogue Scale of pain intensity, the Roland-Morris Disability Questionnaire, the Patient Specific Functional Scale were collected at baseline and periodically during the trial. These measures have previously been reported on [10].

Measurement of costs

An estimate of productivity was developed using participant self-reported industry field (18 possible codes) based on gender-specific data provided by the Australian Bureau of Statistics [15]. The Australian Bureau of Statistics provides mean income (based on 2015 data) for these classifications. These industry estimates were pro-rated against the degree to which participants reported they could perform the duties of their occupation. An item from the Fear Avoidance Beliefs Questionnaire was used to gauge the degree to which back pain limited participation in their occupation [16]. This item was worded as "I cannot do my normal work with my present pain" and was scaled on a 0 to 6 scale with zero being "completely disagree", three being "unsure" and six being "completely agree".

Use of pain medications was estimated based on self-reported medication use captured at baseline and any change in medication use captured using the daily pain diary. The daily pain diary was scheduled for completion over the first 3 months of the trial. Medications to treat unrelated conditions (eg. heart disease) were not captured as these were assumed to have little variance over the follow-up period from baseline attributable to the management of back pain. Medication costs were valued using market prices based on the Australian Pharmaceutical Benefits Schedule and market rates for medications that are not subsidized under this scheme.

Use of imaging and general practitioner visits for back pain complaints were captured from participant self-report at the 3, 6, 9 and 12 month assessments. These costs were valued using market prices based on the Australian Medical Benefits Schedule (eg. item 63557 is $492.80 AUD for magnetic resonance image of lumbar spine). Use of medical or therapies (eg. physiotherapy, chiropractic) received for management of low back pain in addition to the intervention or control services provided were captured from participant self-report at the 3, 6, 9 and 12 month assessments. These services were valued using market prices based on locally advertised rates for private practitioner services (i.e. $77.95 AUD per visit). The use of medical services and therapies provided as a part of the intervention and control conditions were captured directly by project data collectors based on attendance at treatment sessions. These services were valued using the same local market prices ($77.95 AUD per visit). We added a cost per session for intervention group participants for having access to the ViMove system and the consumables required for its use. There is an annual fee of $5000 AUD per year for the software license and one set of equipment. In clinical practice, it may be feasible to use one set of equipment for up to 33 patients per year if applied in the same manner as in the randomised controlled trial ("in clinic" and "at home" monitoring with 6–8 sessions per patient). However, for this economic evaluation, we have conservatively estimated that one set of equipment could be used for ~12 patients in 1 year. This creates a "per-participant" cost of $416.67, which is approximately $60 per session if seven sessions are booked on average. DorsaVi specific adhesives were used to attach the motion analysis sensors and electromyography sensors in the trial. We have conservatively added a $20 per session cost to cover the price of adhesives and other consumables required to apply this equipment. This resulted in a total $80 cost per session per participant. However, electromyography sensors may not be required for all assessments subsequent to the initial assessment, which in real life would reduce the consumables cost to ~ $9 per session.

All costs were calculated in Australian dollars ($AUD) at 2015 values.

Measurement of outcome

The clinical outcome used for this economic evaluation was the Patient Global Impression of Change measured at the 12 month follow-up assessment [17]. This scale measures improvement relative to participant recall of their condition at baseline on a seven-point ordinal Likert scale (Very much improved, Much improved, Minimally improved, No change, Minimally worse, Much worse, Very much worse). The Patient Global Impression of Change has shown high levels of reliability and construct validity [18, 19].

Procedure

Clinics and clinicians were recruited by staff administering the trial. Patients were then recruited by their treating clinicians. All participants provided written informed consent. Participants were provided with their respective treatments and data for the economic evaluation was collected via the baseline assessment, the daily pain diaries (first 3 months of trial) and assessments conducted with a research assistant blinded to group allocation at 3 months, 6 months and 1 year.

Analyses

Measures of productivity and medication use for low back pain were calculated as change scores relative to baseline. These change scores were calculated over a 12 month follow-up time horizon using an area under the curve approach. Only participants who completed the final follow-up assessment (which included the only assessment of clinical outcome measure for this economic evaluation) were included in these analyses, making this a form of "complete case" analysis approach. If a participant missed a particular follow-up prior to the 12 month assessment, then the area under the curve approach was used to impute the missing data for change scores based on the adjacent assessment points. Measures of clinical visits and imaging for management of low back pain were calculated as absolute values consumed over the 12 month follow-up period. No participants reported use of hospitals or surgery for management of low back pain, thus these costs did not affect our estimate of direct health costs. A total cost figure was calculated for each participant, being the sum of productivity loss (or gain) over the 12 month follow-up period relative to baseline, the increase (or decrease) in medication use cost over the 12 month follow-up period relative to baseline, and the absolute cost of clinical visits outside of the trial therapy visits, imaging, and cost of clinical visits as a part of the trial protocol. The total cost figure was used to form the numerators in the incremental cost effectiveness ratio.

The dichotomous measure of effect used to form the denominator in the incremental cost effectiveness ratio was generated by merging participants who rated themselves as very much improved or much improved into one category, with all other responses being merged into the other category. The incremental cost effectiveness ratio was then able to be calculated as being:

$$\text{Incremental cost effectiveness} = \frac{\text{Total Cost (Intervention Group)} - \text{Total Cost (Control Group)}}{\%\text{Very or Much Improved (Intervention Group)} - \%\text{Very or Much Improved (Control Group)}}$$

$$(1)$$

The numerator of this ratio was calculated using linear regression analyses of the total cost variable so that the difference between groups in their geometric mean of the total cost variable could be calculated. We used Huber White "sandwich" variance estimators and clustered data based on the site from which the participant was recruited in keeping with best practice for analyses of cluster randomised trials (so that the units of analyses are equivalent to the units of randomisation) [20]. We used a similar approach to calculate the difference between groups in proportion of participants who were very or much improved according to their reported Patient Global Impression of Change. We used bootstrap resampling to calculate a 95% confidence ellipse to visually represent the uncertainty surrounding the incremental cost effectiveness estimate generated [21]. We conducted 2000 replications of the original sample, based on the original sample size that was collected within allocated groups. The analyses were repeated for each bootstrap replication, and the ensuing results plotted. Cost-effectiveness acceptability curve analyses were pursued to identify the probability that the intervention program was more effective and less costly from the societal perspective than the control program [22].

Two sensitivity analyses were pursued to examine the impact of key assumptions made for the primary analysis. First, we changed the threshold for dichotomization of our clinical outcome, so that we now combined those with a response of very much improved, much improved, or minimally improved into the one category. This is a justifiable sensitivity analysis to pursue as there are no universally accepted guidelines determining how much improvement in the Patient Global Impression of Change scale is necessary to be clinically significant. In the second sensitivity analysis, we excluded the cost of providing "trial" therapy to control group participants. This is a more controversial choice, though can be justified under the reasoning that those in the control group may not ordinarily have pursued the amount and duration of trial therapy sessions included in this trial in a real life context, yet still achieved the same clinical outcome. This sensitivity analysis intentionally has the effect of providing a more conservative estimate of the cost-effectiveness of the intervention.

Results

There were $n = 9$ sites assessed for eligibility of which eight met study inclusion criteria and were recruited into the study. These sites recruited $n = 112$ participants of whom $n = 38$ (intervention) and $n = 45$ (control)

completed the Patient Global Impression of Change at the final assessment. These numbers are lower than the total number who completed the final assessment in the pilot trial as the Patient Global Impression of Change was added to the study protocol after the first 11 patients were scheduled to have completed their 12 month follow-up. A description of participant demographics and their use of medication and productivity data at baseline is presented (Table 1). Other demographics of this sample have previously been reported [10]. The mean (sd) change in medication use and productivity costs, along with mean (sd) absolute costs for use of imaging, medical and therapy services (within the trial and external to the trial) over the follow-up period are presented (Table 2). Three participants in the intervention group had a total of four MRI scans of their lumbar spine compared to six participants in the control group each having one over the follow-up period. Thirteen participants in the intervention group had an additional 67 therapy or medical appointments for their back pain over the follow-up whereas twenty participants in the control group had an additional 88 therapy or medical appointments. We identified significant difference between groups in term of productivity changes (intervention group participants became more productive relative to baseline compared to control), in the resources consumed in trial based medical and therapy services (intervention group consumed more) and in resources consumed in non-trial based medical and therapy services (control group consumed more). Table 2 also presents the break-down of responses to the Patient Global Impression of Change scale across intervention and control groups where there were significant differences in favour of the intervention group.

The incremental cost-effectiveness of the intervention compared to the control condition for the primary analysis revealed that both total costs and clinical effects favoured the intervention group compared to the control. If there were 100 patients treated with the intervention, 41 more would have been 'very much improved' or 'much improved' than had those 100 patients been provided with the control condition. There would also have been a net saving of $478,100. Much of this saving however was driven by improved productivity costs. Thus it is not a direct saving to the health care system, rather, a gain for insurers, employers and society through participants being able to work more after receiving intervention with ViMove. The 95% confidence ellipse for the primary analysis revealed that the intervention dominated over the control condition (Fig. 2). Cost-effectiveness acceptability analysis was not pursued as the intervention dominated

Table 1 Participant demographics and baseline data from participants who completed the 12 month assessment

	Intervention	Control
n	38	45
Age	39 (14)	49 (12)
Gender	18 (47%) female	26 (58%) female
Pain intensity (QVAS) (0–100 scale, mean)	61.4 (16.0)	61.0 (12.0)
Pain episode duration (weeks, median)	52 (IQR: 17.5, 62.5)	52 (IQR: 16, 364)
Fear of movement (Fear Avoidance Beliefs Questionnaire: Physical Activity subscale) (0–24 scale, mean)	14.4 (6.4)	14.2 (6.6)
Activity limitation (Patient Specific Functional Scale) (0–100 scale, mean)	3.9 (1.7)	4.4 (2.4)
Activity limitation (Roland-Morris Disability Questionnaire) (0–100 scale, mean)	52.6 (19.9)	45.6 (26.4)
$AUD medication use per day at baseline	$1.03 ($0.91)	$0.96 ($0.75)
$AUD weekly income estimate based on gender and industry codes	$1467 ($265)	$1433 ($301)
Employment industry codes		
Professional, Scientific and Technical services	10 (26%)	5 (11%)
Health Care and Social Assistance	4 (11%)	10 (22%)
Agricultural, Forestry and Fishing	4 (11%)	5 (11%)
Administrative and Support services	4 (11%)	3 (7%)
Education and Training	2 (5%)	5 (11%)
Transport, Postal and Warehousing	2 (5%)	3 (7%)
Other categories	12 (32%)	14 (31%)

Data are mean (sd) or n (%) unless otherwise indicated

over the control condition with >99% certainty. Sensitivity analyses undertaken did not affect the conclusion of dominance of the intervention condition over the control condition, nor the degree of certainty of dominance of the intervention compared to the control condition being >99%.

Discussion

This economic evaluation based on a pilot cluster randomised controlled trial indicates that use of a motion-sensor biofeedback system to augment guidelines-based care dominates (is both more effective and less costly)

Table 2 Comparison of cost and clinical outcome measures between groups that were included in the economic evaluation

	Intervention	Control	Regression coeff (robust 95% CI)
$AUD lost productivity (total over 12 months)	$-6081 ($19, 627),	$-958 ($20,364)	$-5123 ($-10,174, $-72)
$AUD increase in medication use (total over 12 months)	$81 ($170)	$166 ($293)	$-85 ($-238, $68)
$AUD absolute imaging use	$52 ($191)	$66 ($169)	$-14 ($-125, $97)
$AUD absolute non-trial medical & therapies use	$137 ($232)	$170 ($285)	$-53 ($-105, $-0)
$AUD absolute trial medical & therapies use	$993 ($217)	$516 ($71)	$477 ($447, $508)
$AUD total cost (primary analysis)	$-4822 ($19,667)	$-40 ($20,278)	$-4781 ($-9748, $186)
$AUD total cost (sensitivity analysis)	$-4822 ($19,667)	$-557 ($20,277)	$-4265 ($-9221, $691)
Patient Global Impression of Change	8 Very much improved	2 Very much improved	
	15 Much improved	7 Much improved	
	10 Minimally improved	3 Minimally improved	
	5 No change	21 No change	
	0 Minimally worse	10 Minimally worse	
	0 Much worse	1 Much worse	
	0 Very much worse	1 Very much worse	
n (%) very or much improved on Patient Global Impression of Change (primary analysis)	23 (61%)	9 (20%)	0.41 (0.27, 0.54)
n (%) very or much or minimally improved on Patient Global Impression of Change (sensitivity analysis)	33 (87%)	12 (26%)	0.60 (0.46, 0.74)

Data are mean (sd)

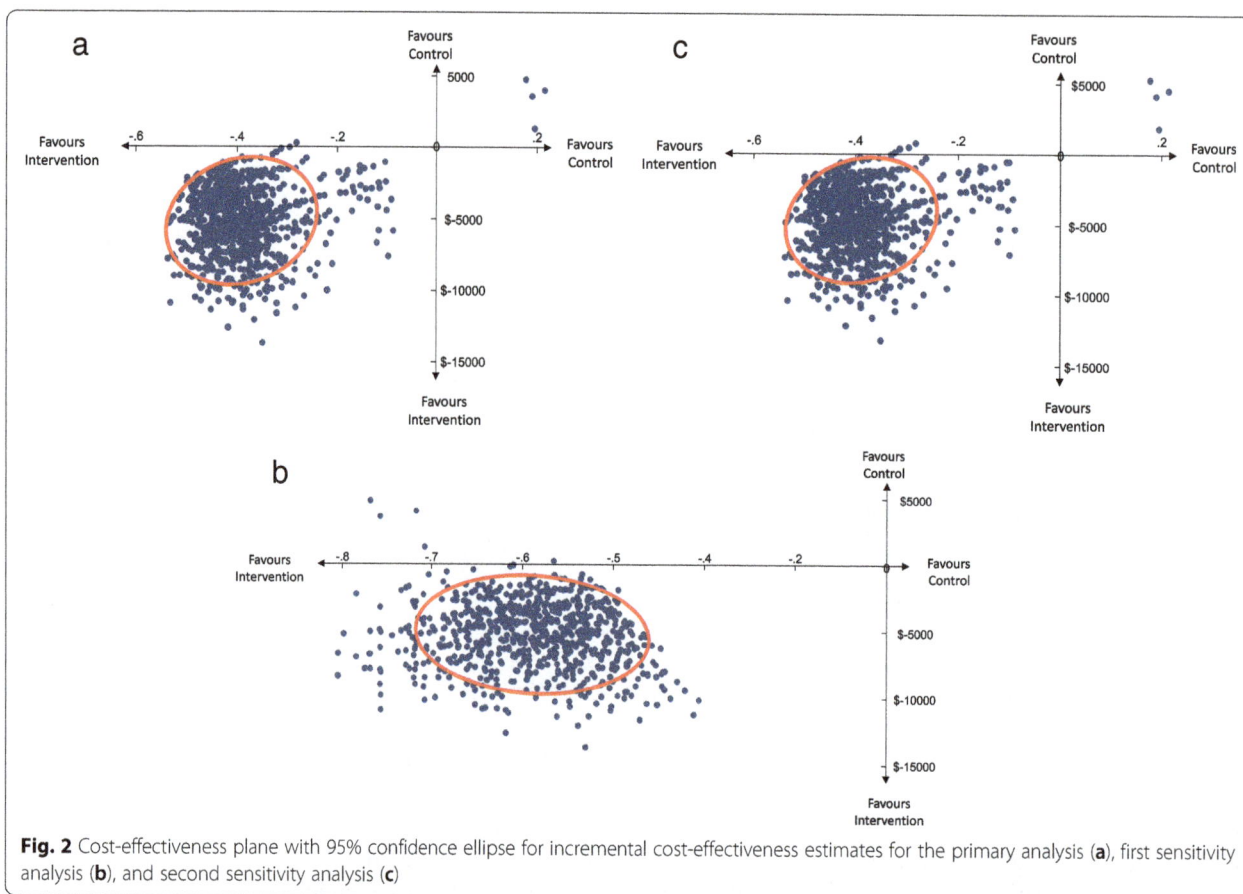

Fig. 2 Cost-effectiveness plane with 95% confidence ellipse for incremental cost-effectiveness estimates for the primary analysis (**a**), first sensitivity analysis (**b**), and second sensitivity analysis (**c**)

compared to guidelines-based care alone. It is important to be clear in this finding that the costs of providing the intervention was greater than providing the control in this study, but that the intervention group became more productive over the 12 month follow-up period and used fewer non-trial medical and therapy resources. This culminated in an overall saving to society, estimated to be $478,100 for every 100 patients treated to go with an additional 41 patients being classified as much or very much improved in relation to their low back pain. This finding of dominance was robust to the two key sensitivity analyses undertaken, where the costs of providing guidelines based care to the control group was eliminated, and where the threshold for classifying participants as being improved or not was changed.

The finding of dominance (both being less costly and more effective) with 95% confidence is particularly notable given the rarity of such a finding in this field. A review of economic evaluations for guideline endorsed interventions to reduce low back pain published in 2011 [8] included 26 studies, but identified only six studies where the intervention was thought to "dominate" over the control condition when considering cost-effectiveness [23–29]. In one, the follow-up period was only 3 months post-intervention and did not include costs of medical

services outside the trial protocol [23]. Another did not formally undertake an incremental cost effectiveness analysis [24, 25]. Another did not examine the 95% confidence interval ellipse surrounding the incremental cost-effectiveness estimate. This was important for this study given the highly skewed cost data they reported [26]. Of the studies that examined the 95% confidence ellipse that surrounded the incremental cost effectiveness estimate, none demonstrated dominance with 95% confidence [27–29].

Some caution should be employed when using these findings to guide clinical decision making and policy formation. Data used to build this economic evaluation were derived from a single, pilot (though of reasonable size) randomized trial. It is the nature of "concurrent economic evaluations" that any design-related issues or concerns of bias or imprecision in effect size estimates relating to the original randomized trial equally apply to the economic evaluation. In the same way that authors of the original trial recommended that a fully powered trial was warranted to be clear on the effectiveness of this intervention [10], further research is also required to confirm the results of this economic evaluation. This trial has demonstrated that the motion-sensor biofeedback approach appears to be a viable intervention from both a clinical and economic perspective, and that future research using this approach should be a priority.

Productivity costs were a key driver of the outcome of this economic evaluation. This was not surprising given that productivity costs are the key driver of burden of disease estimates in this condition [3]. Our approach to calculating productivity was relatively indirect in that we estimated income based on occupation and industry rather than directly capturing income from the participant. We also estimated presenteeism by using a linear extrapolation of the participants reported ability to perform their occupation. Using indirect methods to calculate productivity in economic evaluations conducted alongside clinical trials is common [30] and is often necessary given the threat to broader trial viability that more intensive data collection methods for these outcomes may create. These concerns may have introduced random error into our productivity estimates, but as these categorisations were undertaken by an investigator blinded to group allocation status (KB) we do not believe this would have created a systematic bias between groups that would have had a substantial effect on our results or conclusions. We also ignored the potential for productivity losses in one individual to negatively affect co-workers' productivity in case of team-dependent production. The productive output of a full team can be jeopardized by one member's illness [30]. This is more likely to have affected the group with more productivity losses (the control group in our case), which would make our cost effectiveness estimate more conservative.

Further research in this field is clearly indicated. First, to conduct a larger randomized trial and economic evaluation. Second, to understand potential mechanisms of action between the motion-sensor biofeedback intervention and improved productivity. Such research should consider whether it is purely changes in pain and function that drive improved occupational performance, or whether there are additional psychological benefits from wearing the device. The function of the motion-sensor biofeedback system to be able to alert the wearer when they remain in a particular position for too long or if they move in a way that may compromise their musculoskeletal health may reassure them and make them feel as if they can perform their work with less risk of injury. This may enhance their willingness and motivation to participate in their occupation. Understanding potential mechanisms of action may be useful for refining treatment protocols that optimise the value of this approach.

Conclusion

Low back pain continues to have a major impact on occupational productivity around the world, despite years of research to address this problem. The motion-sensor biofeedback treatment approach investigated in this research appears to be both more clinically effective and economically efficient than guidelines based care alone. This approach appears to be a viable means to manage low back pain that may enhance productivity. Further research in this area should be a priority as these data have been drawn from a pilot randomised trial.

Abbreviations
CI: Confidence interval; sd: Standard deviation

Acknowledgements
Not applicable.

Funding
Funding for this study was equally provided by (i) a grant from the Department of Business and Innovation (Market Validation Program), Victorian Government, Australia, and (ii) dorsaVi P/L (the Australian company who manufactures the ViMove motion-sensor system used in this study). The Department of Business and Innovation helped in the governance of the trial. DorsaVi supplied the motion-sensor equipment and coordinated the trial, assisted by a contract research organisation (Kendle P/L, Oakleigh, Victoria, Australia). All data and trial-related documentation were independently audited by Paul L Clark and Associates (Beaumaris Victoria, Australia). The authors analysed the results and wrote this paper independently of both funders, and neither funder had any influence over how these data were presented and the conclusions reached.

Authors' contributions
TH and KB contributed to the design of the economic evaluation, analysis of data and interpretation of results. TH wrote the initial draft of the manuscript while KB undertook blinded analyses of cost data. TH takes responsibility for writing of the manuscript and both authors for analyses and interpretation. Both authors read and approved the final manuscript.

Competing interests
Both authors were paid from the funding provided by the Victorian State Government and dorsaVi. The authors analysed the results of this research independently of both funders and neither funder had any influence on how these data were presented or conclusions reached. TH has previously been paid to undertake analyses and report preparation for the pilot randomized controlled trial that this economic evaluation was based upon.

Consent for publication
Not applicable.

References

1. Hoy D, March L, Brooks P, Blyth F, Woolf A, Bain C, Williams G, Smith E, Vos T, Barendregt J, et al. The global burden of low back pain: estimates from the Global Burden of Disease 2010 study. Ann Rheum Dis. 2014;73(6):968–74.
2. Maniadakis N, Gray A. The economic burden of back pain in the UK. Pain. 2000;84(1):95–103.
3. Dagenais S, Caro J, Haldeman S. A systematic review of low back pain cost of illness studies in the United States and internationally. Spine J. 2008;8(1):8–20.
4. Maas E, Juch J, Groeneweg J, Ostelo R, Koes B, Verhagen A, et al. Cost-effectiveness of minimal interventional procedures for chronic mechanical

low back pain: design of four randomised controlled trials with an economic evaluation. BMC Musculoskelet Disord. 2012;13:260.

5. Chou R, Qaseem A, Snow V, Casey D, Cross JT, Shekelle P, Owens DK. Diagnosis and treatment of low back pain: a joint clinical practice guideline from the American College of Physicians and the American Pain Society. Ann Intern Med. 2007;147(7):478–91.

6. Savigny P, Watson P, Underwood M. Early management of persistent non-specific low back pain: summary of NICE guidance. BMJ. 2009;338:b1805.

7. Koes BW, van Tulder MW, Ostelo R, Burton AK, Waddell G. Clinical guidelines for the management of low back pain in primary care: an international comparison. Spine. 2001;26(22):2504–13.

8. Lin CW, Haas M, Maher CG, Machado LA, van Tulder MW. Cost-effectiveness of guideline-endorsed treatments for low back pain: a systematic review. Eur Spine J. 2011;20(7):1024–38.

9. Jones AL, Wolf SL. Treating chronic low back pain. EMG biofeedback training during movement. Phys Ther. 1980;60(1):58–63.

10. Kent P, Laird R, Haines T. The effect of changing movement and posture using motion-sensor biofeedback, versus guidelines-based care, on the clinical outcomes of people with sub-acute or chronic low back pain-a multicentre, cluster-randomised, placebo-controlled, pilot trial. BMC Musculoskelet Disord. 2015;16:131.

11. Drummond M, O'Brien B, Stoddart G, Torrance G. Methods for the economic evaluation of health care programmes. 2nd ed. New York: Oxford Medical Publications; 1993.

12. Blumenthal D, Stremikis K, Cutler D. Health care spending–a giant slain or sleeping? N Engl J Med. 2013;369(26):2551–7.

13. Australian Acute Musculosekeltal Pain Guidelines Group. Evidence-based management of acute musculoskeletal pain. Bowen Hills, Queensland, Australia: Australian Academic Press; 2003.

14. Airaksinen O, Brox JI, Cedraschi C, Hildebrandt J, Klaber-Moffett J, Kovacs F, Mannion AF, Reis S, Staal JB, Ursin H, et al. Chapter 4. European guidelines for the management of chronic nonspecific low back pain. Eur Spine J. 2006;15 Suppl 2:S192–300.

15. Australian Bureau of Statistics. Average weekly earnings, industry, Australia (dollars) http://www.abs.gov.au/AUSSTATS/abs@.nsf/DetailsPage/6302. 0May%202015?OpenDocument. Last accessed 3 Jan 2016.

16. Waddell G, Newton M, Henderson I, Somerville D, Main CJ. A Fear-Avoidance Beliefs Questionnaire (FABQ) and the role of fear-avoidance beliefs in chronic low back pain and disability. Pain. 1993;52(2):157–68.

17. Hurst H, Bolton J. Assessing the clinical significance of change scores recorded on subjective outcome measures. J Manip Physiol Ther. 2004;27(1):26–35.

18. Costa LO, Maher CG, Latimer J, Ferreira PH, Ferreira ML, Pozzi GC, Freitas LM. Clinimetric testing of three self-report outcome measures for low back pain patients in Brazil: which one is the best? Spine. 2008;33(22):2459–63.

19. Farrar JT, Young Jr JP, LaMoreaux L, Werth JL, Poole RM. Clinical Importance of changes in chronic pain intensity measured on an 11-point numerical pain rating scale. Pain. 2001;94(2):149–58.

20. Freedman DA. On the so-called "Huber sandwich estimator" and "robust standard errors". Am Stat. 2006;60(4):299–302.

21. Efron B, Tibshirani R. An introduction to the bootstrap. New York: Chapman and Hall; 1993.

22. Fenwick E, O'Brien B, Briggs A. Cost-effectiveness acceptability curves - facts, fallacies and frequently asked questions. Health Econ. 2004;13:405–15.

23. Herman PM, Szczurko O, Cooley K, Mills EJ. Cost-effectiveness of naturopathic care for chronic low back pain. Altern Ther Health Med. 2008; 14(2):32–9.

24. Karjalainen K, Malmivaara A, Mutanen P, Roine R, Hurri H, Pohjolainen T. Mini-intervention for subacute low back pain: two-year follow-up and modifiers of effectiveness. Spine. 2004;29(10):1069–76.

25. Karjalainen K, Malmivaara A, Pohjolainen T, Hurri H, Mutanen P, Rissanen P, Pahkajarvi H, Levon H, Karpoff H, Roine R. Mini-intervention for subacute low back pain: a randomized controlled trial. Spine. 2003;28(6):533–40. discussion 540–531.

26. Loisel P, Lemaire J, Poitras S, Durand MJ, Champagne F, Stock S, Diallo B, Tremblay C. Cost-benefit and cost-effectiveness analysis of a disability prevention model for back pain management: a six year follow up study. Occup Environ Med. 2002;59(12):807–15.

27. Niemisto L, Rissanen P, Sarna S, Lahtinen-Suopanki T, Lindgren KA, Hurri H. Cost-effectiveness of combined manipulation, stabilizing exercises, and physician consultation compared to physician consultation alone for chronic low back pain: a prospective randomized trial with 2-year follow-up. Spine. 2005;30(10):1109–15.

28. Schweikert B, Jacobi E, Seitz R, Cziske R, Ehlert A, Knab J, Leidl R. Effectiveness and cost-effectiveness of adding a cognitive behavioral treatment to the rehabilitation of chronic low back pain. J Rheumatol. 2006;33(12):2519–26.

29. van der Roer N, van Tulder M, van Mechelen W, de Vet H. Economic evaluation of an intensive group training protocol compared with usual care physiotherapy in patients with chronic low back pain. Spine. 2008;33(4):445–51.

30. Krol M, Brouwer W, Rutten F. Productivity costs in economic evaluations: past, present, future. Pharmacoeconomics. 2013;31(7):537–49.

Permissions

The contributors of this book come from diverse backgrounds, making this book a truly international effort. This book will bring forth new frontiers with its revolutionizing research information and detailed analysis of the nascent developments around the world.

We would like to thank all the contributing authors for lending their expertise to make the book truly unique. They have played a crucial role in the development of this book. Without their invaluable contributions this book wouldn't have been possible. They have made vital efforts to compile up to date information on the varied aspects of this subject to make this book a valuable addition to the collection of many professionals and students.

This book was conceptualized with the vision of imparting up-to-date information and advanced data in this field. To ensure the same, a matchless editorial board was set up. Every individual on the board went through rigorous rounds of assessment to prove their worth. After which they invested a large part of their time researching and compiling the most relevant data for our readers.

The editorial board has been involved in producing this book since its inception. They have spent rigorous hours researching and exploring the diverse topics which have resulted in the successful publishing of this book. They have passed on their knowledge of decades through this book. To expedite this challenging task, the publisher supported the team at every step. A small team of assistant editors was also appointed to further simplify the editing procedure and attain best results for the readers.

Apart from the editorial board, the designing team has also invested a significant amount of their time in understanding the subject and creating the most relevant covers. They scrutinized every image to scout for the most suitable representation of the subject and create an appropriate cover for the book.

The publishing team has been an ardent support to the editorial, designing and production team. Their endless efforts to recruit the best for this project, has resulted in the accomplishment of this book. They are a veteran in the field of academics and their pool of knowledge is as vast as their experience in printing. Their expertise and guidance has proved useful at every step. Their uncompromising quality standards have made this book an exceptional effort. Their encouragement from time to time has been an inspiration for everyone.

The publisher and the editorial board hope that this book will prove to be a valuable piece of knowledge for researchers, students, practitioners and scholars across the globe.

List of Contributors

Marc Perron and Marianne Roos
Department of Rehabilitation, Faculty of Medicine, Université Laval, Pavillon Ferdinand-Vandry, Local 4445, 1050, avenue de la Médecine, Québec, QC G1V 0A6, Canada

Chantal Gendron
Department of Rehabilitation, Faculty of Medicine, Université Laval, Pavillon Ferdinand-Vandry, Local 4445, 1050, avenue de la Médecine, Québec, QC G1V 0A6, Canada
Canadian Forces Health Services Group, Valcartier Garison, Quebec City, Canada

Pierre Langevin
Department of Rehabilitation, Faculty of Medicine, Université Laval, Pavillon Ferdinand-Vandry, Local 4445, 1050, avenue de la Médecine, Québec, QC G1V 0A6, Canada
Physio Interactive, Quebec City, Canada

Jean Leblond
Centre for Interdisciplinary Research in Rehabilitation and Social Integration (CIRRIS), Quebec City, Canada

Jean-Sébastien Roy
Department of Rehabilitation, Faculty of Medicine, Université Laval, Pavillon Ferdinand-Vandry, Local 4445, 1050, avenue de la Médecine, Québec, QC G1V 0A6, Canada
Centre for Interdisciplinary Research in Rehabilitation and Social Integration (CIRRIS), Quebec City, Canada

Jenny Setchell, Nathalia Costa, Mandy Nielsen and Paul W. Hodges
School of Health and Rehabilitation Sciences, St Lucia, QLD 4072, Australia
Institute of Bone and Joint Research/The Kolling Institute, Sydney Medical School, The University of Sydney, St Leonards, NSW 2065, Australia

Manuela Ferreiram and Joanna Makovey
Institute of Bone and Joint Research/The Kolling Institute, Sydney Medical School, The University of Sydney, St Leonards, NSW 2065, Australia

Kjersti Storheim
Research and Communication unit for musculoskeletal disorders (FORMI), Oslo University Hospital Ullevål, Nydalen 0424, Oslo, Norway
Faculty of Medicine, University of Oslo, Blindern 0316, Oslo, Norway

Linda Berg
Department of Radiology, Haukeland University Hospital, 5021 Bergen, Norway
Section for Radiology, Department of Clinical Medicine, University of Bergen, N-5020 Bergen, Norway
Department of Radiology, Nordland Hospital, 8092 Bodø, Norway
Institute of Clinical Medicine, UiT, The Arctic University of Norway, Langnes 9037, Tromsø, Norway

Christian Hellum
Department of Orthopaedics, Oslo University Hospital Ullevål, Nydalen 0424, Oslo, Norway
Øivind Gjertsen
Department of Radiology and Nuclearmedicine, Oslo University Hospital Rikshospitalet, Nydalen 0424, Oslo, Norway

Gesche Neckelmann
Department of Radiology, Haukeland University Hospital, 5021 Bergen, Norway

Ansgar Espeland
Department of Radiology, Haukeland University Hospital, 5021 Bergen, Norway
Section for Radiology, Department of Clinical Medicine, University of Bergen, N-5020 Bergen, Norway

Anne Keller
Department of Physical Medicine and Rehabilitation, Oslo University Hospital Ullevål, Nydalen 0424, Oslo, Norway
Center for Rheumatology and Spine Diseases, National Hospital, 2600 Glostrup, Denmark

Romain Shanil Perera
Department of Allied Health Sciences, Faculty of Medicine, University of Colombo, 25, Kynsey Road, Colombo 8, Sri Lanka

Poruwalage Harsha Dissanayake
Department of Anatomy, Faculty of Medical Sciences, University of Sri Jayewardenepura, Gangodawila, Nugegoda, Sri Lanka

Upul Senarath
Department of Community Medicine, Faculty of Medicine, University of Colombo, 25, Kynsey Road, Colombo 8, Sri Lanka

Lalith Sirimevan Wijayaratne
National Hospital of Sri Lanka, Colombo 10, Sri Lanka

Aranjan Lional Karunanayake
Department of Anatomy, Faculty of Medicine, University of Kelaniya, Annasihena Road, Ragama, Sri Lanka

Vajira Harshadeva Weerabaddana Dissanayake
Department of Anatomy, Faculty of Medicine, University of Colombo, 25, Kynsey Road, Colombo 8, Sri Lanka

Shinji Tanishima and Hideki Nagashima
Department of Orthopedic Surgery, Faculty of Medicine, Tottori University, 36-1 Nishi-cho, Yonago, Tottori 683-8504, Japan

Hiroshi Hagino
School of Health Science, Tottori University Faculty of Medicine, 86 Nishi-cho, Yonago, Tottori 683-8503, Japan
Rehabilitation Division, Tottori University Hospital, 36-1 Nishi-cho, Yonago, Tottori 683-8504, Japan

Hiromi Matsumoto
Rehabilitation Division, Tottori University Hospital, 36-1 Nishi-cho, Yonago, Tottori 683-8504, Japan

Chika Tanimura
School of Health Science, Tottori University Faculty of Medicine, 86 Nishi-cho, Yonago, Tottori 683-8503, Japan

Vasoontara Yiengprugsawan
Centre for Research on Ageing, Health and Wellbeing and Department of Global Health, Research School of Population Health, The Australian National University, Canberra, Australia

Damian Hoy
Research, Evidence and Information Programme, Public Health Division, Secretariat of the Pacific Community, Noumea, New Caledonia

Rachelle Buchbinder
Department of Epidemiology & Preventive Medicine, School of Public Health and Preventive Medicine, Monash University, Melbourne, Australia
Monash Department of Clinical Epidemiology, Cabrini Institute, Melbourne, Australia

Chris Bain
QIMR Berghofer Medical Research Institute, Brisbane, Australia

Sam-ang Seubsman
School of Human Ecology, Sukhothai Thammathirat Open University, Nonthaburi, Thailand

Adrian C. Sleigh
National Centre for Epidemiology and Population Health, Research School of Population Health, The Australian National University, Canberra, Australia

Ko Matsudaira
Department of Medical Research and Management for Musculoskeletal Pain, 22nd Century Medical and Research Center, Faculty of Medicine, The University of Tokyo, Tokyo, Bunkyo-ku, Japan
Department of Pain Medicine, Fukushima Medical University School of Medicine, Fukushima, Japan

Hiroyuki Oka
Department of Medical Research and Management for Musculoskeletal Pain, 22nd Century Medical and Research Center, Faculty of Medicine, The University of Tokyo, Tokyo, Bunkyo-ku, Japan

Yasushi Oshima, Yuki Taniguchi, Yoshitaka Matsubayashi and Sakae Tanaka
Department of Orthopaedic Surgery, The University of Tokyo, Tokyo, Bunkyo-ku, Japan

Hirotaka Chikuda
Department of Orthopaedic Surgery, The University of Tokyo, Tokyo, Bunkyo-ku, Japan
Department of Orthopedic Surgery, Gumma University Graduate School of Medicine, Maebashi, Japan

Mika Kawaguchi, Emiko Sato, Haruka Murano and Thomas Laurent
Clinical Study Support, Inc., Nagoya, Japan

Anne F. Mannion
Spine Center Division, Department of Teaching, Research and Development, Schulthess Klinik, Zürich, Switzerland

Mika Kawaguchi, Takayuki Sawada and Akiko Ishizuka
Clinical Study Support, Inc., 2F Daiei Bldg., 1-11-20 Nishiki, Naka-ku, Nagoya 460-0003, Japan

Ko Matsudaira
Department of Medical Research and Management for Musculoskeletal Pain, 22nd Century Medical and Research Center, Faculty of Medicine, The University of Tokyo, Tokyo, Japan

Tadashi Koga
Clinical Study Support, Inc., 2F Daiei Bldg., 1-11-20 Nishiki, Naka-ku, Nagoya 460-0003, Japan
Shin Nippon Biomedical Laboratories, Ltd., Kagoshima, Japan

Tatsuya Isomura
Clinical Study Support, Inc., 2F Daiei Bldg., 1-11-20 Nishiki, Naka-ku, Nagoya 460-0003, Japan
Institute of Medical Science, Tokyo Medical University, Tokyo, Japan

David Coggon
MRC Lifecourse Epidemiology Unit, Southampton General Hospital, University of Southampton, Southampton, UK
Arthritis Research UK/MRC Centre for Musculoskeletal Health and Work, University of Southampton, Southampton, UK

Tom Petersen
Back Center Copenhagen, Mimersgade 41, 2200 Copenhagen N, Denmark

Mark Laslett
PhysioSouth Ltd, 7 Baltimore Green, Shirley, Christchurch 8061, New Zealand
Southern Musculoskeletal Seminars, Christchurch, New Zealand

Carsten Juhl
Research Unit for Musculoskeletal Function and Physiotherapy, Department of Sports Science and Clinical Biomechanics, University of Southern Denmark, Odense, Denmark

Department of Rehabilitation, University Hospital of Copenhagen, Herlev and Gentofte, Niels Andersen Vej 65, 2900 Hellerup, Denmark

Markus Hildebrandt
Physio Hildebrandt, Sickingerstrasse 4, 3014 Bern, Switzerland

Gabriela Fankhauser
Hauptstrasse 26, 3254 Messen, Switzerland

André Meichtry and Hannu Luomajoki
Institute of Physiotherapy, School of Health Professions, Zurich University of Applied Sciences, Technikumstrasse 71, 8401 Winterthur, Switzerland

Linzette Deidrè Morris
Division of Physiotherapy, Department of Health and Rehabilitation Sciences, Faculty of Medicine and Health Sciences, Stellenbosch University, Cape Town 8000, South Africa
Division of Epidemiology and Biostatistics, Faculty of Medicine and Health Sciences, Stellenbosch University, Tygerberg, South Africa

Kurt John Daniels and Quinette Abegail Louw
Division of Physiotherapy, Department of Health and Rehabilitation Sciences, Faculty of Medicine and Health Sciences, Stellenbosch University, Cape Town 8000, South Africa

Bhaswati Ganguli
Department of Statistics, University of Calcutta, Kolkata, India

Arnela Suman
Amsterdam Public Health research institute, Department of Public and Occupational Health, VU University Medical Centre, MB Amsterdam, The Netherlands

Frederieke G. Schaafsma and Johannes R. Anema
Amsterdam Public Health research institute, Department of Public and Occupational Health, VU University Medical Centre, MB Amsterdam, The Netherlands
Department of Public and Occupational Health, Research Centre for Insurance Medicine, Collaboration between AMC-UMCG-UWV-VUmc, VU University medical centre, MB Amsterdam, The Netherland

Jiman Bamarni
Faculty of Earth & Life Sciences, Department of Health Sciences, Student Health Sciences at the VU University Amsterdam, De Boelelaan 1085, 1081 HV Amsterdam, The Netherlands

Maurits W. van Tulder
Amsterdam Public Health research institute, Faculty of Earth & Life Sciences, Department of Health Sciences, VU University Amsterdam, De Boelelaan 1085, 1081 HV Amsterdam, The Netherlands

Adrian Bamford, Andy Nation and Susie Durrell
Gloucestershire Hospitals NHS Foundation Trust, Gloucester, UK

Lazaros Andronis and Hugh McLeod
University of Birmingham, Birmingham, UK

Ellen Rule
Gloucestershire Clinical Commissioning Group, Gloucester, UK

Mélanie Cogné
Service de Médecine Physique et de Réadaptation, hôpital Raymond Poincaré, 92380 Garches, France
Service de Médecine Physique et de Réadaptation, CHU de Bordeaux, 33076 Bordeaux, France
EA4136 Handicap, Activité, Cognition, Santé, Bordeaux University, Bordeaux, France
Hervé Petit and Alexandre Creuzé Service de Médecine Physique et de Réadaptation, CHU de Bordeaux, 33076 Bordeaux, France

Dominique Liguoro
Neurosurgical Unit, University Hospital, Bordeaux, France

Mathieu de Seze
Service de Médecine Physique et de Réadaptation, CHU de Bordeaux, 33076 Bordeaux, France
EA4136 Handicap, Activité, Cognition, Santé, Bordeaux University, Bordeaux, France

Lisbeth Hartvigsen
Department of Sports Science and Clinical Biomechanics, University of Southern Denmark, Odense, Denmark

Lise Hestbaek and Alice Kongsted
Department of Sports Science and Clinical Biomechanics, University of Southern Denmark, Odense, Denmark

Nordic Institute of Chiropractic and Clinical Biomechanics, Odense, Denmark

Charlotte Lebouef-Yde
Research Department, Spine Center of Southern Denmark, Hospital Lillebælt, Middelfart, Denmark
Institute for Regional Health Research, University of Southern Denmark, Odense, Denmark

Werner Vach
Institute for Medical Biometry and Statistics, Faculty of Medicine and Medical Center, University of Freiburg, Freiburg, Germany

Monica Unsgaard-Tøndel
Department of Neuromedicine and Movement Science (INB), NTNU, Faculty of Medicine and Health Sciences, N-7491 Trondheim, Norway
Department of Public Health and Nursing, Norwegian University of Science and Technology, Faculty of Medicine and Health Sciences, Trondheim, Norway

Ingunn Gunnes Kregnes
Department of Physical Medicine and Rehabilitation, St. Olav's Hospital, Trondheim University Hospital, Trondheim, Norway

Tom I. L. Nilsen
Clinic of Anaesthesia and Intensive Care, St Olavs Hospital, Trondheim University Hospital, Trondheim, Norway
Department of Public Health and Nursing, Norwegian University of Science and Technology, Faculty of Medicine and Health Sciences, Trondheim, Norway

Gunn Hege Marchand
Department of Neuromedicine and Movement Science (INB), NTNU, Faculty of Medicine and Health Sciences, N-7491 Trondheim, Norway
Department of Physical Medicine and Rehabilitation, St. Olav's Hospital, Trondheim University Hospital, Trondheim, Norway

Torunn Askim
Department of Neuromedicine and Movement Science (INB), NTNU, Faculty of Medicine and Health Sciences, N-7491 Trondheim, Norway

Shanthi Ramanathan
Hunter Medical Research Institute, New Lambton Heights, Newcastle 2305, Australia Faculty of Health and Medicine, University of Newcastle, Newcastle, Australia
Centre for Healthcare Resilience and Implementation Science, Australian Institute of Health Innovation, Macquarie University, Sydney, Australia

Peter Hibbert and William Runciman
Centre for Healthcare Resilience and Implementation Science, Australian Institute of Health Innovation, Macquarie University, Sydney, Australia
Centre for Population Health Research, Sansom Institute for Health Research, The University of South Australia, Adelaide, Australia
Australian Patient Safety Foundation, Adelaide, Australia

Louise Wiles
Centre for Healthcare Resilience and Implementation Science, Australian Institute of Health Innovation, Macquarie University, Sydney, Australia
Centre for Population Health Research, Sansom Institute for Health Research, The University of South Australia, Adelaide, Australia

Christopher G. Maher
Institute for Musculoskeletal Health, Sydney, Australia
Sydney School of Public Health, Sydney Medical School, University of Sydney, Sydney, Australia

Terry Haines and Kelly-Ann Bowles
Allied Health Research Unit & Physiotherapy Department, School of Primary Health Care, Monash University and Monash Health, Kingston Rd, Cheltenham 3192, Australia

Index